A few letters in support of Dr. Goldman's writings and practice

"Dr. Goldman's book is novel and revolutionary. I recommend this book as a common sense approach to pain management. At last, an author who ties together biomechanics and the important foot/ankle and spine relationship. This is required reading!"

Mark A. Young MD, Fellow, American College of Pain Management

Physical Medicine & Rehabilitation

Professor, Dept of Orthopedic Sciences & Rehabilitation New York College of Podiatric Medicine

Editor, Physical Medicine and Rehabilitation Secrets Editions 1,2 and 3

Author, *"Women & Pain: Why it Hurts and What You Can do?"* (Hyperion)

"This book is a treasure-trove of insights and expertise from a master clinician. Dr. Goldman's approach to physical diagnosis changed the way I think about low back pain. Instead of resorting to medications, injections, or surgery, many people can benefit from improved gait mechanics. **This book is a step-by-step guide to identifying specific problems and implementing practical solutions. Your patients will thank you!"**

Beth B. Murinson, MD, PhD

Diplomate, American Board of Psychiatry and Neurology

Diplomate, American Board of Pain Medicine

Associate Professor and Director of Pain Education

Department of Neurology Johns Hopkins School of Medicine

Author, *"Take Back Your Back"* (Fair Winds Press, 2011)

"Dr. Goldman's work serves as a reminder that all medical progress starts with impeccable observation. **His presentation of the association of spinal stenosis, pseudo stenosis and peripheral neuropathy expands the traditional view and provides a new structure for practitioners to diagnose and treat disorders of the peripheral nervous system.**

This text provides clinicians and patients a novel vision for abetting suffering from these disorders by explaining precise symptom complaints, examination findings, treatments and testable outcomes. The patient case format allows accessibility for patients and reminds practitioners that we serve to holistically improve the lives of people by treating body, mind, and spirit."

Marian Lamonte, MD Chief of Neurology, St Agnes Hospital Baltimore.

Clinical Associate Professor, Neurology, University of Maryland School of Medicine

"Dr. Goldman's new book will be found illuminating to many doctors and patients alike. This book provides a delightfully written overview of techniques, many of which Dr. Goldman has developed himself. These approaches have often enabled him to resolve chronic or severe arthritis and neuropathy pain that had resisted prior care. Over the years many patients of mine have been the beneficiaries of his care. **Readers will take away valuable information that may lead to the same great improvement that so many satisfied patients have already.**

Successful implementation of this book will provide a path to living a more active life with much less pain for many people. I highly recommend it."

Julian Jakobovits MD, Diplomate American Board of Internal Medicine

Associate Professor of Medicine Johns Hopkins University School of Medicine

As a surgical podiatrist by training who purchased Dr Goldman's previous practice, I am in a unique position to comment on his techniques. I was fortunate to spend time with Dr Goldman seeing patients. My skepticism on his unusual techniques proved unfounded as numerous patients told me that their pain had been relieved. I have been able to help quite a few people thanks to the time spent with Dr Goldman and, as a surgical residency director, I am proud to pass this school of thought on to my surgical residents.

Through this revolutionary book, the podiatry and medical community at large will be fortunate as I was to learn and implement these discoveries in their practices. **This book reveals the links between Spinal Stenosis / Pseudo-Stenosis and painful arthritis, peripheral neuropathy, and the many other medical conditions addressed in this book, and presents innovative paths for successful treatment.**

The timing for this book could not be better. The ART of medical practice is being lost. Too many patients have treatment failure based on tests and imaging, without thorough evaluation. An equally important message to take home from Dr Goldman's wonderful book is the imperative need to ask the right general and specific questions, to listen, to touch the patient, and to watch them walk! How else can we honestly attempt to help our patients with lower extremity pain, and to "Do no harm?"

Kyle J. Kinmon, MS, DPM, FACFAS
Director of Residency Training Podiatric Medicine and Surgical Residency
Bethesda Memorial Hospital Boynton Beach Florida

"I have had many patients over the years who have had the privilege of excellent diagnosis and treatment of their foot problems by Dr. Goldman. He has applied his insights and experience in treating peripheral neuropathies in the foot and illuminating their relationships to spinal stenosis. **All readers should benefit from his knowledge, as well as following Dr Goldman's holistic and common sense approach to help his patients.**"

Allen Friedman MD Diplomate American Board of Internal Medicine

"I have known Dr. Goldman for many years and have shared many patients with him. He has a wonderful ability to help people with chronic pain of various etiologies with his non-invasive holistic approach. **He has save many patients from risky procedures and spared them from life with chronic pain.** I highly recommend considering his evaluation and treatment techniques."

Elliot Rothschild MD Diplomate American Board of Internal Medicine
CEO Baltimore Suburban Health

"Dr. Goldman has been taking care of my patients for years. **His diagnostic and therapeutic techniques are applicable for patients with arthritis of the spine, hip, knee, and feet as well as patients with spinal stenosis.** Dr. Goldman's research and resultant techniques have helped many of my patients with these conditions significantly reduce their suffering. The great majority of my patients achieved rapid improvement in their symptoms in an average of 1-2 days. Additionally, use of his therapies reduces cost, as more expensive imaging studies such as MRIs are not needed and referrals to other specialty providers are greatly reduced. I strongly recommend this book for both patients and practitioners."

Miguel Sadovnik MD Diplomate American Board of Internal Medicine

"I am a Geriatric Nurse with 38 years of experience who became crippled by spine and leg pain that was not helped by physical therapy, medicines, or injections, despite efforts by many specialists over 7 years.

Dr. Goldman rapidly relieved all of my symptoms without medication or therapy, and helped me to resume a normal lifestyle, including going back to work full time, without pain, at the age of 68! I recommend that anyone treating geriatric patients study his book, and use his original insights and approaches to Pain Management of Spinal Stenosis, Arthritis, and Neuropathy symptoms. Your patients will thank you!»

Francis Shultz RN BS Geriatric Nurse.

As a Physician Assistant working in Internal Medicine, I see how many patients suffer from chronic neuropathic and degenerative, arthritic pain. Conventional treatment often provides limited or only temporary relief. Through sharing patients with Dr. Goldman, I have been fortunate enough to see many patients reap the benefits from his techniques, rapidly, with greater effect and duration than conventional treatment. **It is my opinion that the practices presented in this book should be considered in the primary care setting as an initial mode of investigation and treatment for neuropathic and arthritic pain, before pharmacotherapy.**

Rachel Richards, PA-C

PAIN FREE Walking, Standing, Sleeping & Sitting
Frequent Relief in 1-3 Days

Walking Well Again
Neutralize the Hidden Causes of Pain

**A GUIDE FOR PATIENTS & CLINICIANS to
Abolish Symptoms Associated with**

*Arthritis   Fibromyalgia   Spinal Stenosis
PseudoStenosis   Diabetic Neuropathy   Peripheral Neuropathy
Leg Length Discrepancy   Restless Leg Syndrome   Painful Swollen Legs
Poor Circulation   Poor Balance   Flat Feet   & other conditions.*

Stuart M Goldman DPM

Fellow, American College of Foot and Ankle Surgeons
Diplomate, American Board of Foot & Ankle Surgery
Facilitation Press LLC

Walking Well Again
Neutralize the Hidden Causes of Pain

A GUIDE FOR PATIENTS & CLINICIANS to *abolish symptoms associated with Arthritis, Fibromyalgia, Spinal Stenosis, PseudoStenosis, Diabetic Neuropathy, Peripheral Neuropathy, Leg Length Discrepancy, Restless Leg Syndrome, Painful Swollen Legs, Poor Circulation, Poor Balance, Flat Feet, & other conditions*

Publisher's Cataloging-in-Publication data

Names: Goldman, Stuart, 1955-, author.

Title: Walking well again : neutralize the hidden causes of pain / Dr. Stuart Goldman, DPM, DABPS, FACFAS.

Description: First edition | Baltimore [Maryland] : Facilitation Press LLC, 2016 | Includes bibliographical references and index.

Identifiers: ISBN 978-0-9961119-0-4 (Hardcover) | ISBN 978-0-9961119-1-1 (pbk.) | LCCN 2015919418.

Subjects: LCSH Chronic pain--Treatment. | Chronic pain--Alternative treatment. | Backache. | Spinal canal--Stenosis. | Diabetic neuropathies. | Fibromyalgia. | Arthritis. | BISAC HEALTH & FITNESS / Pain Management | MEDICAL / Pain Medicine.

Classification: LCC RB127 .G65 2016. | DCC 616/.0472—dc23.

Attention: Quantity discounts are available for purchases by corporations, medical groups, educational institutions, state or local associations for resale, teaching, incentives, gifts, or fundraising. Institutions interested in books or excerpts should contact Facilitation Press at FacilitationPress@Gmail.com

Table of Contents

You MUST read this first

Do you, or does someone you care for, have any of these concerns:

Spinal Stenosis	Low back pain or arthritis	Pain radiating from the back
Diabetic or Peripheral Neuropathy	Burning or tingling feet or legs	Numbness of the feet or legs
Poor circulation, causing symptoms	Claudication of the legs	Painful swollen legs
Improved walking with a grocery cart	Poor balance	Fibromyalgia
Arthritis of the hip, knee, ankle, or foot	Overall discomfort that persisted or got worse after joint surgery	Feet that are different from each other
Tendonitis of the ankle	Lack of success with orthotics	Restless Leg Syndrome
Leg cramps, day or night	Aching or tired feet	Inability to walk well
Inability to stand well	Inability to sleep well	Inability to sit well
Difficulty arising from a seated position	Difficulty bending over to pick things up	

If so, welcome to *Walking Well Again*.

Believe me when I say that this book is a labor of love. Whether you are a patient seeking help, a family member trying to help a loved one regain the pain-free living and mobility that he or she enjoyed in years past, or a medical professional investigating, welcome.

I am not an academician. I did not spend years in an intellectual ivory tower, hatching theories and testing them. The approaches shared on these pages that can rapidly conquer foot, leg, and back symptoms, were developed "in the trenches" of private practice. I was desperate to help people who were desperate to be helped. You might say that necessity was the mother of invention in the formulation of all my ideas, but I know that I have also had Divine assistance. The result? With these techniques, in the last 15 years, well over 3500 people have been freed of chronic painful symptoms and disability that had defied previous diagnosis or care.

Through the rigors of my private practice and by preparing many articles for publication, my ideas have been refined and improved, and their uses expanded. I now understand the basics of how these approaches work, although I'm sure there is still much to learn. The most important point is that they *do* work. For some conditions, these approaches are effective about *70% of the time*.

If they work, they always work within 1–3 days.

When you attend a live acrobatic performance or view one on TV, you might hear the announcer open with the disclaimer "Don't try this at home." In contrast, the goal of this book is to provide direction that may help overcome problems–and that often can be implemented without medical guidance–at home.

Before you try any suggested treatment, it is important to adequately understand the symptoms. People often do not know the details of the symptoms that cause so much of their suffering and limitation. Heroically struggling to cope, they do their best to ignore the pain. They resign themselves. They adjust. Some have almost given up hope of ever living pain free again.

For your own benefit, it is valuable to take stock of your symptoms first. Chapter 3 contains a questionnaire that you can fill out before and after treatment, allowing you to follow the status of your symptoms. The comparison will help you clearly grasp the benefits or limitations of treatment.

There are, however, circumstances under which you MUST obtain a professional evaluation rather than try the techniques I will share on these pages. While these techniques *might* be helpful for an acute flare-up of a long-standing problem, they are primarily designed to treat chronic problems, not new and sudden ones.

Acute problems involving the back or leg may be dangerous. An extreme but fortunately rare example is a condition called "Cauda Equina Syndrome." Symptoms include severe back pain that may radiate to the legs and may be accompanied by a loss of bladder or bowel control, constipation, and numbness in the genital or anal area. If such a severe change occurs, it's important to be seen by emergency room personnel as soon as possible, and *not* to try to relieve your symptoms at home.

A fracture of a vertebra (bone of the back), a slippage of a vertebra, an abdominal aneurism (enlarged artery), a spinal infection, a kidney stone, or even shingles can appear present with acute low-back pain, which may or may not radiate into the legs. If you have any such symptoms that develop suddenly, seek emergency evaluation as soon as possible. **With sudden or severe back pain, the rule is better safe than sorry. Get it checked out.**

Sudden weakness in a foot or leg could be a sign of a stroke. Coolness or coldness in a foot or leg could be a sign of a circulation blockage, which must be addressed quickly. Redness or swelling on a leg could be caused by an infection, a blood clot, a fracture or tendon problem, or a flare-up of a form of arthritis such as gout—all of which require immediate medical attention.

All sudden changes must be checked out by a competent medical specialist, and quickly. This book is not intended to replace that kind of care.

In contrast, *chronic* symptoms—whether constant or intermittent—in the back, thighs, knees, legs, or feet, can be investigated with the approaches described here. However, I repeat that before you try the approaches I provide, you should properly investigate and document your symptoms by filling out the questionnaire in Chapter 3.

Here ends the mandatory section of this introduction.

The remainder will help you better understand and use this book

By now, you may have noticed that I tend to repeat myself. This is intentional. There are four reasons for repetition in this book.

1. You might not read the whole book! I anticipate that many people will skip to the chapter focusing on their particular problem. Each chapter must therefore be able to stand somewhat independently. Throughout the book, I reinforce basic or essential ideas, as well as refer the reader to the relevant chapters for in-depth understanding.

2. It will help you really "get it." It is well known among medical professionals that important information must be repeated to ensure the best chance that the patient will understand and comply. A visit to the doctor's office induces a natural amount of stress, and if you are in need of help, you may also experience stress while reading this book. Under such conditions, people don't always remember everything they've been told or have read.

3. What I present here is very different from standard medical practice. Please consider the repetition of these ideas as a sign of my commitment to the approaches presented here. I do not make any recommendation frivolously. These ideas and approaches are the product of 14 years of investigation, contemplation, and successful use. Repetition is meant as a reinforcement of my commitment to them, and of my belief in the hope they hold out to so many long-time sufferers.

4. The fourth and final reason is specifically for medical professionals. Repetition and the large numbers of stories included here may induce a new way of investigation and management of the many conditions addressed in this book. Repetition may help clinicians internalize and easily access the approaches I find so helpful.

The ideas and techniques presented in this book are exactly as used in my day-to-day practice. The communication style presented is the kind I employ in my office as well—casual, but hopefully clear and convincing. It is my job as a doctor to make sure the patient understands the potential benefit of my suggested treatment, to the point where he or she is willing to comply with some behavioral changes. It is therefore essential to communicate well enough to bring the patient on board. I hope that in your case, I will succeed.

By writing and sharing this book, I am not claiming to be a world expert in biomechanics, neuropathy, or arthritis. I do not have all the answers. What I do claim is that the information and guidelines shared in this book can help both patients and clinicians get a better handle on the cause of many common symptoms, and can provide guidance on how to improve symptoms rapidly—with a high likelihood of success.

Meet My Website

On my website, WalkingWellAgain.com, **you'll also find interviews of over 120 people who have benefitted greatly from the techniques in this book, many of whom were interviewed both before and after treatment.** I hope you also take pleasure when you see the great changes that these people have experienced. You may find encouragement in their stories, many of which are shared in the relevant chapters of this book.

WalkingWellAgain.com is also a way for you to communicate with me. Writing this book, as well as writing the articles I've published in medical journals over the years, has been a lonely and time-consuming process. One shares information but rarely knows if it accomplishes the desired goal. Please share your story with me. I always enjoy hearing of successful cases. These stories strengthen my resolve. As such, they are a real contribution to my work.

In addition, I may add new recommendations through this site that I could not otherwise share.

Eventually, on the website, I will share many of the ideas in this book, presented as videos, as if we were together in my office. **Because some people (especially the elderly) learn better by listening than by reading, the website may help them better understand their symptoms, and may motivate and guide them to undertake the treatment best suited to provide the relief they crave.** However, since this book has been written in my "free time," I am not sure when that project will be completed.

StoryTime

Throughout the book the phrase *StoryTime* introduces a story that shares important details and lessons learned or confirmed by the treatment of one of my patients. Detailed stories of over 85 patients are included in this book. Those patients identified by their first name and the first letter of their last name also have interviews shared on the website. Not all *StoryTime* stories will be found on the website. Some occurred prior to my obtaining a video camera to record the interviews. Some stories included information that I felt might be embarrassing to either the patient or the clinicians who treated them. Those individuals are identified only by first name.

How This Book Was Written

When patients walk into my office, they want to know what can be done to help them with whatever concerns brought them there.

The problem presented may be something simple, such as a foot problem that came up a few days ago, or it might involve a severe walking limitation that has been present for years or even decades. I listen to the description of the symptoms, ask a number of questions, and then conduct a physical examination. During the course of the exam I often identify additional concerns that can be addressed and hopefully resolved.

Occasionally I need some sort of testing—such as circulation or nerve testing, blood tests, X-rays, or spinal imaging such as MRIs or CT scans—to diagnose and treat. Although much of the medical establishment here in the United States regularly employs such tests, I find that with age (mine!) and experience I order tests less frequently than I used to. In the great majority of cases, a focused discussion with the patient and a thorough examination are all that are necessary to make the probable diagnosis, and to allow direction of the proper treatment. As long as the treatment relationship is established for the sole purpose of helping the patient get better, rather than for research purposes, that's what is really important: **getting the right working diagnosis and guiding the patient to the desired improvement**.

That's the way this book was written, with the expectation that you have purchased it in order to receive clear direction for your particular situation, leading to a treatment plan that will help relieve your symptoms. I begin by focusing on the symptoms themselves, based on the diagnosis that you believe is causing the problems. I then try to help you (the patient, caregiver, or physician) confront and understand the true nature of those symptoms.

One must then address symptoms that may be caused by spinal nerve compression. By eliminating the symptoms that arise from Spinal Stenosis and what I have dubbed "PseudoStenosis" (to be explained in depth in later chapters)—something that is often astonishingly easy to do—it is then easier to understand which symptoms stem from other conditions. Direction is provided for addressing remaining symptoms.

The book is divided into four sections.

Section 1 includes three chapters that introduce the concepts of the book and that guide you to understand your symptoms.

Section 2, Chapters 4–14, presents a detailed understanding of both Spinal Stenosis (SS) and PseudoStenosis (PS) and mechanisms for evaluation and treatment of these conditions.

Section 3, Chapters 15–26, addresses medical conditions or activities that either SS or PS can mimic or impact. Details are provided on each particular condition or activity, and on how to identify and manage the possible SS/PS component contributing to the symptoms.

Section 4 includes just two chapters, one presenting interesting cases and more lessons learned, and one that summarizes, entitled "Final Thoughts."

For better or for worse, reading this book is quite a bit like speaking to me in person. My wife says that she can hear me saying the words as she reads them. This is how I communicate, and I believe that it is an important key to the success of the approaches I use.

Because of the effort I put into questioning and evaluating my patients, they perceive that I am trying my best to understand and guide them to the right approach. Once a patient knows that his doctor is committed and dedicated, he becomes more willing to cooperate. An old saying has it right: "Patients don't care how much you know until they know how much you care."

This book is directed to patients as well as medical professionals. I deliberately chose editors with no medical background to ensure that the most essential information I provide does not require a medical education to be able to follow.

I have taken certain liberties in format. I make liberal use of modified fonts, having certain phrases in **bold** or *italics*, to draw attention to them. I capitalize certain conditions, testing protocols, and treatment protocols to draw attention that I treat the capitalized phrase as a specific condition or protocol, and not just a description. One such example is "Positional Testing," which is a very specific set of behaviors. I believe that use of the capitalization will help patients recognize these terms as distinct names, which must be understood to be properly addressed. I use spelled-out numbers some **one hundred times**, but also numerals over **100 times** to attract attention to certain details. The way I have done it may not always be grammatically or stylistically correct, but I sacrifice that ideal in order to make the book more readable for the lay public.

In a similar vein, the pictures of this book are not of professional quality, as they were not done by a professional! Similar to the 120-plus videos on my website, they were primarily taken by me in the office, to try to clearly present the details contained in the picture. Some pictures have too much clutter in the background, and some are not of great quality. I ask that you tolerate the imperfections of the pictures in order to allow them to do their job—to convey information and ideas. I hope that the end result justifies the means.

For the Clinician and the Very Curious

Some sections of this book go into greater detail and will be most useful to clinicians, but they may be of interest to anyone looking for a deeper understanding. I try to present them in layman's language, even though they are primarily for clinicians. These sections are often identified in advance as "For the Clinician and the Very Curious," so if you are not interested in such detail, simply skip those sections.

Be aware that much of the practical information in this book is completely original. Some of it I have already published in peer-reviewed journals. These journals, including the research journals of the American Podiatric Medical Association, the American Diabetes Association, and the British Diabetes Association, as well as the *Journal of Family Practice*, are strict about the data and observations that they publish. Some of the observations and techniques that allow me to help people have not been previously published, in part because of a lack of controlled data. **My observations and suggestions must therefore be taken "with a grain of salt."** Though the treatments presented have proved helpful for some 3500 patients, this treatment has taken place within private practice and not within the parameters of research that has been clinically documented well enough to publish.

This is how I practice in my office; my patients reap the benefits of real-life experience and empirical knowledge. It is my hope that you, the reader, will do the same.

Some of the information presented in this book is not original. A number of ideas and articles have been published by others over the years, which has helped me greatly in developing the protocols that I present here. I share these protocols the way I use them, and I fully acknowledge that I stand on the shoulders of giants in the fields of biomechanics, orthopedics, physical medicine, and other specialties. Specifically, some of the guidance provided in Chapters 12 and 19 is based upon great information I have learned from literature or lectures—much of which, unfortunately, has not yet become integrated into mainstream medicine. In the *Appendix* at the end of the book here is a list of excellent resources.

Why This Book Was Written

In my opinion this information is necessary for the optimal practice of not only podiatry, but also primary care, geriatrics, vascular medicine, orthopedics, rheumatology, neurosurgery, endocrinology, neurology, physiatry, sleep medicine, cardiology, chiropractic, and physical therapy. All of these fields commonly deal with individuals who have Lumbar Spinal Stenosis or PseudoStenosis. Both conditions greatly affect a patient's quality of life, in recognized and, quite frequently, unrecognized ways.

The approaches shared here allow easy, inexpensive, safe, and rapid identification and management of Lumbar Spinal Stenosis and PseudoStenosis for so many people, that I am convinced they should become part of standard medical practice. This book is meant to provide an ordered set of answers to the questions that could be asked in all of the medical fields listed above.

The information contained in *Walking Well Again* has the potential to help millions of Americans as well as millions of others around the world. For many years my practice has enjoyed good-to-excellent improvement in approximately 70% of our patients with Spinal Stenosis and PseudoStenosis, but closer to a 50% success rate with individuals suffering from many of the other conditions addressed in the later chapters. These figures are in part based on small, retrospective, in-house studies, some of which I have published, and they are reflective of the overall success seen in my practice. **As I will repeat throughout this book, almost all patients who improve with these methods do so in just 1, 2, or possibly 3 days.**

I have tried many times to get universities and top researchers to partner with me in investigating some of my approaches, so far without success. The lack of randomized controlled studies of these approaches is not because I am avoiding them, but rather because I cannot conduct them without help, and as of today—December of 2015—I have not yet been able to obtain that help.

My lack of success in the research end of this endeavor stands in glaring contrast to the incredible and frequent success I've seen in my clinical work. Such success obligates me to share this information. That obligation, I hope, is fulfilled with this book.

How do I know these things that other doctors don't? I certainly do not claim to be smarter than the next doctor. However, because of my family upbringing and time spent with some wonderful, sincere physicians, I try to approach every patient with a deep desire to help him or her. As I became known for putting in the time and effort to try to solve long-term problems, more patients with similar problems came to me, often referred by their physicians, family, or friends. Their desperation, combined with their expectation and hope that I would be the one to help them, drove me to think—and, at times, obsess—about the common, unresolved problems that I saw repeatedly in my practice.

I hope the reasons why this book was written are now clear. I believe that the insights and techniques I use can guide clinical improvement for millions of people. I have worked hard at understanding—not as a researcher, but as a clinician who pays attention to details and strives to help my patients. Theory has followed practical success, as much as the other way around. I firmly believe that Heaven has helped me greatly in the areas that have brought about the greatest success. To date, I believe that I have helped bring about dramatic improvement in the quality of life of some 3500 people with the techniques presented in this book.

My hope is that this book results not only in individual success stories and in clinicians being brought on board to make use of the information I've presented, but also in the beginning of the sort of medical research, thus far lacking, needed to support this approach. I hope that any such investigation will be embraced by top-quality researchers and will not be held back because of its humble beginnings or the limitations of its originator.

* * * * *

On a personal note, allow me to share something that still amuses me, 39 years after the fact. While I never aspired to write articles or books, I've always enjoyed dabbling in music. In my first year of podiatry school, impressed by the intensity of the studies that were meant to prepare us completely as medical professionals (for which I am grateful), I wrote a song called "The Finals Lullaby," patterned after Tom Lehrer's "MLF Lullaby." One of the verses went as follows: "A doctor is a doctor; / You must know it all. / One day you'll have to help / The neurologist down the hall."

And so, with that unwitting prophecy fulfilled, welcome to *Walking Well Again*.

Stuart Goldman, 2015

Confronting the Challenges of Individuals

Walk Well, Stand Well, Sleep Well, and Sit Well

I smiled in welcome, as I've done every day for over thirty-three years in my podiatry practice, and said, "Tell me why you're here today."

The woman sitting opposite me was a new patient, aged 45, referred by her internist. I saw from the history she'd filled out that she'd been suffering from Lupus for the past three decades.

"Well," she began, "my right heel has been hurting for several months."

I looked at her feet for a moment, and familiar warning bells went off in my head. I nodded encouragingly. "Anything else?"

"My feet and legs really hurt when I walk."

Knowing the potential of her particular problems to cause other symptoms, I asked another question—a common one. "Any back pain, neck pain, jaw pain, or headaches?"

She hesitated. "I know you're a foot doctor, so I didn't think to write it down . . . but my back aches something awful when I walk, too. And my jaws hurt—TMJ."

"Actually, that's not at all uncommon. And I'm interested in *all* your symptoms." I leaned forward. "Approximately how long after you start walking do you have to stop because of the pain?"

"After just a few minutes usually." She grimaced. "And it gets worse as the day goes on. By midafternoon," she said with simple resignation, "I can barely walk at all."

"Really? How do you get around the house?"

She looked me right in the eye, resigned to the pain, but seeming to be relieved to be finally discussing it. "Afternoons and evenings, I get up the stairs . . . by crawling."

The picture she painted made me wince. "How long has this been going on?"

"Almost 5 years now."

I asked some other questions, and then examined my patient carefully. Afterward, she listened intently as I outlined my plan of action.

Within 3 days, she was Walking Well Again. Everywhere. All day long. Up the stairs and down.

A miracle?

Not at all. Just good, solid medicine.

* * * * *

At least several times each week, someone comes into my office with symptoms that have held them back from enjoying life, often for many years. Each of them describes difficulty walking, standing, and even sleeping, usually associated with foot, leg, or back problems. After I treat them, these symptoms, which may have been present for a long period of time—and which, interestingly, are often not even the reason the patient came to my office in the first place—are usually much improved within a few days, and often as early as the next day.

The positive results that I've had by combining original insights and techniques with methods I've learned from other practitioners and publications have become the impetus for this book and the corresponding website. For years, I have actively sought out patients who were unable to find relief elsewhere. And with most of them, I've had a very high success rate—as I hope to share on these pages.

Welcome to *Walking Well Again*.

The Art of Investigation

The first thing I do upon meeting a new patient is ask what brought him or her to my office. I listen attentively to the complaint that impelled them to make the appointment. Then, after hearing the patient's initial concern and conducting a brief physical examination, I ask a few simple questions: Do you have any other problems with your feet and legs? Do you have difficulty standing or walking? How far are you able to walk before you have to stop for any reason?

Sometimes it is difficult for patients to open up. If they are especially hesitant, I ask them to humor me. "Pretend that all your problems can be solved, if only I could get a clear description of them." With this encouragement, I am usually treated to a narrative that includes a great many additional woes. Many of my patients have been suffering with their symptoms—which cause difficulty not only in their walking, but also in their ability to stand or even sleep—for months, years, or even decades.

Over the years, I've become a bit smarter, incorporating additional questions into my patient history form. Here is a sequence from that form:

Chief complaints or concerns at this time:

1. _____ 2. _____
3. _____ 4. _____
5. _____

Duration of problems:

1. _____ 2. _____ 3. _____
4. _____ 5. _____

Have you been treated for this by another clinician? ___No ___Yes

Prior Treatment: _____

Please circle current concerns:

Bunions	Burning feet	Morton's Neuroma	Foot or leg pain of
Hammertoes	Arthritis of:	Ulcers or infections	unknown cause
Tendon pain	Foot Ankle Knee	Walking limitations	Difficulty:
Corns & calluses	Hip Back Neck	from foot or leg	Standing Sitting
Ingrown & fungus nails	Flat Feet	pain	Getting up
Skin growths	High-Arched Feet	Foot or leg pain or	Poor balance
Neuropathy	Heel & arch pain	cramps at night	Spinal Stenosis
	Diabetic foot care		Back pain

Other _____

Call me a medical detective. Through these and other questions, and by taking the time to encourage and build upon the answers and doing a detailed but specific physical examination, I investigate the symptoms that have been afflicting my patient for a very long time. I "attack" each case as if it were a fascinating medical mystery—which, indeed, it often is. By eliminating possibilities and peeling away irrelevant or erroneous conclusions, I usually come to the crux of the matter—the source of the patient's pain or discomfort that is hampering his or her ability to walk and live well.

Only when the mystery has been solved does it become possible to properly treat the problem. Using the insights and techniques presented in this book, I can usually reduce or eliminate the symptoms within a matter of days.

The Kinds of Symptoms and Problems Addressed

Here is a smattering of case histories, each presented in detail later in this book, many of which seem hopeless at first glance. In my office, such cases are frequently resolved on a daily basis.

- A 74-year-old woman with diabetes, whose severe leg and foot pain prevented her, over a period of 14 months, from walking for even a few minutes, and who was told that her only option was Spinal Stenosis surgery (which had a good chance of failing).

- An 82-year-old woman with severely swollen legs from Lymphedema, for years unable to stand or walk for more than a few minutes without pain.

- A 90-year-old man who experienced a burning sensation in his feet every night in bed from idiopathic neuropathy, as well as difficulty walking—all this for over a decade.

- A 25-year-old woman with foot and leg pain, knee pain, hip pain, back pain, and headaches dating back to her junior high school days, and who had not improved with anti-inflammatory medication, physical therapy, acupuncture, or chiropractic manipulation.

- A 48-year-old man with burning, tingling, and aching in his feet and legs for 16 years, attributed to neuropathy caused by either HIV/AIDS or the medication used to control that condition.

- A 22-year old woman with moderate foot and leg pain but worse neck and shoulder pain that had bothered her for several years.

- An 80-year-old woman diagnosed with Diabetic Neuropathy, who for more than 5 years suffered severe foot pain in bed at night and while walking, and who did not improve with medicine.

- A 16-year-old high school runner who for 18 months suffered back and leg pain brought on by running and even extensive walking.

- A 70-year-old man who suffered hip and back pain for 25 years despite extensive medications and physical therapy.

- A 70-year-old man with balance problems that had developed gradually over the prior 2 years, with no help from neurology or physical therapy management.

- A 60-year-old man with difficulty walking because his legs got tired, often after only one block. He was told his problem was due to poor circulation and that surgery was not an option. He became inactive and gained a great deal of weight during his years of a forced sedentary lifestyle.

- A woman in her 40s diagnosed with Fibromyalgia, suffering back, leg, and ankle pain for over 15 years, causing difficulty standing, walking, sitting sleeping, with an inability to pick things off of the floor.

- A 68-year-old woman with severe Flat Feet, who underwent surgery with perfect-looking results by a world-class foot and ankle surgeon—but who continued to experience the same foot pain she'd had for the previous 10 years.

- A 68-year-old man suffering back pain that radiated down his left leg when he was sleeping, who, as a result, had slept very poorly for more than 5 years.

- A 68-year-old woman with chronic back and knee pain that caused difficulty walking or standing for even a few minutes, despite knee replacement surgery and a total of 20 spinal and knee steroid injections.

- A 74-year old woman who suffered a minor stroke, and subsequently experienced back and leg pain that prevented her from standing or walking for more than 5 minutes, and from climbing stairs at all—all this for 1½ years.

- A 49-year old woman who had back and leg pain frequently present while sitting or lying down, and who had back and leg stiffness that usually lasted for several minutes when she arose from sitting or sleeping.

And, of course, there was our 45-year-old woman with Lupus, who'd been forced to crawl upstairs every day for 5 long years.

Each of these patients saw dramatic improvement in his or her symptoms after just one or two visits to my office. In each case, a simple treatment protocol proved far more effective than the medications, injections, therapies, or surgeries they'd had in the past. Even more importantly, each patient maintained the improvement once it was achieved. **I believe this was because we addressed** *the cause of the problems*, **rather than simply using something to** *mask the symptoms.*

This book is dedicated to providing some new insights and combining them with medical information that is published but underutilized, to help patients, their families, and their physicians understand, recognize, and solve these kinds of problems. This chapter will serve as an introduction, outlining the basics of what this book will do, and how, and why.

The Value and Challenges of Walking

Walking has many benefits. As we age, walking is, for most people, our primary form of exercise. Whether a person remains strong, grows weaker, or regains lost strength is to a great extent determined by his or her pattern of walking. Walking well—or, for many, Walking Well Again—is the gateway to independence, work, good health, and the ability to fully enjoy life.

I'm not suggesting that people who cannot walk well are doomed. Many people who are unable to walk well, or at all, still lead rich and full lives. They work, have families, and may live either with loved ones or independently. Many have learned to cope in remarkable ways, to their credit and to the credit of those who help them.

And yet the ability to walk well is an integral part of living. The loss of this vital ability can have a host of negative effects. The root of this loss of mobility—which may include back pain, foot or leg pain, arthritic pain, neuropathy symptoms, poor endurance, overall weakness, poor balance, and even Shortness of Breath—can quickly or gradually change so many aspects of the life that many of us regard as normal. Losing the ability to walk well, for a person accustomed to walking well, may lead to depression, weight gain, increased inflammation in the body, loss of strength, loss of self-esteem, diminished thinking ability, and even loss of independence. Inability to walk also reduces an individual's ability to combat chronic illnesses, such as heart disease and diabetes.

In the recent past, dozens of scientific articles have documented the enormous physiological and psychological values of active walking. For this reason, striving to keep that ability, and taking advantage of methods aimed at maintaining or regaining it, are key components to aging gracefully, successfully, and independently.

I am belaboring this point to encourage all my readers to take full advantage of what this book has to offer. My approaches are certainly not typical, nor are they standard, facts which may lead some people to resist them. By emphasizing information that most of us already know instinctively, but which has also been validated in numerous medical studies and scholarly articles, I hope to encourage you to open yourself to a whole new set of approaches.

Approaches that work. Approaches that will hopefully lead you, and a great many others who pick up this book, to resume Walking Well Again.

* * * * *

If you are a patient, reading this section will reinforce the value of walking and the importance of regaining your ability to walk. It should urge you to seek the relief available, even at the cost of a little inconvenience. The effort will be more than worthwhile, if it results in your being able to walk well again.

If you are a clinician, this initial chapter is designed to accomplish two goals. First, it is a reminder of the importance of being able to walk well and of the effect walking ability has on the life and lifestyle of your patient. **Second, it stresses the vital need to routinely and aggressively investigate certain details.** As we will discuss in Chapter 5, taking a thorough and exacting walking and Positional History—learning the details of how well your patients walk, how far they walk, what assists them in walking, and what limits them—is essential to helping the patients to the best of your ability. By asking these questions and following up on the details, you will identify a great many people who have previously unaddressed walking difficulty—most of whom can be helped easily. This book provides the necessary information for you to help the great majority of these people.

For both groups, *Walking Well Again* will introduce you to techniques that I use on a regular basis with my patients, techniques that have already helped thousands of people.

* * * * *

Despite its title, this book deals not only with walking, but also with the associated areas of standing, sleeping, and even sitting. Though I will touch on various other issues, these are the primary focal points.

Before addressing the main point of this chapter, I'd like to lay some groundwork.

Let me share something that all clinicians know: medicine is an art as well as a science. The diagnosis of the cause of specific symptoms is often unclear or uncertain. When practicing medicine, even the most sincere and dedicated doctor does best with a correct diagnosis upon which to base his treatment. Unfortunately, sometimes a doctor is presented with a previous diagnosis of a condition that is incorrect. At times, the diagnosed condition is not really present at all. Frequently, the condition *is* present but is not the primary cause of the presenting symptoms.

Again, a correct diagnosis is essential for treatment success. Having the right antibiotic for the wrong bacteria does not work. Similarly, the right treatment for the wrong diagnosis in the area of walking difficulty is not likely to provide more than partial and temporary help for the patient.

Some causes of difficulty walking (not a complete list)	
Alcoholic Neuropathy	Lumbar Spinal Stenosis
Anemia	Muscular Dystrophy
Arterial insufficiency (ASO)	Multiple Sclerosis
Arthritis, tendonitis, or bursitis	Myopathy
Cervical Myelopathy/ Stenosis	Normal-Pressure Hydrocephalus
COPD causing Shortness of Breath	Obesity
	Old Age
Congestive Heart Failure causing Shortness of Breath	Peripheral Arterial Disease (PAD)
Dermatomyositis	Peripheral Neuropathy
Demyelinating Peripheral Neuropathy such as CIDP or MGUS	Parkinson's Disease
	Pernicious Anemia
	Poor conditioning
Amyotrophy	Popliteal Entrapment Syndrome
Diabetic Peripheral Neuropathy	Polymyositis
	PseudoStenosis
Equinus (tight leg muscles)	Sickle Cell Anemia
Flat Feet	Stroke
Fibromyalgia	Spinal Stenosis
Hypothyroidism	Venous insufficiency
Lymphedema	Vitamin B$_{12}$ deficiency

There are many conditions that are diagnosed as the cause of walking difficulty. Any could possibly be associated with a significant reduction in a patient's ability to walk.

The Challenges of Standing and Sleeping

Standing is an essential skill, an effort requiring endurance and balance that we take for granted from the time we are very young. With age, or after an injury or illness, standing can become a chore for many people. They find themselves shifting from side to side, needing a cane for balance, or having to sit down frequently for no apparent reason. This sort of thing is not necessarily addressed in standard medical practice. Yet an inability to stand is a trap, because it prevents a person from feeling secure when walking, and it retards the independent performance of those daily activities that may give life meaning.

There are many factors and conditions that are diagnosed as the cause of difficulty standing. Any of these conditions could possibly be associated with a significant reduction in a patient's ability to stand.

Perhaps you have been diagnosed or the person you seek help for has been diagnosed with one of these conditions as the cause of the difficulty in walking or standing. That diagnosis may be either totally correct, partially correct, or completely incorrect.

The third symptom we will look at is the inability to sleep comfortably and effectively. As a podiatrist, I was never taught to address this issue, and yet it has become something that I frequently address in my patients. This will be addressed in Chapters 21 and 22.

There are many factors and conditions that are diagnosed as the cause of difficulty sleeping. Any of these conditions could possibly be associated with nighttime foot or leg symptoms that make it hard to get a good night's sleep.

Some causes of difficulty standing (not a complete list)

Alcoholic Neuropathy	Multiple Sclerosis
Anemia	Muscular Dystrophy
Arthritis, tendonitis, or bursitis	Myopathy
Baker's cyst	Orthostatic Hypotension
Lymphedema	Parkinson's disease
Cervical Myelopathy/ Stenosis	Peripheral Neuropathy
Deep Vein Thrombosis	PseudoStenosis
Inner ear disorder	Spinal Stenosis
	Venous insufficiency

Some causes of nighttime foot or leg symptoms (not a complete list)

Arterial insufficiency (ASO/ PAD)	Hypothyroidism
Arthritis, tendonitis, or bursitis	Restless Leg Syndrome
Baker's cyst	Peripheral Neuropathy
Charley horse (leg cramps)	Polymyalgia Rheumatica
Electrolyte imbalance	PseudoStenosis
Fibromyalgia	Sciatica
Growing pains	Sleep Apnea
	Spinal Stenosis
	Venous insufficiency

Of course, Sleep Apnea is well recognized as a common cause of sleep pathology. As we will see, this can actually have a strong relationship to lower-back and lower-extremity symptoms.

The Twin Culprits: The Common Hidden Causes of Pain

You will note some overlap on the above lists. Several conditions appear in all three lists and can interfere with a person's ability to walk, stand, and sleep well. **It is my opinion, and a major emphasis of this book, that one certain pair of conditions is the primary culprit.** Understanding this is the key to helping improve the health of millions of Americans and saving our wonderful country $10 billion or perhaps even $20 billion in health care costs each year.

Spinal Stenosis and PseudoStenosis

A great many people are told that the difficulty they have walking, standing, and sleeping is caused by one of the many conditions listed above—when the actual sole cause, or a strongly contributing cause, is either Spinal Stenosis or PseudoStenosis. When a diagnosis is incorrect or incomplete, the resultant treatment plan is most likely doomed to failure.

Similarly, a great many people are told that their difficulty walking, standing, and even sleeping is caused by Spinal Stenosis, when the real cause—or a strongly contributing one—is what I have termed "PseudoStenosis." **I feel strongly that every Spinal Stenosis patient should be investigated for possible PseudoStenosis.**

Traditional treatment for Spinal Stenosis, such as physical therapy, epidural injections, and surgery (including implants, laminectomy, or even fusion), may provide a patient with only temporary or incomplete relief because PseudoStenosis contributes to the problems, making the original diagnosis either erroneous or incomplete. **PseudoStenosis, as we will see, is a fairly deep and involved subject, but it is often easy to identify and treat.** Sometimes it can even be treated at home by the patient, without professional help.

Even if the diagnosis of Spinal Stenosis is indeed correct, extensive research has shown that standard treatment often provides incomplete or temporary relief, and that even invasive treatments such as injections or surgery may provide only limited help. There is therefore a great need for successful conservative treatment for true Spinal Stenosis.

"Spinal Stenosis" refers to a condition in which there is narrowing of a pathway within lower spine structures that can cause local or referred symptoms. "PseudoStenosis" is a term I have selected for a condition in which lower-extremity dysfunction causes the spinal canal to function as if Spinal Stenosis is present.

This book will aid you in differentiating these conditions from each other and from other conditions, help you understand their effect on the spine and on a variety of lower-extremity symptoms—and will direct treatment that often provides relief in 1–3 days.

*Most important, by identifying and addressing the fundamental problem of either Spinal Stenosis or PseudoStenosis, we can usually achieve the goal: a **sustainable fundamental alignment**, that allows the person to heal, and maintain the improvement long term.*

What is needed is a protocol that is safe, rapidly effective, and inexpensive. A protocol that does not interfere with other possible treatments and that can help clarify the diagnosis. **After experiencing success with over two thousand patients over the last thirteen years, I have developed just such a diagnostic and treatment protocol for true Spinal Stenosis.**

* * * * *

How do you arrive at a proper diagnosis? How do you separate the causes of symptoms in patients suffering from multiple problems? How do you test to see if your suspicion is correct? If your diagnosis is validated, how do you treat the condition? How can you guide the patient to long-term management to prevent or address recurrence of symptoms and to eliminate the need for additional expensive and disruptive tests and treatments?

For patients with difficulty walking (or standing, sleeping, or even sitting), as well as for the clinicians and caretakers of such individuals, this book promises to provide some answers. In the next chapter, we will discuss how the use of symptoms as "clues" can serve as a basis for suspecting and differentiating the different conditions that may cause the lower-extremity symptoms that interfere with walking.

Seeking the Best Options

There are many ways to skin a cat. While I find that my methods are frequently effective, quick, and safe, and that they help differentiate the causes of the symptoms, there are, of course, other ways to treat those symptoms. If the root of the problem is Spinal Stenosis, standard treatments may be successful. However, in my experience, physical therapy often provides only limited and temporary relief and often requires weeks or months and thousands of dollars to bring about even this limited success. Epidural injections often provide real relief, but their effect is usually temporary. Surgery often helps, but it has its share of failures and complications.

The most insidious interventions, perhaps, are the medications used to treat pain. According to a report published by the American Gastroenterological Association, each year the side effects of NSAIDs (non-steroidal anti-inflammatory medication)—including aspirin and ibuprofen—hospitalize over 100,000 people and kill 16,500 in the United States, mostly due to bleeding stomach ulcers. Many sources report that use of NSAIDs increases risk of stroke or heart attack. Many articles report that narcotics and antidepressant medications significantly increase the likelihood of falls in senior citizens.

I am not condemning the use of medications when necessary, but merely stressing that they come with common risks and side effects. In my opinion, they are warranted only if a successful outcome cannot be obtained with safer, readily available treatment.

The approaches described in this book can help millions of people achieve significant clinical improvement without the risks, costs, and ongoing demands of the other treatment options, including medications, therapy, injections, and surgery. These approaches need to be given full clinical-research evaluation. Until that happens, I encourage patients and clinicians to use the information provided on these pages to the best of their ability.

Relief in 1–3 Days

An essential point: Any positional or mechanical management that I describe in this book, when effective, will provide relief of symptoms within 1–3 days. The intervention should never be physically uncomfortable.

To see if you will benefit from these approaches, it is best to undertake the following steps:

1. Understand your symptoms.
2. Document your symptoms.
3. Investigate whether you may have Spinal Stenosis or PseudoStenosis contributing to your symptoms.
4. Try treating the symptoms, usually with the appropriate Mechanical Testing or Positional Testing.
5. Follow up based on the results of testing, and deal with your remaining symptoms, guided by the appropriate chapters.

The following chapters will start you on your journey.

Supplemental Information

Throughout the book, you will often find a summary or supplemental paragraph at the end of a chapter, or even at the end of an individual section. Its purpose is to reinforce or emphasize important points or to qualify a point to prevent any misunderstanding. Here are a few points that I'd like to make right now, to wind up this initial chapter:

1. I want to be clear on expectations. **In my practice, we achieve good (50%–74%) to excellent (75%–100%) improvement in about 70% of patients with either Spinal Stenosis or PseudoStenosis, usually within 1-2 visits, with success within 1–3 days of proper treatment.** I believe that the guidance provided in this book can help clinicians, and often even individuals, achieve similar improvement. Bear in mind, however, that *only* about 70% of such patients will be quickly helped by treatment, and not 100%. In addition, although these techniques have helped many people with "Failed Back Syndrome," in which pain persists despite spine surgery, the success rate for this group is lower than in those who have not had back surgery.

   In addition, symptoms associated with other conditions such as neuropathy, or circulation or swelling problems, or lower-extremity or spine arthritis, are helped less frequently with these approaches, closer to 50% of the time, also within 1–3 days of appropriate treatment. You may be able to treat yourself with the techniques I provide on these pages, or you may require follow-up with a good podiatrist or physician. However, even if you need to seek help from a professional, success may be far more likely when their efforts are combined with information from this book.

2. **More than 85 stories are presented in detail in this book.** They make up an interesting variety of case histories and give both patients and clinicians an insider's view of the great results I enjoy. Over 55 of these people are identified by name, and sections of interviews they gave are available **on the website, WalkingWellAgain.com**. They are among the 120-plus patients whose interviews are also shared there. These are not interviews recorded in a studio, rather in my office—with my patients talking to me and the camera during office visits.

   Many people gave multiple interviews, sharing their stories and symptoms at the initial visit, and then reporting on their improvement days, weeks, or months later. In most cases, I have follow-up confirming persistent success.

   Lesley J, the young woman whose story is found at the beginning of this chapter, has interviews from her initial visit and three subsequent visits shared on WalkingWellAgain.com.

3. **This book is not a substitute for medical care but a supplement to it.** I communicate with my readers the same way I do with patients in my office. Nevertheless, patients should continue overall management of their condition with a qualified clinician.

4. **This book is not meant to address significant or sudden changes.** If sudden, significant changes in spine or lower-extremity symptoms occur, they might signify a major problem in the spine (tumor, fracture, infection, etc.) or in the circulation (blood clot, arterial blockage, etc.), or they might signify other problems that need to be addressed by a medical or surgical specialist. Please discuss this sort of development with your primary care provider and seek emergency help if recommended.

   With these points understood, on to the journey.

CHAPTER 2

Symptoms: Understanding Them and Using Them

Symptoms are actually a double-edged sword. On the one hand, pain, burning, or numbness can drain away a patient's quality of life. These symptoms can make it hard to stand or walk, hard to sleep or sit, and hard to concentrate. Sometimes they prompt people to take pain medications that may have serious consequences. As such, the symptoms can truly take the wind out of the sails of a person trying to lead a normal life.

On the other hand, pain and other symptoms are often important warning signs. After all, a child only learns to avoid touching a hot stove because the heat causes pain, which can serve to prevent any real harm from being done. Pain, unpleasant as it is, is an essential part of life in that it frequently stops people from seriously damaging themselves.

Nevertheless, as useful as pain is, we often spend a great deal of effort and money—sometimes taking dangerous medications or submitting to difficult surgical procedures—in our effort to avoid it.

It's important to understand the difference between pain that serves as a warning signal and pain that develops because of an illness or other pathology. Obviously, we want to retain the "warning signal" kind of pain that prevents us from damaging ourselves. We also want to eliminate the discomfort that keeps us from our normal activities. Reducing or even eliminating chronic pain by addressing the root causes is a primary goal of the protocols presented in *Walking Well Again*.

Medication: Friend or Foe

One problem with strong pain medication is that it can block warning pain from being perceived and thereby prevent people from knowing when they're harming themselves. Another problem, more common, involves the complications that can be caused by taking such medications. Anti-inflammatory medications can cause gastric ulcers and increase likelihood of heart attack or stroke. Narcotics, antidepressants (such as Elavil or Cymbalta), and anticonvulsants (such as Neurontin [Gabapentin] or Lyrica) can also lead to problems—the most serious of which, for older patients, might include loss of mental function or loss of balance, which can lead to falls, fractures, and other serious complications.

While I *occasionally* use such medications in my practice, I strive to avoid them just as I strive to avoid surgery. Instead, I attempt to deal with the **cause** of the symptoms whenever possible, to obviate the need for medications that can cause such severe complications.

Use of Medications as You Evaluate Your Symptoms

In this stage, as you are evaluating your symptoms in order to understand and treat them, there *may* be value in reducing your use of medication for a few days. Here are some thoughts on this matter.

If the medication is blocking all or almost all of your symptoms and your goal is to reduce your use of the medication, then it may be necessary to stop the medication before evaluating your symptoms or trying any treatment. Why? If medication is blocking your symptoms, then you will not know what your symptoms currently are, and will not be able to perceive any improvement with treatment.

If, however, the medication for symptoms provides only limited help and you are still aware of details of symptoms, you will be able to perceive improvement with treatment. If this is the case, you can wait to decrease your use of medication until after you see improvement with the treatment.

That is the basic approach I use in my office.

One qualifier: Medications such as anti-inflammatory medicine or narcotic painkillers can usually be stopped and resumed without significant risk. Some other medicines used to treat pain need to be dosed carefully and reduced gradually to prevent complications. For example, incorrectly stopping anticonvulsant medications such as Neurontin (Gabapentin) or Lyrica may cause seizures. Other commonly used medications, such as antidepressants, or the pain medication Tramadol (Ultram), may require gradual changes or close monitoring. **Therefore, talk with your doctor before adjusting your prescription medication.**

Paying Close Attention to Symptoms: Is That Giving In?

Many people, striving to maintain their independence, do their best to ignore their symptoms. I must confess that I find this heroic. Such patients live with arthritic or neuropathic symptoms or weakness and do whatever they can for themselves, struggling mightily not to be a burden on other people.

Just as there is heroism (all too infrequently recognized) in the everyday lives of people who work to support their families, parents who take care of their children, children who take care of their parents, and individuals who volunteer to help others despite their own challenges in life, there is also heroism in living with symptoms believed to be untreatable with a minimum of fuss and complaint. These heroes of everyday life cope valiantly with the challenges that come with their reality. For those who struggle to maintain their ability to be active and independent despite significant symptoms—hats off to you!

The sad thing about this is that symptoms once believed to be untreatable often *are* treatable—a vital fact that was the impetus for this book.

Although I applaud the heroism of a stoic attitude and recognize the logic in trying to ignore symptoms while going about your lives, in this chapter I ask you to change your approach, at least temporarily. While many of you have struggled to ignore your symptoms in an effort to keep them from affecting your quality of life or the scope of your activities, **I now ask you to pay close attention to the details of your symptoms.**

In the following chapter, you will find a scale developed for the specific purpose of identifying as completely as possible all the symptoms present in the lower extremities and back that affect your ability to stand, sleep, walk, or perform everyday activities of almost any type.

At first, this new approach may feel like a burden. It may seem draining or un-heroic to pay attention to your pain and limitations. However, there are very important reasons for doing so.

The Importance of Details

It is important for both the patient and the physician to be able to track improvement in specific symptoms in order to judge the success of treatment. A person who initially reports severe foot pain seven nights a week—a "10" on a scale of 1–10—while trying to sleep on his back, has a clear picture about the intensity of his symptoms and their effect on his quality of life. If, after treatment, he still experiences symptoms, but his pain level is now only a "2" on a scale of 1–10 and occurs only a few times a week, we understand that there has been an excellent but not perfect improvement. The fact that there are still symptoms present would not mean that the treatment was unsuccessful and should be terminated; it just means that the improvement has been great but not perfect.

I have occasionally had patients come into my office and express dissatisfaction because they were still symptomatic. However, when they reviewed their own evaluation of their symptoms before treatment, they realized that the treatment had brought about significant improvement and was worth continuing. The best way to successfully track improvement in symptoms is to clearly define the level and type of symptoms before treatment begins. This is a primary reason for the detailed questionnaire that I share in the next chapter.

Details can guide the doctor's understanding of the symptoms' underlying cause. Many people present with foot, leg, or back symptoms that derive from multiple causes. If a patient reports a level-9-out-of-10 burning pain in the feet after standing or walking for more than 5 minutes, and suffers level-2-out-of-10 pins and needles in the feet when sitting, these symptoms would strongly suggest that the burning pain is caused by Spinal Stenosis or PseudoStenosis, while the pins-and-needles sensation could be caused by neuropathy. If, after treatment for the spine, all the burning is gone, but the pins-and-needles sensation lingers, then I would suspect a separate condition and try to treat that in its turn.

In other words, if after treating one condition there is excellent overall improvement in terms of eliminating or reducing one set of symptoms, it is likely that whatever symptoms remain are due to a second condition. This is the approach that I have used so successfully in my practice and which I would like you to be able to use successfully for your own symptoms. For this reason, I believe it's important to have clarity about the symptoms before any treatment is started—and then again after each treatment is implemented.

Understanding the particulars of your symptoms can be very helpful for you and your relationship with family, friends, physicians, and caregivers. Once you've filled out the questionnaire, the people in your support system will be better able to understand your symptoms and how they affect your quality of life and independence. While I hope that the recommendations in this book will help relieve those symptoms and turn back the hands of time, understanding the symptoms you have had and whatever symptoms remain will enable the people in your life to understand you better, and to help you better as well.

I believe that many people with the symptoms addressed in this book do not receive the support they need—in part, because there is often no obvious physical deformity present. If you had a broken ankle or severe arthritis, people would understand your pain and limitation. But pain or discomfort stemming from Spinal Stenosis, PseudoStenosis, or neuropathy is not accompanied by obvious deformity, so most people do not grasp the extent of your symptoms. Using the questionnaire will help those who love you do just that.

I therefore strongly suggest that before you begin any treatment protocol you complete the symptom questionnaire in the following chapter. It may be quite helpful to fill it out again after trying the different treatment protocols outlined in this book or after treatment by another physician. In this way, you will truly understand your symptoms and be better prepared to overcome them.

The next chapter is divided into three sections. After the introduction, there is a shortened LuSSSExt questionnaire that deals with overall limitations, without specifying the location of the symptoms. For those with limited or straightforward symptoms, this may be enough to give you a feel for where you are starting from.

Next is a section on how to move forward once you are armed with that basic information. PLEASE read that section for guidance.

Finally, the chapter concludes with a more complete questionnaire that deals with symptoms in much greater detail. Originally designed for research, it provides greater insight into which symptoms need to be addressed. For those with extensive symptoms affecting multiple parts of the body, this section can provide direction for you as well as for your doctor. I hope you find it helpful.

CHAPTER 3

The LuSSSExt Scale

Having read the previous chapter, you now know why it's so important to understand your symptoms. Having a good grasp of exactly what symptoms you are experiencing is the vital first step in being able to treat them.

Introducing the LuSSSExt Scale

As medical detectives, it is our job to garner the clues that will help us do some super-sleuthing and track down the source of your pain. This means closely observing your symptoms and describing them accurately. **To help you do this, I've drawn up an easy-to-answer but detailed questionnaire that will help you become very closely acquainted with your symptoms.** I call it the "LuSSSExt scale." "LuSSSExt" stands for **Lu**mbo**S**acral **S**pinal **S**tenosis **Ex**tremopathy.

This tool, which I designed for research purposes, is meant to identify every common symptom in the feet, legs, thighs, and lower back that could be related to Spinal Stenosis or PseudoStenosis. At times, these symptoms can also be caused by other conditions. Filling out this questionnaire may take only 15–30 minutes or so. Afterwards, you will have a clear understanding of the symptoms that have been afflicting you and of the effect that those symptoms have on your overall activity level.

To give you a "heads-up," the symptoms that will be addressed include **pain, aching, burning, numbness, pins and needles, arthritic pain, loss of sensation; and how they affect your ability to stand, walk, sleep, or sit will also be addressed.** Knowing that these questions will be asked, you may want to simply try to be active for a day or two and then take the test. Another option would be to look the test over in detail, and then spend a day or two trying to be active, while paying close attention to what your body is telling you. After you've gone out of your way to become aware of your symptoms, you will be ready to take the test.

Don't be overwhelmed by the test length. First of all, the questions will be easy for you to answer. It's important to understand that you are not contrasting your level of symptoms with that of another person. You are only trying to understand *your* symptoms as they affect *you*, with the goal of being able to compare them to the severity of symptoms you have after treatment.

After you have filled out the LuSSSExt scale, you will know what symptoms you have in detail. Armed with that knowledge, seek clarity and improvement with the guidance of the chapters on both Spinal Stenosis and Pseudo-Stenosis in Section 2 of this book. Regarding any symptoms that remain, or that are attributed to specific medical conditions, you can refer to the appropriate chapters of Section 3 with greater clarity and direction.

Since you will fill out the scale more than once, you have two choices. You can either make copies of the LuSSSExt scale, or you can use the same scale more than once by using different color pencils, or perhaps different symbols. For example:

First time, circle the answer.   **Second time, box the answer.**

Third time, triangle the answer.   **Fourth time, star the answer.**

Hopefully, you will see a dramatic improvement with the "box." In any case, you will obtain a much greater understanding of the symptoms that you have been living with, which can help guide treatment.

If you would like to take a shortcut, you can fill out the first two pages only. This is the section called "Abbreviated Scale of Overall Symptoms." I believe it helpful to fill out the whole form, to best understand symptom details, but even the first section would be helpful.

Patient instructions

1. Please fill out this form slowly and carefully. Please take your time and properly identify the symptoms you have had.

2. Only record your symptoms or limitations that have been present on a fairly consistent basis. It is only such symptoms that can be followed.

    a. For example, if you think that, despite being active, you rarely have a burning sensation on the top of your foot (less frequently than every week), do not mention it. Only mention symptoms that are clearly present and fairly common. Symptoms must be common enough for you to notice that they have improved!

    b. If, however, the symptom is present whenever you try to do any activity, such as walking as far as you would like, and you avoid the symptom by avoiding the activity, then you should record the symptom and describe how the symptom presents itself when you try to be active.

3. The following guide will be present at the top of each left-hand page to guide you. It presents two categories: LEVEL OF SYMPTOMS and LEVEL OF EFFECT.

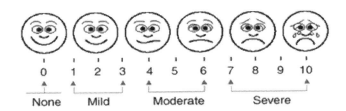

Level of symptoms

- **0**   *No symptoms*
- **1-3**   *Mild definite symptoms*
- **4-6**   *Moderate symptom*
- **7-9**   *Severe symptoms*
- **10**   *Completely disabling symptoms*

Level of effect

- **0**   *None*
- **1**   *Mild occasional effect*
- **2**   *Mild frequent effect*
- **3**   *Mild constant effect*
- **4**   *Moderate occasional effect*
- **5**   *Moderate frequent effect*
- **6**   *Severe occasional effect*
- **7**   *Moderate constant effect*
- **8**   *Severe frequent effect*
- **9**   *Severe constant effect*
- **10**   *Severe disabling constant effect*

When filling out this form, use your own judgment. These answers will not be compared to other people's, but will allow you to understand your situation and to understand the amount of improvement you see with the treatment that is provided.

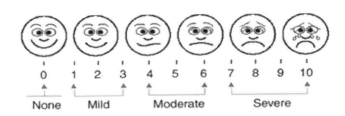

Level of symptoms

0 *No symptoms*

1-3 *Mild definite symptoms*

4-6 *Moderate symptom*

7-9 *Severe symptoms*

10 *Completely disabling symptoms*

Level of effect

0 *None*

1 *Mild occasional effect*   **2** *Mild frequent effect*

3 *Mild constant effect*   **4** *Moderate occasional effect*

5 *Moderate frequent effect*   **6** *Severe occasional effect*

7 *Moderate constant effect*   **8** *Severe frequent effect*

9 *Severe constant effect*   **10** *Severe disabling constant effect*

Abbreviated Scale of Overall Symptoms

1. Overall, when you try to do normal activity, how severe is the level of symptoms in your back, thighs, legs, or feet?

   0 1 2 3 4 5 6 7 8 9 10

2. Overall, how do your symptoms in your back, thighs, legs, or feet affect your ability to care for your daily needs?

   0 1 2 3 4 5 6 7 8 9 10

3. Overall, how do the symptoms in your back, thighs, legs, or feet affect your quality of life?

   0 1 2 3 4 5 6 7 8 9 10

4. Overall, how do the symptoms in your back, thighs, legs, or feet affect your mood?

   0 1 2 3 4 5 6 7 8 9 10

5. Overall, how do the symptoms in your back, thighs, legs, or feet affect your ability to be active?

   0 1 2 3 4 5 6 7 8 9 10

6. Overall, how do the symptoms in your back, thighs, legs, or feet affect your ability to engage in activity as you could many years ago?

   0 1 2 3 4 5 6 7 8 9 10

7. Overall, how would you describe the arthritis pain in your back, hips, knees, or feet (any of above)?

   0 1 2 3 4 5 6 7 8 9 10

8. Overall, how do the symptoms in your back, thighs, legs, or feet affect your ability to get a full night's sleep?

   0 1 2 3 4 5 6 7 8 9 10

9. Overall, how do the symptoms in your back, thighs, legs, or feet affect your ability to get in and out of a bed or chair easily?

   0 1 2 3 4 5 6 7 8 9 10

10. Overall, how far are you usually able to **walk comfortably, without any device or help**?

    0 Well over 1 mile   **1** About 1 mile   **2** About ¾ of a mile (7 blocks)

    3 About ½ mile (5 blocks)   **4** About ¼ mile (2½ blocks)   **5** About 1½ blocks

6 About 1 block (500 feet)   **7** About ½ block   **8** About ¼ block (125 feet)

9 Less than 100 feet (40 steps)   **10** Less than 50 feet (20 steps)

11. How much do your back, thigh, leg, or foot symptoms interfere with your ability to sleep?

    0 My sleep is never disturbed.

    2 My sleep is only occasionally disturbed by back, foot, or leg symptoms.

    4 Because of back, foot, or leg symptoms, I often have less than 6 hours of uninterrupted sleep.

    6 Because of back, foot, or leg symptoms, I often have less than 4 hours of uninterrupted sleep

    8 Because of back, foot, or leg symptoms, I often have less than 2 hours of uninterrupted sleep.

    10 Because of back, foot, or leg symptoms, I often have less than 1 hour of uninterrupted sleep.

    Follow-up question: Have you had NEW significant symptoms develop since the treatment began?

    NO   YES   ____Back   ____Thighs   ____Legs   ____Feet

12. **How long can you stand before you want to sit** because of back, thigh, leg, or foot discomfort?

    0 over 30 minutes   **2** 21–30 minutes   **4** 11–20 minutes

    6 6–10 minutes   **8** 3–5 minutes   **10** Less than 3 minutes

13. **How long can you walk before you want to** sit because of back, thigh, leg, or foot discomfort?

    0 over 30 minutes   **2** 21–30 minutes   **4** 11–20 minutes

    6 6–10 minutes   **8** 3–5 minutes   **10** Less than 3 minutes

14. How far can you walk before you have **some increased discomfort** in your back, thighs, legs, or feet?

    0 Well over 1 mile   **1** About 1 mile   **2** About ¾ of a mile (7 blocks)

    3 About ½ mile (5 blocks)   **4** About ¼ mile (2½ blocks)   **5** About 1½ blocks

    6 About 1 block (500 feet)   **7** About ½ block   **8** About ¼ block (125 feet)

    9 Less than 100 feet (40 steps)   **10** Less than 50 feet (20 steps)

15. Overall, how far are you usually able to walk comfortably without any device or help **before you must stop** because of symptoms in your back, thighs, legs, or feet?

    0 Well over 1 mile   **1** About 1 mile   **2** About ¾ of a mile (7 blocks)

    3 About ½ mile (5 blocks)   **4** About ¼ mile (2½ blocks)   **5** About 1½ blocks

    6 About 1 block (500 feet)   **7** About ½ block   **8** About ¼ block (125 feet)

    9 Less than 100 feet (40 steps)   **10** Less than 50 feet (20 steps)

16. **How long can you sit before you want to get up** because of back, thigh, leg, or foot discomfort?

    0 over 30 minutes   **2** 21–30 minutes   **4** 11–20 minutes

    6 6–10 minutes   **8** 3–5 minutes   **10** Less than 3 minutes

17. Overall, when you sit too long, how severe is the level of symptoms in your back, thighs, legs, or feet?

    0 **1** **2** **3** **4** **5** **6** **7** **8** **9** **10**

Should I do the full LuSSSExt scale?

Those who want only a basic understanding of their symptoms may stop after this first section of the LuSSSExt scale is completed and proceed with "The Next Step." Those who want a more detailed understanding of their symptoms, especially if they have multiple locations of symptoms, should complete the full LuSSSExt scale, presented later in this chapter. In either case, there may be value in repeating the questionnaire after treatment that you do yourself or get from a medical professional.

The Next Step

Now that you have a clearer handle on your symptoms, how do you proceed?

If after completing this questionnaire you find that your symptoms are *absolutely consistent* and do not get worse with walking, standing, sitting, or lying down, then I am afraid my main approaches will likely not help you a great deal. Much of my success comes from modifying the function and position of the feet, legs, and back. **If your symptoms are not at all affected by position or activity, there is less likelihood of success using the methods outlined here.**

Two Outliers–Difficulty Sitting

Many people have greater back or leg discomfort while walking, standing, or lying down. If, however, your symptoms are often worse while sitting, there are two common possibilities to consider.

First, it is quite possible that you have a problem with a herniated disc. Modifying sitting position may be helpful. I advise people to sit on a pillow or two and see if that helps. If it does, they should use a pillow for sitting all the time (even in a car) for at least a few days.

Second, it is also common that such symptoms are affected by PseudoStenosis, with the most common cause being Limb Length Discrepancy. Such individuals often have discomfort both while sitting and upon arising from a seated position. Guidance on evaluation and treatment is provided in Chapters 12 and 19.

If symptoms do not resolve, follow up with an orthopedist or physiatrist.

You can certainly go to the section of this book that concerns your diagnosis, such as arthritis, neuropathy, circulation problems, nighttime symptoms, etc. You may find valuable information there, but probably not the quick or dramatic source of healing that may be obtained with other presentations. I am sorry.

If you find that your symptoms are constantly present but become much worse with walking, standing, or even lying down, then you should read the chapters on Positional History and Positional Testing for Spinal Stenosis. These may guide you to quick relief.

If you've already been diagnosed with Spinal Stenosis, read the next section on the traditional approaches for this condition, and read the sections on Positional History and Positional Testing. I have included the section on the traditional treatment of Spinal Stenosis, but I only use those approaches if mine have not worked. Because they *do* work more than 70% of the time, I send people for traditional therapy, injections, or surgery fairly infrequently.

EVEN IF you have good results with treatment for Spinal Stenosis, it is essential to read the sections on PseudoStenosis. Many people with Spinal Stenosis, even those who've seen good results with Positional Testing, also have PseudoStenosis, and the management of that condition is often absolutely necessary for long-term success.

If you have a diagnosis of Peripheral Neuropathy, poor circulation, arthritis, painful swollen legs, or Restless Leg Syndrome, you should read the chapter on your particular diagnosis, but you should still read the chapter on Positional History. There is a great deal of overlap between all of these conditions and either Spinal Stenosis or PseudoStenosis.

When it comes down to Positional Testing, which you will soon understand, I advise as strongly as possible to put your heart and soul into trying all the advice. Remember, relief may be obtained in just 1, 2, or at most 3 days—if you do it right!

Following is the remainder of the full version of the LuSSSExt scale. Those who fill this out will obtain a far greater clarity as to the details of their symptoms.

The Full LuSSSExt Scale Questionnaire

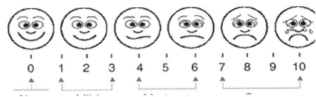

Level of symptoms		Level of effect	
0 No symptoms		**0** None	
1-3 Mild definite symptoms		**1** Mild occasional effect	**2** Mild frequent effect
4-6 Moderate symptom		**3** Mild constant effect	**4** Moderate occasional effect
7-9 Severe symptoms		**5** Moderate frequent effect	**6** Severe occasional effect
10 Completely disabling symptoms		**7** Moderate constant effect	**8** Severe frequent effect
		9 Severe constant effect	**10** Severe disabling constant effect

Spine symptoms

18. Overall, how would you describe your arthritis pain of the lower spine?

    0   1   2   3   4   5   6   7   8   9   10

19. When you try to do normal activity, how severe is the level of symptoms in your back?

    0   1   2   3   4   5   6   7   8   9   10

20. Overall, how do the symptoms in your back affect your ability to care for your daily needs?

    0   1   2   3   4   5   6   7   8   9   10

21. Overall, how do the symptoms in your back affect your quality of life?

    0   1   2   3   4   5   6   7   8   9   10

22. Overall, how do the symptoms in your back affect your ability to sleep a full night's sleep?

    0   1   2   3   4   5   6   7   8   9   10

23. Overall, how do the symptoms in your back affect your mood?

    0   1   2   3   4   5   6   7   8   9   10

24. Overall, how do the symptoms in your back affect your ability to be active?

    0   1   2   3   4   5   6   7   8   9   10

25. Overall, how do the symptoms in your back affect your ability to get in and out of a bed or chair easily?

    0   1   2   3   4   5   6   7   8   9   10

26. Overall, how do the symptoms in your back affect your ability to engage in activity as you could many years ago?

    0   1   2   3   4   5   6   7   8   9   10

27. Overall, how do the symptoms in your back affect urination or moving your bowels?

    0   **1**   **2**   **3**   **4**   **5**   **6**   **7**   **8**   **9**   **10**

28. How long can you stand before you want to sit because of back discomfort?

0 over 30 minutes	**2** 21–30 minutes	**4** 11–20 minutes
6 6–10 minutes	**8** 3–5 minutes	**10** Less than 3 minutes

29. How long can you walk before you want to sit because of back discomfort?

0 over 30 minutes	**2** 21–30 minutes	**4** 11–20 minutes
6 6–10 minutes	**8** 3–5 minutes	**10** Less than 3 minutes

30. How far can you walk before you have some **increased discomfort** in your back?

0 Well over 1 mile	**1** About 1 mile	**2** About ¾ of a mile (7 blocks)
3 About ½ mile (5 blocks)	**4** About ¼ mile (2½ blocks)	**5** About 1½ blocks
6 About 1 block (500 feet)	**7** About ½ block	**8** About ¼ block (125 feet)
9 Less than 100 feet (40 steps)	**10** Less than 50 feet (20 steps)	

31. Overall, how far are you able to usually walk comfortably without any device or help **before you must stop** because of symptoms in your back?

0 Well over 1 mile	**1** About 1 mile	**2** About ¾ of a mile (7 blocks)
3 About ½ mile (5 blocks)	**4** About ¼ mile (2½ blocks)	**5** About 1½ blocks
6 About 1 block (500 feet)	**7** About ½ block	**8** About ¼ block (125 feet)
9 Less than 100 feet (40 steps)	**10** Less than 50 feet (20 steps)	

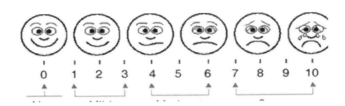

<table>
</table>

Level of symptoms

0   *No symptoms*

1-3 *Mild definite symptoms*

4-6 *Moderate symptom*

7-9 *Severe symptoms*

10 *Completely disabling symptoms*

Level of effect

0   *None*

1   *Mild occasional effect*   *2*   *Mild frequent effect*

3   *Mild constant effect*   *4*   *Moderate occasional effect*

5   *Moderate frequent effect*   *6*   *Severe occasional effect*

7   *Moderate constant effect*   *8*   *Severe frequent effect*

9   *Severe constant effect*   *10* *Severe disabling constant effect*

Thigh symptoms

32. Overall, how would you describe the discomfort in your thighs?

   0   1   2   3   4   5   6   7   8   9   10

33. Overall, how would you describe arthritis pain in your hip or hips?

   0   1   2   3   4   5   6   7   8   9   10

34. Overall, when you try to do normal activity, how severe is the level of symptoms in the front of your thighs?

   0   1   2   3   4   5   6   7   8   9   10

35. Overall, when you try to do normal activity, how severe is the level of symptoms in the back of your thighs?

   0   1   2   3   4   5   6   7   8   9   10

36. With activity, what is the level of aching or cramping in your thighs?

   0   1   2   3   4   5   6   7   8   9   10

37. What is the level of burning sensation in your thighs?

   0   1   2   3   4   5   6   7   8   9   10

38. What is the level of sharp or shooting pain in your thighs?

   0   1   2   3   4   5   6   7   8   9   10

39. When you try to be active, what is the level of weakness you feel in your thighs?

   0   1   2   3   4   5   6   7   8   9   10

40. What is the level of uncomfortable tingling sensation (paresthesias) in your thighs?

   0   1   2   3   4   5   6   7   8   9   10

41. What is the level of a sensation of numbness in your thighs?

   0   1   2   3   4   5   6   7   8   9   10

42. Overall, how do your symptoms in your thighs affect your ability to care for your daily needs?

   0   1   2   3   4   5   6   7   8   9   10

43. Overall, how do the symptoms in your thighs affect your quality of life?

 0   1   2   3   4   5   6   7   8   9   10

44. Overall, how do the symptoms in your thighs affect your ability to get a full night's sleep?

 0   1   2   3   4   5   6   7   8   9   10

45. Overall, how do the symptoms in your thighs affect your mood?

 0   1   2   3   4   5   6   7   8   9   10

46. Overall, how do the symptoms in your thighs affect your ability to be active?

 0   1   2   3   4   5   6   7   8   9   10

47. Overall, how do the symptoms in your thighs affect your ability to get in and out of a bed or chair easily?

 0   1   2   3   4   5   6   7   8   9   10

48. Overall, how do symptoms in your thighs affect your ability to engage in extensive activity as you could many years ago?

 0   1   2   3   4   5   6   7   8   9   10

49. **How long can you stand before you want to sit** because of thigh discomfort?

| **0** over 30 minutes | **2** 21–30 minutes | **4** 11–20 minutes |
| **6** 6–10 minutes | **8** 3–5 minutes | **10** Less than 3 minutes |

50. How long can you walk before you **want to sit** because of thigh discomfort?

| **0** over 30 minutes | **2** 21–30 minutes | **4** 11–20 minutes |
| **6** 6–10 minutes | **8** 3–5 minutes | **10** Less than 3 minutes |

51. How far can you walk before you experience some **increased discomfort** in your thighs?

0 Well over 1 mile	**1** About 1 mile	**2** About ¾ of a mile (7 blocks)
3 About ½ mile (5 blocks)	**4** About ¼ mile (2½ blocks)	**5** About 1½ blocks
6 About 1 block (500 feet)	**7** About ½ block	**8** About ¼ block (125 feet)
9 Less than 100 feet (40 steps)	**10** Less than 50 feet (20 steps)	

52. Overall, how far are you able to usually walk comfortably without any device or help **before you must stop** because of symptoms in your thighs?

0 Well over 1 mile	**1** About 1 mile	**2** About ¾ of a mile (7 blocks)
3 About ½ mile (5 blocks)	**4** About ¼ mile (2½ blocks)	**5** About 1½ blocks
6 About 1 block (500 feet)	**7** About ½ block	**8** About ¼ block (125 feet)
9 Less than 100 feet (40 steps)	**10** Less than 50 feet (20 steps)	

53. Are the symptoms overall

a. Not significant at all in the thighs **b.** About the same in both thighs

c. Worse in the right thigh   **d.** Worse in the left thigh

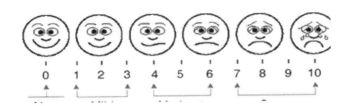

Level of symptoms		**Level of effect**	
0 No symptoms	**0** None	
1-3 Mild definite symptoms	**1** Mild occasional effect	**2** Mild frequent effect
4-6 Moderate symptom	**3** Mild constant effect	**4** Moderate occasional effect
7-9 Severe symptoms	**5** Moderate frequent effect	**6** Severe occasional effect
10 Completely disabling symptoms	**7** Moderate constant effect	**8** Severe frequent effect
	9 Severe constant effect	**10** Severe disabling constant effect

Leg symptoms

54. Overall, how would you describe the discomfort in your LEGS?

   0   1   2   3   4   5   6   7   8   9   10

55. Overall, how would you describe arthritis pain of your knee or knees?

   0   1   2   3   4   5   6   7   8   9   10

56. Overall, when you try to engage in normal activity, how severe is the level of symptoms in the front of your legs?

   0   1   2   3   4   5   6   7   8   9   10

57. Overall, when you try to engage in normal activity, how severe is the level of symptoms in the back of your legs?

   0   1   2   3   4   5   6   7   8   9   10

58. With activity, what is the level of aching or cramping in your legs?

   0   1   2   3   4   5   6   7   8   9   10

59. What is the level of burning sensation in your legs?

   0   1   2   3   4   5   6   7   8   9   10

60. What is the level of sharp or shooting pain in your legs?

   0   1   2   3   4   5   6   7   8   9   10

61. When you try to be active, what is the level of weakness your legs feel?

   0   1   2   3   4   5   6   7   8   9   10

62. What is the level of the uncomfortable tingling sensation (paresthesias) in your legs?

   0   1   2   3   4   5   6   7   8   9   10

63. What is the level of a sensation of numbness in your legs?

   0   1   2   3   4   5   6   7   8   9   10

64. Overall, how do the symptoms in your legs affect your ability to care for your daily needs?

   0   1   2   3   4   5   6   7   8   9   10

65. Overall, how do the symptoms in your legs affect your quality of life?

    0   1   2   3   4   5   6   7   8   9   10

66. Overall, how do the symptoms in your legs affect your ability to get a full night's sleep?

    0   1   2   3   4   5   6   7   8   9   10

67. Overall, how do the symptoms in your legs affect your mood?

    0   1   2   3   4   5   6   7   8   9   10

68. Overall, how do the symptoms in your legs affect your ability to be active?

    0   1   2   3   4   5   6   7   8   9   10

69. Overall, how do the symptoms in your legs affect your ability to get in and out of a bed or chair easily?

    0   1   2   3   4   5   6   7   8   9   10

70. Overall, how do the symptoms in your legs affect your ability to engage in extensive activity as you could many years ago?

    0   1   2   3   4   5   6   7   8   9   10

71. **How long can you stand before you want to sit** because of leg discomfort?

    0 over 30 minutes   **2** 21–30 minutes   **4** 11–20 minutes

    6 6–10 minutes   **8** 3–5 minutes   **10** Less than 3 minutes

72. **How long can you walk before you want to** sit because of leg discomfort?

    0 over 30 minutes   **2** 21–30 minutes   **4** 11–20 minutes

    6 6–10 minutes   **8** 3–5 minutes   **10** Less than 3 minutes

73. How far can you walk before you have **some increased discomfort** in your legs?

    0 Well over 1 mile   **1** About 1 mile   **2** About ¾ of a mile (7 blocks)

    3 About ½ mile (5 blocks) **4** About ¼ mile (2½ blocks) **5** About 1½ blocks

    6 About 1 block (500 feet) **7** About ½ block   **8** About ¼ block (125 feet)

    9 Less than 100 feet (40 steps) **10** Less than 50 feet (20 steps)

74. Overall, how far are you able to usually walk comfortably without any device or help **before you must stop** because of symptoms in your legs?

    0 Well over 1 mile   **1** About 1 mile   **2** About ¾ of a mile (7 blocks)

    3 About ½ mile (5 blocks) **4** About ¼ mile (2½ blocks) **5** About 1½ blocks

    6 About 1 block (500 feet) **7** About ½ block   **8** About ¼ block (125 feet)

    9 Less than 100 feet (40 steps) **10** Less than 50 feet (20 steps)

75. Are the symptoms overall

    a. Not significant at all in the legs   **b.** About the same in both legs   **c.** In the right leg only.

    d. In the left leg only   **e.** In both legs, but worse in the right **f.** In both legs, but worse in the left

    h. In both legs, but with very different discomfort patterns in the two legs

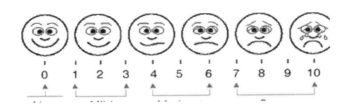

Level of symptoms		**Level of effect**	
0 No symptoms		**0** None	
1-3 Mild definite symptoms		**1** Mild occasional effect	**2** Mild frequent effect
4-6 Moderate symptom		**3** Mild constant effect	**4** Moderate occasional effect
7-9 Severe symptoms		**5** Moderate frequent effect	**6** Severe occasional effect
10 Completely disabling symptoms		**7** Moderate constant effect	**8** Severe frequent effect
		9 Severe constant effect	**10** Severe disabling constant effect

Foot symptoms

76. Overall, how would you describe the discomfort in your feet?

0   1   2   3   4   5   6   7   8   9   10

77. Overall, how would you describe arthritis pain in your ankle or ankles?

0   1   2   3   4   5   6   7   8   9   10

78. Overall, how would you describe arthritis pain in your foot or feet?

0   1   2   3   4   5   6   7   8   9   10

79. Overall, when you try to engage in normal activity, how severe is the level of symptoms in the top of your feet?

0   1   2   3   4   5   6   7   8   9   10

80. Overall, when you try to engage in normal activity, how severe is the level of symptoms in the bottom of your feet?

0   1   2   3   4   5   6   7   8   9   10

81. With activity, what is the level of aching or cramping in your feet?

0   1   2   3   4   5   6   7   8   9   10

82. What is the level of burning sensation in your feet?

0   1   2   3   4   5   6   7   8   9   10

83. What is the level of sharp or shooting pain in your feet?

0   1   2   3   4   5   6   7   8   9   10

84. When you try to be active, what is the level of weakness in your feet?

0   1   2   3   4   5   6   7   8   9   10

85. What is the level of uncomfortable tingling sensation (paresthesias) in your feet?

0   1   2   3   4   5   6   7   8   9   10

86. What is the level of a sensation of numbness in your feet?

0   1   2   3   4   5   6   7   8   9   10

87. Overall, how do the symptoms in your feet affect your ability to care for your daily needs?

    0   1   2   3   4   5   6   7   8   9   10

88. Overall, how do the symptoms in your feet affect your quality of life?

    0   1   2   3   4   5   6   7   8   9   10

89. Overall, how do the symptoms in your feet affect your ability to get a full night's sleep?

    0   1   2   3   4   5   6   7   8   9   10

90. Overall, how do the symptoms in your feet affect your mood?

    0   1   2   3   4   5   6   7   8   9   10

91. Overall, how do the symptoms in your feet affect your ability to be active?

    0   1   2   3   4   5   6   7   8   9   10

92. Overall, how do the symptoms in your feet affect your ability to get in and out of a bed or chair easily?

    0   1   2   3   4   5   6   7   8   9   10

93. Overall, how do symptoms in your feet affect your ability to engage in extensive activity as you could many years ago?

    0   1   2   3   4   5   6   7   8   9   10

94. **How long can you stand before you want to sit** because of foot discomfort?

0 over 30 minutes	**2** 21–30 minutes	**4** 11–20 minutes
6 6–10 minutes	**8** 3–5 minutes	**10** Less than 3 minutes

95. **How long can you walk before you want to** sit because of foot discomfort?

0 over 30 minutes	**2** 21–30 minutes	**4** 11–20 minutes
6 6–10 minutes	**8** 3–5 minutes	**10** Less than 3 minutes

96. How far can you walk before you have some **increased discomfort** in your feet?

0 Well over 1 mile	**1** About 1 mile	**2** About ¾ of a mile (7 blocks)
3 About ½ mile (5 blocks)	**4** About ¼ mile (2½ blocks)	**5** About 1½ blocks
6 About 1 block (500 feet)	**7** About ½ block	**8** About ¼ block (125 feet)
9 Less than 100 feet (40 steps)	**10** Less than 50 feet (20 steps)	

97. Overall, how far are you usually able to walk comfortably without any device or help **before you must stop** because of symptoms in your feet?

0 Well over 1 mile	**1** About 1 mile	**2** About ¾ of a mile (7 blocks)
3 About ½ mile (5 blocks)	**4** About ¼ mile (2½ blocks)	**5** About 1½ blocks
6 About 1 block (500 feet)	**7** About ½ block	**8** About ¼ block (125 feet)
9 Less than 100 feet (40 steps)	**10** Less than 50 feet (20 steps)	

98. Are the symptoms overall

a. Not significant at all in the feet	**b.** About the same in both feet	**c.** In the right foot only.
d. In the left foot only	**e.** In both feet, but worse in the right	**f.** In both feet, but worse in the left
h. In both feet, but with very different discomfort patterns in the two feet		

Now that you have filled out the complete questionnaire, please proceed to use the information available in this book as guided by "The Next Step," presented earlier in this chapter.

Spinal Stenosis and PseudoStenosis:

Everything you Need to Know

CHAPTER 4

Spinal Stenosis: The Classic Approach

Know your enemy—a sound piece of advice for anyone with a battle to fight. It is an especially useful tip when dealing with a medical "villain." A major focus of this book is the recognition and treatment of two culprits that are behind a high percentage of the painful symptoms I see in my practice: Lumbar Spinal Stenosis and PseudoStenosis. Accordingly, I will present here a brief, basic overview of the classic approach to the recognition and treatment of the first of these conditions—Spinal Stenosis.

The positional approach, which often makes it so easy to identify and treat stenosis symptoms, will be dealt with in Chapters 7–10. PseudoStenosis will be addressed in Chapters 11 and 12.

Our two villains are like a wily pair of nearly identical twins. PseudoStenosis symptoms are often exactly the same as those of Spinal Stenosis. In their respective chapters, I will also explain how to differentiate between the two, something that is essential for anyone who has Spinal Stenosis symptoms that have not been resolved with treatment.

If you have been diagnosed with Spinal Stenosis, some of what follows may be a review of the condition and the treatment protocols that you have already undergone. The treatment approaches presented here are not the ones I usually use, but rather what I recommend for symptoms of Spinal Stenosis if my own approaches fail.

An Overview of Spinal Stenosis

"Stenosis" means "narrowing." When stenosis is present, there is a narrowing of structures of the spine, which can cause either local arthritic pain or pressure on the nerves that can lead to symptoms in the parts of the body that are controlled, or innervated, by those nerves. Depending on where the nerve is compressed in the lower back, you may experience symptoms in your buttocks, thighs, legs, or feet. Sometimes only one area is affected, while at other times, two or even all of the areas come into play.

Stenosis can affect the central canal of the spinal area, or it can involve the areas where individual nerves leave the spinal canal. These areas are called the "foramen," which means "window." A person can have either *central canal stenosis* or *lateral-recess / foraminal stenosis.*

The most common location of classic central canal Spinal Stenosis is the L4/L5 area of the lumbosacral spine. This most frequently causes symptoms in the legs, with the classical symptom known as "neurogenic claudication." You can recognize this condition by an aching, tired, or weak feeling in the legs, a sensation which is aggravated by standing and walking and which is best relieved by sitting or leaning forward. These symptoms, based upon the location of the narrowing, can also be present in the feet or thighs.

Symptoms of spinal-induced (neurogenic) claudication are somewhat similar to those caused by poor arterial circulation, as will be presented in great detail in Chapter 16.

Symptoms of Spinal Stenosis may be aggravated by fully extending the lumbosacral spine—for example, when a person stands up and looks at the sky. The pain is often worse at night in bed and may even be exacerbated by coughing.

Walking may actually be easier going uphill than downhill, because of the effect that the gradient may have on the spine position and on spinal nerve compression.

Lateral stenosis, in which the compression occurs where the nerve leaves the central canal, may cause symptoms similar to those of central canal stenosis, but may also be consistent with the classical nerve compression that sometimes accompanies a herniated disc. There can be sharp pain, burning, or aching following a specific nerve root distribution. It may be the cause of sciatica symptoms.

Here's a fact that may throw the medical detective off the scent: **People with Spinal Stenosis may or may not experience significant back pain.** There may be a history of low-grade arthritic back pain aggravated by activity or changes in the weather, but there may be absolutely *no* significant or disabling back pain at the time of extremity symptoms—or, indeed, any history of back pain at all. **It is essential to understand that the absence of back pain does not rule out a diagnosis of Spinal Stenosis (or PseudoStenosis) as the cause of the symptoms.**

Standard Approach to Treating Spinal Stenosis

I recommend physical therapy, medications, epidural injections, and consideration for surgery only if the *mechanical approaches* for PseudoStenosis and the *positional approaches* for Spinal Stenosis do not prove adequate for a specific patient. While I sometimes resort to these traditional methods, I feel that when I do, it represents a failure of my own approaches. I am grateful not to have to resort to what are for me "the old ways" very often.

Treatment for Spinal Stenosis in the classic manner can either be conservative or surgical in nature. Conservative treatment includes anti-inflammatory medications, antidepressant or anticonvulsant medications, or narcotic pain medications to control the pain. Some clinicians recommend acupuncture. Topical medications, such as Lidoderm patches or Diclofenac patches, may be used. A back brace can be utilized. Physical therapy can be brought into play, involving modalities to reduce local inflammation as well as exercises to strengthen the abdomen—also known as "strengthening the core"—in an attempt to stabilize the spine.

Conservative care also includes epidural injections, having a specialist inject cortisone into the area around the nerves in the spine. **Conventional wisdom directs that these epidural injections should be administered under fluoroscopy, a mechanism whereby the spine is evaluated on a radiology unit at the time of injection.** This facilitates the application of the cortisone to the correct place.

Finally, if conservative care is not helpful in restoring an adequate quality of life to the individual, surgery may be an option. This could involve a laminectomy, in which bone and soft tissue are removed to allow greater room in the spine, or it could involve a fusion, in which vertebrae are fused together in such a way as to provide adequate room in the spine. There are newer procedures, whereby surgery is done with small incisions, or even the insertion of an implant such as the X-stop to try to restore proper spinal alignment. A discussion of the details of these surgeries is beyond the scope of this book.

Management of Spinal Stenosis with these techniques is best done by a physiatrist, a pain management specialist, or either an orthopedic spine surgeon or a neurosurgeon.

The Next Step

Many people who suffer from Spinal Stenosis have success with these treatments and experience enough resolution of their symptoms to restore the quality of life that they seek.

HOWEVER, I believe it likely that people who are reading this book and know that they have Spinal Stenosis have either already tried standard protocols or have chosen to avoid some of the more extensive or invasive treatments. In either case, they are looking for another approach.

The approaches that I use, which have proved helpful to some 3500 of my patients with Spinal Stenosis and PseudoStenosis symptoms, are described in the next chapters. For those who have read in detail thus far, I repeat the caveat that these methods—positional management for Spinal Stenosis and mechanical management for PseudoStenosis—have been helpful for "only" about 70% of the people that I have treated for Spinal Stenosis symptoms. If treatment works, it always works within a few days. If it does not work, it does not interfere with the patient's exploring other treatment.

Nearly three-quarters of my patients suffering with Spinal Stenosis symptoms have benefitted from the methods you are about to become acquainted with in the next several chapters. These methods reduced or eliminated pain and disability from their lives and allowed them to embrace a slew of activities and pleasures that they'd written off—sometimes for years.

Move on to the next chapters and see what you can do to join their satisfied club.

For the clinician and the very curious

The following three sections, "Radiologic Testing," "Nerve Testing," and "Radiologic Findings," are presented for those who want additional understanding of the process of diagnosing Spinal Stenosis. Those who are interested only in moving on to sections on identifying and managing Spinal Stenosis symptoms may skip these sections.

Radiologic Testing for Spinal Stenosis

The gold-standard test for confirming the presence of Spinal Stenosis is magnetic resonance imaging, or MRI. This is a safe test, and it is usually accurate. However, it is also a test with limited value. Because the presence of Spinal Stenosis as an anatomic pathology does not mean that Spinal Stenosis is actually causing the symptoms in question, it is common for a patient to have a positive MRI in which stenosis is identified, but to still suffer symptoms caused by another condition.

This is similar to having a person take a foot X-ray that identifies arthritis, a heel spur, or a bunion, while in fact the identified problem is not the cause of the patient's pain. This concept is supported by findings reported in a recent article in the highly respected journal *SPINE* (Kalichman, L., et al. 2009. "Spinal stenosis prevalence and association with symptoms: The Framingham Study." *SPINE* 9 (7): 545–50.).

The authors reported that among people over 60 years old, 47.2% were found to have at least some Spinal Stenosis. Many, even with severe changes, did not have any stenosis symptoms. Thus, an MRI is a very valuable test but one that is often inconclusive and not necessary. As will be detailed in Chapter 14, on radiology, the American College of Physicians opines that an MRI should usually not be ordered for Spinal Stenosis unless there is strong doubt as to the diagnosis, or unless there is strong consideration of invasive treatment such as spinal injections or surgery.

Other published research studies have reported that standard MRI examinations often fail to identify the Spinal Stenosis that is actually present. There are two modifications that may be done to the MRI, one in which a flexion/extension MRI is taken, and another in which there is axial loading, which may reveal spine pathology not identified in the standard MRI.

One large study, published in *SPINE*, reported that 250 out of 500 patients who had symptoms strongly suggestive of Spinal Stenosis but negative or unimpressive MRI findings, had those findings appear much more definitive if axial loading was used to simulate the effect of weight-bearing on the spine.

Another article in *SPINE* highlighted a significant failure of inter-reader reliability. In other words, some radiologists do not identify Spinal Stenosis pathology that is picked up by other radiologists using the exact same images.

Therefore, the MRI, which is the gold standard in identifying Spinal Stenosis, sometimes shows significant pathology when Spinal Stenosis is not the cause of symptoms, and it certainly can fail to report stenosis even if stenosis is present and is the cause of symptoms. It is the best test that we have at this time for Spinal Stenosis, according to standard medical protocol, but it is only part of the puzzle.

X-rays can, at times, also be helpful in recognizing a cause of Spinal Stenosis, involving either disc pathology, severe arthritis, or an unstable spine in which there is shifting of one vertebra onto another (a condition called "Spondylolisthesis"). Again, anatomic abnormalities can be suspected and confirmed, but this does not always clarify whether Spinal Stenosis is the cause of the presenting symptoms.

More detail, for those interested, is presented in Chapter 14.

Nerve Testing for Spinal Stenosis

Nerve studies are commonly used to test for Spinal Stenosis, specifically nerve-conduction and electromyographic studies. These tests are often quite painful, involving needles and electrical jolts. While often used to evaluate patients with neuropathy, the test can also be useful in evaluating possible spinal nerve compression. **This test often has good value, and can show changes that are consistent with the presence of spinal nerve compression. However, it is not uncommon for these studies to show signs of BOTH spinal nerve compression and Peripheral Neuropathy.** In these situations the nerve study may not clarify which condition is causing the symptoms. In addition, this test does not have value in evaluating the presence or effect of PseudoStenosis. Thus, this test is occasionally of great value, but too often it does not provide help. In my opinion, it should be used only if full clinical evaluation and testing does not provide the needed clarity.

Radiologic Findings for Spinal Stenosis

What follows is a list and brief explanation of anatomic conditions that are recognized as causing symptoms of Spinal Stenosis. If you are a clinician, this may remind you that many conditions can cause symptoms of stenosis. If not a clinician, but interested in in-depth understanding, this may enhance your background and vocabulary. Feel free to skip it if it bogs you down.

#1 Congenital Spinal Stenosis. This involves either bony- or soft-tissue enlargement, causing narrowing of the spinal canal or the foramen. The symptoms of congenital Spinal Stenosis usually do not present until the patient is in the third decade.

#2 Acquired Spinal Stenosis. This stenosis is the most common presentation, with a wide variety of anatomic etiologies. It most commonly develops when a person is in the fifth or sixth decade.

#3 Central canal stenosis. This is associated with enlargement or calcification of soft-tissue structures, significant bulging of the intervertebral discs, or a bony narrowing of the central canal. It is currently divided into relative (mild-to-moderate) Spinal Stenosis, and absolute (more severe) Spinal Stenosis.

#4 Lateral stenosis. This involves a narrowing of the lateral recess of the foramen and causes compression of the individual nerve roots after they branch off the spinal canal. This may be the common cause of Spinal Stenosis symptoms that are asymmetrical, affecting one side of the body more than the other.

#5 Intervertebral disc resorption. This happens when the disc between two vertebrae becomes compressed and narrow. It often causes symptoms of a lateral or foraminal stenosis and is usually bilaterally symmetrical, although it can also produce asymmetric symptoms.

#6 Spondylolisthesis. This is a shifting of one vertebra onto another, which can cause both central-canal and lateral narrowing. This instability may be picked up on X-rays taken in both a flexion and an extension position and can also, according to some articles, be better identified on an MRI that is modified with axial compression.

#7 Ischemic Spondylolisthesis (Spondylolysis). A defect of pars interarticularis can cause an enlargement of a joint portion of the vertebrae and cause narrowing.

#8 Scoliosis. This is a lateral curve of the spine that can cause compression, whether or not there are significant degenerative changes.

#9 Spondylosis. This is a degenerative change of the bony structure of the spine, with enlargements that can cause nerve irritation.

#10 Tumor. An actual growth, either benign or malignant, can cause compression of the spinal cord or nerve root by taking up space, leaving the section of the spinal area involved narrower than usual.

CHAPTER 5

Spinal Stenosis: The Positional History

Spinal Stenosis mimics or worsens the symptoms of so many conditions in the lower extremity. A good history can help one suspect or support a diagnosis. But what is the key to understanding the role of Spinal Stenosis (and PseudoStenosis) that can guide both layperson and clinician to seriously consider this possibility?

It's all about the shape of the spine.

The internal shape of the spinal canal actually changes based upon the spine's position—in other words, depending on whether the person is leaning backward, standing straight, leaning forward, or sitting. **Making use of these changes can be used to suspect, corroborate, and often successfully treat Spinal Stenosis or PseudoStenosis symptoms affecting both the lower extremities and the spine.**

Although this scientific understanding of changes in spinal position is well recognized in the medical community, it is my observation that it is underutilized for either the diagnosis or management of Spinal Stenosis. Proper use of positional management is one of the major keys to helping millions of people resume Walking Well Again.

I repeat this basic and essential information. "Stenosis" means "narrowing." Therefore, Spinal Stenosis is a narrowing of the spine. This most frequently involves the lumbosacral (lower) spine, which is all that this chapter deals with. Both the central canal and the outside sections of the spine (called the lateral recess and foramen) can be made narrow because of changes in the anatomy.

The narrowness of the spine causes pressure on the spinal nerves, which become irritated and/or inflamed, and which then cause the abnormal sensations of pain, aching, weakness, tiredness, shooting pain, burning, numbness, or pins and needles in the feet, legs, or thighs. Local degenerative changes can cause the localized low-back pain which is often, but not always, present.

Although the disabling symptoms in the legs and feet may come from the spine, there may be no back pain present. While some patients may have a history of back pain, others with severe symptoms from Spinal Stenosis never experience significant back pain. For many, this may be the reason the proper diagnosis was missed.

The Role of Lumbosacral Flexion

The key to positional management is the fact that lumbosacral flexion—leaning forward—increases the diameter (opens) the spine.

The spine can usually flex to the point that the narrow section is adequately opened to eliminate nerve pressure. This knowledge, if used properly, can provide the relief that so many people are looking for. This concept was long ago reported in a clinically useful manner by Drs. Goldsmith and Wiesel in the *Journal of Clinical Rheumatology*. They reported that walking while pushing a grocery cart greatly improved the ability to walk in their patients with Spinal Stenosis. This concept is well known by spine surgeons, physiatrists, physical therapists, and many astute physicians of different specialties.

The aggressive use of this information is the key to recognizing Spinal Stenosis, both to distinguish its symptoms from those of other conditions and often to allow total or nearly total resolution of those symptoms. **It does not, however, distinguish symptoms of Spinal Stenosis from those of PseudoStenosis.** Remember, as you read these next chapters, that the chapters on PseudoStenosis must also be read and understood.

How do we use this information? The positional protocol is divided into three sections:

1. Positional History (Chapter 5)
2. Positional Testing (Chapters 7 and 8)
3. Positional Therapy (Chapter 10)
4. Added to this list are two additional investigations:
5. Consideration of possible PseudoStenosis, as explained in Chapters 11 and 12
6. Primarily for clinicians, a physical examination, as presented in Chapter 6

I often use the findings of Chapter 6 to help support my suspicion and to follow up my success, but it is usually not needed by patients.

A Positional History is invaluable. Of the people I've helped using this positional approach, I believe that less than half actually came in to see me because of the SS/PS symptoms. The remainder came in for other foot or leg problems, and the Positional History that I use routinely in the office resulted in a strong suspicion of Spinal Stenosis or PseudoStenosis as a cause of symptoms.

It is one of my goals to have this Positional History become part of standard medical practice for all adults. Having the patient consider the questions and fill out the first section of the LuSSSExt scale makes the attending doctor's job far easier. If you have not yet filled out this questionnaire (Chapter 3), please go back and do so in order to obtain clarity about your symptoms or limitations.

For the Layperson: The Basic Positional History

Individuals are suspected of having Spinal Stenosis (or PseudoStenosis) contributing to or entirely responsible for lower-extremity neuropathic or claudication symptoms if they have a positive Positional History that includes any of the following patterns:

1. Walking or standing difficulty or limitation in which the patient must sit or lean against something to get relief

2. Significant improvement in ambulation when pushing a grocery cart, walker, or baby stroller, or when leaning forward on a treadmill, all of which induce lumbosacral flexion

3. An individual who walks better pushing a grocery cart may have worse symptoms standing in line at the check-out counter

4. Constant, frequent, or occasional lower-extremity symptoms of a neuropathic nature (such as burning, tingling, or shooting pain) with a clear or unclear cause, that is worsened by walking or standing

5. Bedtime worsening neuropathic or other foot or leg symptoms, which are affected by sleep position

6. Finding that relief may also be obtained by holding the hands behind the back or holding the belt along the sides or back of one's clothing, mimicking the "Professor Position," as explained toward the end of Chapter 6

7. A tendency to shift from side to side when standing, or greater difficulty standing than walking (This suggests the presence of a Limb Length Discrepancy, the most common cause of PseudoStenosis, as will be explained in Chapter 12.)

For the Patient: The Next Step

If any of these patterns are present, you may greatly benefit from Positional Testing. Remember, however, that even if you have great success with Positional Testing, you may still have PseudoStenosis that should also be treated.

That is all that is necessary for a patient to know. Any of these patterns can be seen with Spinal Stenosis. This is true even in the presence of other conditions, such as neuropathy, poor circulation, or arthritis. Any of these patterns suggest that Spinal Stenosis or PseudoStenosis plays at least SOME role in the symptoms, and should be evaluated.

The subsequent chapters offer a comprehensive description of Positional Testing and Positional Therapy, as well as direction about how to suspect and investigate PseudoStenosis.

For the Clinician and the Very Curious: The Detailed Positional History

This section is primarily for physicians, other health care professionals, and anyone who would like to understand greater detail on this approach.

In my practice, somewhere around 50% of patients over the age of 60 experience some symptoms of Spinal Stenosis (SS) and/or PseudoStenosis (PS). Of course, my practice is not the norm, as I often have patients come to me because of symptoms that were not successfully treated elsewhere despite good efforts. For these patients, SS/PS is a frequent contributor to their symptoms.

My estimation is that in the general senior population, well over 25% of all patients have SS-/PS-induced symptoms or limitations. I add the concept of limitations in addition to symptoms, as many people restrict their activities in order to avoid symptoms, and thus are greatly affected by SS/PS, even though not symptomatic. The following set of questions is a key to investigating such patients. I therefore present these questions, along with an explanation of the value of each one.

1. **Do you have any other problems with your feet or legs?**

    Many patients with lower-extremity aching or walking limitation do not report these symptoms to their doctor, as they believe that they are a natural part of the aging or disease process, or they have had them previously investigated elsewhere without obtaining relief.

2. **How far can you walk before your feet or legs get tired or have another limiting symptom?**

    Guiding the patient to give a specific answer is necessary to identify whether a limitation is worth investigating, and to allow the patient to confront a limitation he may be doing his best to ignore. Many patients state that they "walk fine" and only recognize the true limitation when asked about a specific distance. Those who say they "walk fine" may think that they are doing well because they can still walk one block, although they may soon

be walking miles after effective management. It is essential to solicit a clear response to this question.

3. **Is that limitation consistent or inconsistent?**

    Patients with claudication (aching in the legs from walking) caused by Peripheral Arterial Disease (PAD) usually have a consistent claudication distance, while those with SS/PS often have an inconsistent claudication distance. This is an important factor. Many people have a mild-to-moderate reduction in circulation, but their actual claudication is neurogenic and will respond to positional management.

4. **When your feet, legs, thighs, or back get(s) tired, heavy, aching, burning, or painful, can you stand erect and rest or must you sit or lean against something in order to get relief?**

    Patients with arterial claudication can stand erect to get relief. Those with SS/PS usually cannot get relief with standing erect, and prefer to sit. Occasionally, a patient will claim that he gets relief by standing without needing to sit, but when questioned in detail he will acknowledge that he has to lean against a counter, cane, or even a wall in order to get relief.

5. **Can you walk better when pushing a grocery cart or baby carriage, or when leaning on a treadmill?**

    Patients with SS can often walk dramatically better while pushing wheeled support that allows lumbosacral flexion. However, some patients with PAD also observe that they walk better with a grocery cart, not understanding that it is the frequent stops involved in shopping that serve to reduce claudication symptoms. Positional Testing is therefore essential for an accurate diagnosis in many cases. The "Grocery Cart Test" clarifies this, and is described at the end of Chapter 7. Patients with neuropathy or other neuromuscular conditions usually report a limited improvement with wheeled support because of improved stability, not because of the elimination of claudication or neuropathic symptoms.

6. **Do you sometimes lean forward with arms crossed along the handle bar when pushing a grocery cart?**

For patients under approximately 5'2", or for those with severe stenosis, this position may induce the flexion needed for adequate opening of the spine to reduce symptoms.

7. Do you find that your symptoms are often much worse at the checkout counter of the grocery store?

This worsening is due to the fact that while walking through the store, patients lean on the cart, but when at the checkout counter they are standing straight, with spinal extension, resulting in intensified symptoms. This may be called a positive "Checkout Counter Sign," a name I thought of while writing this book.

8. Are the painful symptoms you associate with neuropathy made worse with standing and/or walking?

Symptoms that are constantly or almost constantly present, which may be caused by either true neuropathy or severe stenosis, may be exacerbated by standing and walking if SS/PS contributes to the symptoms.

9. Are you more comfortable standing barefoot or in shoes?

Patients with SS may note that the height of the shoe, which can affect spinal stance position, has a significant effect on their foot or leg symptoms. Some patients who are more comfortable barefoot do better in flat or even negative-heel shoes.

10. Are symptoms that are present at night improved by changing your body position?

A reduction of symptoms effected by getting out of bed or sleeping in a recliner suggests that spinal position at night affects symptoms. These patients should be guided in modifying their sleep position, as described in Chapters 8 and 21.

Back in the 1970s, when I went to podiatry school, we were taught to recognize a particular pattern, one that I now disagree with strongly. It involves a person having foot or leg pain in bed that is relieved by sitting up in bed. Often, people with this pattern have adequate large-vessel circulation confirmed by arterial testing and are diagnosed as having symptoms from problems with small blood vessels, a "Microangiopathy." Often, sitting in bed

and placing their legs in a dependent position improves the symptoms. This improvement was attributed to gravity.

This is a pattern that I labeled "nocturnal exacerbation of neuropathic symptoms" and wrote about in 2005 in the journal *Diabetic Medicine.* The patient's suffering actually stems from a positional problem caused by spinal nerve compression, and it suggests SS/PS. Improvement is often achieved by modifying sleep position, without the benefit of gravity!

Some questions point to a Limb Length Discrepancy. Having difficulty standing without shifting from side to side, having difficulty walking straight forward, and having greater difficulty with standing than with walking all suggest Limb Length Discrepancy. A detailed explanation of this condition will be found in Chapter 12, on PseudoStenosis.

These questions can guide you, the clinician, to have a high index of suspicion that either Lumbar Spinal Stenosis or PseudoStenosis is contributing to or is entirely responsible for the symptoms identified. A good Positional History will help clarify the likely diagnosis of SS/PS in your mind. Armed with this strong suspicion, it may be time for you to convince your patient to try . . . Positional Testing.

If I suspect PseudoStenosis, I will usually treat that first. PseudoStenosis is essential to understand, as it is a common reason for the failure of standard treatment for Spinal Stenosis and for the patient's having symptoms of Spinal Stenosis but negative spinal imaging.

If I do not suspect or cannot quickly treat PseudoStenosis, I will utilize Positional Testing. For patients, as well as for clinicians less familiar with PseudoStenosis, Positional Testing allows a quick method to relieve symptoms and confirm SS/PS involvement in symptoms.

I strongly recommend Positional Testing as an initial treatment of true Spinal Stenosis, because the improvement is so rapid, so inexpensive, and so safe. If effective, patients may not need any other treatment! Many of my patients have seen dramatic and rapid improvement with this approach for many years. It can eliminate the deconditioning of benign neglect, avoid the complications of long-term NSAID or narcotic use, and reduce the costs and inconvenience of physical therapy as well as the expenses and risks of spinal imaging and invasive treatment.

My success rate with positional management is about 70%, something you may keep in mind when deciding how to treat patients. Remember, it only takes a few days to know if this approach will work, and this method does not interfere with any other possible treatments.

For patients seeking help, as well as for medical professionals open to investigating this approach, the subsequent chapters offer a comprehensive description of Positional Testing and Positional Therapy.

CHAPTER 6

Physical Findings in SS/PS

What do Spinal Stenosis and PseudoStenosis (SS/PS) actually "look like"? Are there physical clues that can help distinguish them from other conditions that present with similar symptoms, or at least clues that strongly suggest that SS/PS contributes to the overall problem? The answer is yes, but it does require detailed explanation. These clues are not one hundred percent diagnostic, but they are very strongly supportive of a diagnosis of either Spinal Stenosis or PseudoStenosis.

SS and PS are frequently found in people who suffer from other medical problems that can also affect the lower extremities. Most common among these conditions are arthritis, neuropathy, poor arterial circulation,

and swollen legs. Further details about these conditions, including their differentiation from SS/PS, are presented in the relevant chapters.

This chapter has two sections. The first, directed towards patients, is a very basic explanation of the eight clues addressed in greater detail in the second section, which is directed toward clinicians. I am told by editors and readers that the second section would most likely be overly technical for the lay reader, **so I encourage patients to read the first section only and then move on to Chapter 7.** This will give them an introduction to the concepts and allow them to follow stories presented later in the book.

To be honest, this entire chapter could be skipped by individuals just looking to see if Positional Testing can relieve their painful symptoms and allow them to walk, stand, or sleep better. If that is all you are interested in at this time, it is okay to jump to Chapter 7!

Introducing Eight Clues, for the Layperson

1. Patients with SS/PS often have hypersensitivity along certain nerves in the feet as well as in the legs or thighs. I call this clue the **"First Interspace Fine Sign"**. In a patient with this sign, pushing between the first and second metatarsal bones ("1" in Picture 6.1) does not cause tenderness, but each of the other areas shown may be tender. In addition, areas on the inside of the ankle, leg, and thigh may each be tender.

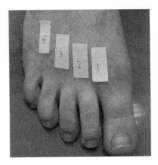

Picture 6.1. Metatarsal interspaces demonstrated.

2. **Loss of sensation** (to light touch) can be seen in multiple conditions, including both Peripheral Neuropathy and SS/PS. There are patterns of loss of sensation that suggest that SS/PS contributes to this problem. If the loss of sensation is worse on one side of the foot or on one side of the body, or if it is higher in the foot than in the toes, it indicates that a nerve compression condition such as SS/PS likely contributes to the problem.

3. The **Extended-Leg Flexion Test** involves flexing legs that are fully extended. This may quickly identify if the symptoms in the feet and legs improve by changing the position of the spine. A good response to this maneuver strongly suggests that spinal position involving SS/PS contributes to symptoms.

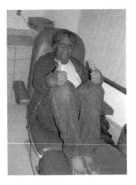

Picture 6.2. Patient indicates that symptoms improve with the legs flexed.

4. The **Professor Position** is a manner of standing with hands behind the back and with the back tilted forward slightly, which opens the spine. Since people with SS/PS usually have symptoms that worsen with standing, which makes them attribute symptoms to bearing weight, relief with this position that flexes the spine suggests that spine position is the cause of pain, and that SS/PS contributes to the symptoms. It is also a therapeutic maneuver that can be helpful for the patient's symptoms, and it is presented in detail in Chapter 8, on the Adjunctive Measures to Positional Testing.

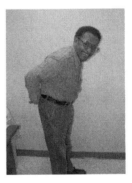

Picture 6.3. Demonstrating the Professor Position.

5. The **Single Stance Flexion Test** is a variant of the Professor Position. If an individual has pain that is worse with standing and is relieved by leaning on a supportive object such as a counter, that suggests that spine position plays a role in pain. However, improvement could also be caused by reducing the weight on the painful leg. In this test, one leans and thus obtains improvement of the pain. Lifting one leg off of the ground, preferably the less uncomfortable extremity, leaves all the weight borne on the remaining leg. If maintaining the spine

position controls the pain, even though the amount of weight is now greater on this leg, it suggests that spine position is the cause of pain and that SS/PS contributes to the symptoms.

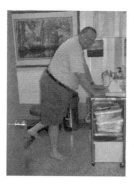

Picture 6.4. Demonstrating the Single Stance Flexion Test.

The next three clues refer specifically to a Limb Length Discrepancy, in which one leg is longer than the other. Many additional clues and physical signs suggestive of a Limb Length Discrepancy will be shared in Chapter 12, but the following three clues are important for you to be aware of as you consider conditions mentioned in this book.

6. **Asymmetric Equinus** refers to a situation in which there is less upward motion in one ankle than in the other. Most often, the shorter leg has less upward motion, although this may improve within just 1-3 days of using a proper lift.

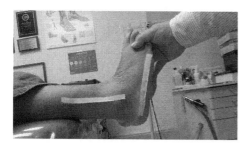

Picture 6.5. This foot does not get to the perpendicular 90-degree position.

7. The **Iliac Crest Pain Resolution Sign** is noted when examining the hips (including the Iliac Crest) of a person with suspected Limb Length Discrepancy. When feeling to see if one hip is higher than the other, as shown, there is frequently increased sensitivity (reported as either discomfort or ticklishness) in areas pressed if there is a discrepancy present and the spinal nerves are irritated.

That sensitivity often resolves immediately when the body is balanced with the proper amount of lift under the short leg. (When the discomfort resolves, I note the patient has **"Happy Hips."**)

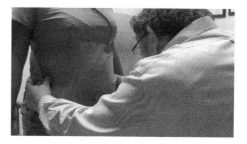

Picture 6.6. Demonstrating examination of the Iliac Crest to the top of the hip bones.

8. **Asymmetric Sensitive Pes Anserinus.** The Pes Anserinus is a spot just below the inside of the knee that is actually the combined tendon of three thigh muscles. While it may be sensitive in both legs in case of arthritis or Flat Feet, it is frequently sensitive only in the longer leg of a patient with a Limb Length Discrepancy. Usually the individual is not aware of this being sensitive unless someone pushes on it, as the knee area may be painless.

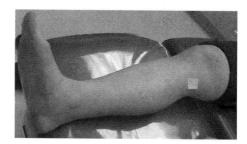

Picture 6.7 Identifying the location of the Pes Anserinus

In addition to these eight clues, it is also essential that every patient with possible Spinal Stenosis or PseudoStenosis have examination for all common causes of PseudoStenosis. These will be addressed in detail in Chapter 12.

IT IS ESSENTIAL for all reading to remember that the methods reported in this book are intended to deal primarily with chronic pain. They are not to be used to treat acute, sudden episodes or any problem that involves nerve changes, such as muscle weakness, change in balance, loss of bladder or rectal control, or any other sudden or serious change in function. Patients who experience such changes should have their care either through an emergency room or in close co-operation with their primary care physician.

Patients and their families can take this basic information and move on to Chapter 7.

* * * * *

The remainder of this chapter is for the clinician and for those who are so very curious that they are willing to put the effort into studying in detail. Given that some non-clinicians will do so, I have tried to present this in a manner that can be understandable for those without a medical background.

Two Catalysts to Investigation

Before presenting the eight clues for clinicians, I want to acknowledge the two potential catalysts that can stimulate investigation. **One is the Positional History as detailed in Chapter 5.** Any clinician who identifies those patterns can be clued in to the need to consider either Spinal Stenosis or PseudoStenosis as a cause of symptoms.

Regarding the physical findings, they can serve three purposes. One is to confirm or at least support the suspicions induced by a positive Positional History. A second is to follow the improvement obtained by appropriate treatment.

The third purpose is primarily for podiatrists, or orthopedists, physical therapists, or any other clinician who makes a thorough examination of the foot an integral part of evaluation visits. The presence of some of these findings can be noted in a quick clinical examination. **The presence of physical findings suggesting either Spinal Stenosis or PseudoStenosis is the second catalyst.** If present, a more aggressive Positional History should be initiated, investigating symptoms that the person may not have come in for or even bother to report when asked in a general manner. Thus, for those who routinely evaluate the foot, identifying these findings, as well as other signs of PseudoStenosis presented in Chapter 12, may open the door to providing life changing assistance for patients. Just as I hope that a Positional History becomes a part of standard medical evaluation, identifying the clues presented here or in Chapter 12 can be the impetus of investigating the potential role of Spinal Stenosis or PseudoStenosis in any of the conditions presented in Section 3 of this book.

Introducing Eight Clues, for the Clinician

The first finding, which is the most versatile and valuable sign, can be used to suggest an SS/PS component under any circumstances. It is the nerve hypersensitivity pattern, which I label the **"First Interspace Fine Sign."** I believe that use of this pattern is one of the most significant original contributions of this body of work.

The second finding is the **Loss of Protective Sensation (LOPS)** pattern. It is most valuable in differentiating SS/PS from Peripheral Neuropathy. It also allows one to follow treatment, as does the First Interspace Fine Sign.

The third finding, the **Extended-Leg Flexion Test**, is something I use only occasionally. It involves the alteration of either the LOPS pattern or symptoms, based upon alteration of seated body position.

The fourth and fifth findings are variants of Positional Testing: the **Professor Position** and the **Single Stance Flexion Test**. The Single Stance Flexion Test, though used infrequently, is absolutely shocking to patients. I use the Professor Position far more frequently, as it not only clearly shows the effect of spinal position on both low-back and lower-extremity symptoms, but it is also a valuable treatment tool. The Professor Position, described in detail in Chapter 8, is an adjunct therapy used therapeutically when external support such as a walker or grocery cart is not available.

The sixth, seventh and eighth findings are specific to Limb Length Discrepancy, the most common cause of PseudoStenosis. They are **Asymmetric Equinus**, the **Iliac Crest Pain Resolution Sign**, and **Asymmetric Sensitive Pes Anserinus**.

Clue 1: The First Interspace Fine Sign: Whetting Your Appetite

What follows is the most dramatic and important physical sign set consistent with Spinal Stenosis/Pseudo-Stenosis. While it is not one hundred percent accurate, it is very common and extremely helpful. This pattern can be used to investigate and follow ALL patients with possible SS/PS symptoms, including patients with symptoms of poor circulation, painful swelling, arthritis, Restless Leg Syndrome, or neuropathy, as well as patients with any other lower-extremity symptom.

This set of signs is useful in four ways:

1. **To identify the SS/PS pattern**

2. **To reassure the patient that I have detailed knowledge of his or her condition, in a manner similar to a convincing Positional History**

3. **To follow progress**

4. **To investigate an asymmetry suggesting Limb Length Discrepancy or another asymmetric condition contributing to a PseudoStenosis component**

Use 1: To Identify the SS/PS Pattern

After I discuss with a patient the spectrum of symptoms and conclude that he may have SS/PS, I ask if certain places that I push in the feet and legs are painful. Insofar as SS/PS causes sensitivity—and often hypersensitivity—of certain nerves, but other common causes of lower-extremity symptoms do not, this pattern supports the likelihood of SS/PS contributing to the problem. This one-minute exam corroborates my suspicion of SS/PS and encourages me to continue investigating that possibility, even if the patient came in for unrelated problems. For example, if a patient came in for an ingrown nail but had a positive Positional History of significant difficulty walking, standing, or sleeping, and/or he had the nerve sensitivity consistent with SS/PS, I would investigate that diagnosis with a great deal of confidence.

Use 2: To Demonstrate Knowledge

It comes as no surprise to me when places in a patient's foot and leg that I expect to be either sensitive or insensitive comply with my expectations. My patients are a different story. When I point out in advance the areas that I expect to be severely sensitive and they are very painful to only moderate pressure, my patients are amazed. They sometimes think I am a foot magician! This is not true. I simply know the locations in the foot and leg that tend to be painful when people have SS/PS.

Combining the Positional History with the First Interspace Fine Sign is a powerful set of tools to help a patient accept that the new diagnosis of SS/PS may be correct. Since patient cooperation is essential for success in managing SS/PS, bringing the patient on board is invaluable.

Use 3: To Follow Progress

The third valuable use of this sign is that it can be used to follow the improvement of SS/PS that can occur in just 1–3 days.

If a patient has Spinal Stenosis or PseudoStenosis and with either Positional Testing or Mechanical Testing obtains relief from symptoms, that person will also usually experience elimination of the nerve sensitivity. As such, elimination of the nerve sensitivity helps the patient understand the process of improvement and helps support my diagnosis and treatment plan.

If they do not have resolution of the nerve sensitivity, it demonstrates that I have not relieved the spinal nerve compression that may be affecting symptoms, and I thus need to alter my treatment approach.

I will address the fourth use, involving asymmetric findings, later in this chapter.

What is this valuable sign? It is called the **"First Interspace Fine Sign."** Here is how it works:

The bones behind the toes in the feet are the metatarsals. The space between two bones is called the "intermetatarsal space," or "interspace." These areas may become sensitive from different foot conditions. I must begin by sharing with you some basic podiatry.

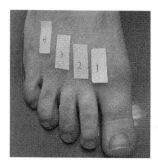

Picture 6.8. The foot with the four interspaces identified

Basic podiatry: Other common nerve sensitivity patterns

The most commonly recognized condition in which there is nerve tenderness is called "Morton's Neuroma," in which there is severe sensitivity between the third and fourth metatarsals—the third interspace. If only the third interspace is very tender, there is often a thickening of the fibrous tissue and the nerve in that area. Morton's Neuroma can cause cramps in the ball of the foot, burning, or sharp pain. The condition usually improves dramatically with cortisone or alcohol injections. Physical therapy and orthotics are useful at times. Surgery to relieve pressure on the nerve or to remove the nerve is an option if conservative care does not prove helpful.

If there is tenderness between the second and third metatarsal—the second interspace—it has been well reported in the literature (and in my experience as well) that this is usually caused by a nerve inflammation associated with an inflammation of the joint behind the second toe. This condition is called "Second Metatarsal Stress Syndrome," with a secondary second intermetatarsal space neuritis. While the symptoms may improve temporarily with a steroid injection, the inflamed joint behind the second toe, which is the primary problem, usually needs to be treated to solve the nerve problem long term.

If the third and the fourth intermetatarsal spaces are hypersensitive, but not the first or second, the cause of symptoms is frequently a Tarsal Tunnel Syndrome involving compression of the Lateral Plantar Nerve. This is an entrapment of the nerve at the level of the ankle, which is the nerve that supplies the third, fourth, and fifth toes. Injecting the intermetatarsal spaces does not provide long-term help. One must treat the condition behind the ankle—with injections, topical medicine, physical therapy, and sometimes mechanical support such as an orthotic or brace. If none of these remedies provide relief, surgery is another option. Also, if the first and second interspaces are hypersensitive, or if all are

hypersensitive, it could be Tarsal Tunnel Syndrome. I have, however, also seen patients—just much less frequently—with sensitivity in these two nerves in which the cause was spinal.

Details of the First Interspace Fine Sign

What is the "First Interspace Fine Sign"? This term refers to a situation in which there is distinct sensitivity in the second, third, and fourth intermetatarsal spaces, but not in the first intermetatarsal space. All the others are sore, but the first interspace is fine! While this could *possibly* be caused by a Lateral Plantar Nerve Tarsal Tunnel Syndrome AND a second intermetatarsal space neuritis, this combination diagnosis is far less likely. (The second metatarsal phalangeal joint would likely be quite sensitive in this case.)

I find that the GREAT majority of people who have moderate-to-severe sensitivity in intermetatarsal spaces 2, 3, and 4 but not in interspace 1 have either Spinal Stenosis or PseudoStenosis contributing to the symptoms. (I have seen a few people who had Cervical (neck) Stenosis, a much less common condition, associated with this pattern, too—as well as a very few in whom the pattern was present for reasons that I never figured out!)

Frequently, the patient also has sensitivity along the course of the posterior tibial nerve, the tibial nerve, and the femoral nerve. These nerves are found along the inner ankle, leg, and thigh. Picture 6.9 shows the areas where those nerves can be checked.

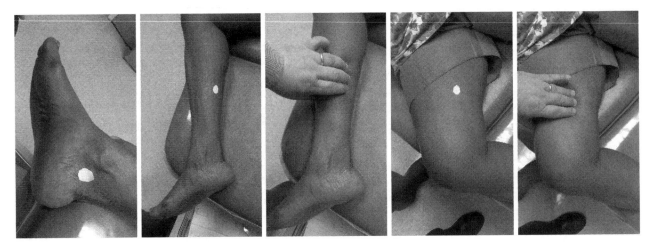

Picture 6.9. Checking the nerves in the inner (medial) ankle, leg, and thigh.

How do I record this? In my Examination Form, I have the following section:

Focused **EXAM**	Left	Right		Left	Right
1. Pulses	DP____ PT____	DP____ PT____	2. CFT	WNL Slow WNL Slow	
3. Skin WNL Shiny Atrophic Hairless Rubor Pallor				_____	
4. **Equinus** (*Leg cramps* Y N OCC) Y N	Y N	5. Significant Biomechanical Problems Y N			
6. **Pain in Interspace**	1 2 3 4	1 2 3 4	7. VPT 1st MPJ	_____ _____	
8. Pain/paresthesias **PT nerve** y L n y R n	**Tib. nerve** y L n y R n	**Fem Nerve** y L n y R n			
9. Sensitive **Pes Anserinus** y L n y R n	**Sinus Tarsi** y L n y R n	**1st MC joint** y L n y R n			
10. **Muscle wasting** None Feet Legs Thigh Hands	11. **Asymmetry of feet** Y N				
12. **Rotation abnormal** Y N _____	**FHL** L R **Significant Pronation** L R **Cavus** L R				
13 **ASIS** Even Higher L R **PSIS** Even Higher L R Iliac Pain Y N **Relief lift** _____ **LLDx** Shorter L _____ R					

Picture 6.10. Part of the physical Examination Form. (This is an old version; the new version is presented in the part of the appendix presenting clinician's tools.)

Recording nerve sensitivity

If there was a positive First Interspace Fine Sign and sensitivity along the higher nerves as well, this is how it would be recorded:

Focused **EXAM**	Left	Right		Left	Right
1. Pulses	DP____ PT____	DP____ PT____	2. CFT	WNL Slow WNL Slow	
3. Skin WNL Shiny Atrophic Hairless Rubor Pallor					
4. **Equinus** (*Leg cramps* Y N OCC) Y Ⓝ	Y N	5. Significant Biomechanical Problems Y N			
6. **Pain in Interspace**	1 ②③④	1 ②③④	7. VPT 1st MPJ	_____ _____	
8. Pain/paresthesias **PT nerve** ⓨ L n ⓨ R n	**Tib. nerve** ⓨ L n ⓨ R n	**Fem Nerve** ⓨ L n ⓨ R n			
9. Sensitive **Pes Anserinus** y L n y R n	**Sinus Tarsi** y L n y R n	**1st MC joint** y L n y R n			
10. **Muscle wasting** None Feet Legs Thigh Hands	11. **Asymmetry of feet** Y N				
12. **Rotation abnormal** Y N _____	**FHL** L R **Significant Pronation** L R **Cavus** L R				
13 **ASIS** Even Higher L R **PSIS** Even Higher L R Iliac Pain Y N **Relief lift** _____ **LLDx** Shorter L _____ R					

Picture 6.11. The form demonstrates a pattern recording a positive "First Interspace Fine Sign."

Sensitivity sometimes occurs primarily in places where there are problematic symptoms present. For example, if the person has aching in the thighs but no discomfort in the feet or lower legs, one might find that none of the intermetatarsal spaces are tender, although there may be severe sensitivity in the thighs with pressure on the femoral nerve. In contrast, if the person has burning, tingling, aching, or hypersensitivity in the feet, then intermetatarsal spaces 2, 3, and 4 are more likely to be very sensitive if the problem is coming from SS/PS. This pattern frequently occurs if there is only leg pain without foot symptoms. **However, I frequently note diffuse nerve sensitivity even when symptoms are more localized.**

Recall what was presented above as Use 3—using this finding to follow improvement. **There is a powerful satisfaction in seeing the elimination of all the diffuse nerve sensitivity in one or even both legs through a single treatment that addresses the cause of spinal nerve involvement.** It guides both clinician and patient to understand with confidence that a major beneficial change has been effected. As you will see in the following chapters, there are many treatments that may induce such improvement in just 1–3 days, depending, of course, upon the cause of the problem!

Of course, besides following success, this method also has value in understanding symptoms. For example, if the sensitivity of the nerves disappeared but the symptoms did not improve, then we would seek another cause of symptoms besides SS/PS. In contrast, if the symptoms improved but the nerve sensitivity persisted, then I would suspect that the spinal nerve irritation that caused this nerve sensitivity had not been completely addressed. **It is a great tool to use to follow success, one that I use on almost every SS/PS patient, frequently until all problems are resolved.**

Use 4: To Investigate the Asymmetric First Interspace Fine Sign

The fourth use of the nerve hypersensitivity pattern is appreciated if there is an Asymmetric First Interspace Fine Sign. In cases of PseudoStenosis from Limb Length Discrepancy, nerve hypersensitivity is often present only in the longer leg—or at least it presents much worse in the longer leg. This is frequently the leg that has greater nerve symptoms, especially if the discrepancy is less than ³⁄₁₆ of an inch. (If the discrepancy is ³⁄₁₆ of an inch or greater, there may be greater sensitivity in the shorter leg, although that pattern is much less frequent.)

Utilizing this awareness of the common pattern of greater nerve sensitivity in the longer leg may guide a quick exam that amazes the patient. Once I've seen signs of a shorter leg, I know where it will hurt to touch and where one leg will hurt more than the other!

This asymmetric nerve sensitivity usually disappears in a day or two with successful compensation for the Limb Length Discrepancy. When both symptoms and nerve sensitivity quickly resolve, the patient becomes aware of the role that the mechanics of the feet play in affecting pain coming from the back, or at least pain that is mediated through the spine.

If there is a Limb Length Discrepancy and there is also nerve hypersensitivity greater in one extremity but present in both, I suspect that there is most likely a problem present in addition to the Limb Length Discrepancy. That problem may be a primary Spinal Stenosis, or another cause of PseudoStenosis, or both. Whatever the case, I have to decide how many of the suspected conditions I should treat at the first visit. In some cases, I will just treat the shorter leg and reevaluate in a few days. If, however, the patient has travelled a long distance, has a high co-pay, is impatient, or is in severe pain, or if I sense that treatment at the first visit

must be successful or else I will not get this patient back for a second visit, I will use multiple approaches at the first visit and then try to decide what is needed long term. Such is the art of management.

Some other patterns

A person may have moderate or even severe symptoms in the feet arising from SS/PS, but no intermetatarsal space sensitivity. This may occur if there is a true and severe loss of sensation due either to neuropathy or to spinal nerve compression. The patient may, for example, have a LOPS score of 7 to 10 (*see below*) and/or a severe reduction in sensitivity to vibration, tested either by tuning fork or Biothesiometer. Because the patient truly cannot feel his feet, compression of the interspaces does not cause pain. Accordingly, the value of the First Interspace Fine Sign is less in the presence of severe loss of sensation. This may be the case even if the person experiences severe symptoms in the feet coming from spinal nerve compression, despite the numbness.

Just to muddy the waters a bit, I have had patients with persistent sensitivity even though they had loss of sensation. Therefore, my regimen includes checking for this pattern and, if present, using it. If, however, there is no sensitivity but there *is* loss of sensation, the lack of sensitivity does not discourage me from considering and treating for SS/PS.

Another less common situation is when a person has great tenderness in all the intermetatarsal spaces. This tenderness may be the result of a Tarsal Tunnel Syndrome (compression of the nerve behind the inside ankle bone), involving the posterior tibial nerve and its two main branches, the Medial Plantar Nerve and the Lateral Plantar Nerve. There is also usually great tenderness in that nerve at the level of the ankle. If there is no tenderness higher up in the leg and thigh along the tibial and femoral nerve, it may be a Tarsal Tunnel Syndrome. Deciding what condition to treat may then be directed by the Positional History.

However, tenderness in all the intermetatarsal spaces and in the tibial and femoral nerves is a pattern I have seen with other conditions, including Cervical Stenosis, as well as other forms of systemic neuropathy.

In patients with these less common patterns, it might be valuable to try Positional Testing or Mechanical

Testing (Chapters 7 and 12) to see how the nerve sensitivity resolves itself. If much of it is resolved (along with elimination of symptoms in just a few days), then the remaining nerve sensitivity patterns and symptoms might be much easier to evaluate.

I have also found a few patients with sensitivity in all the interspaces who had a "space-occupying lesion" in the spine—some sort of growth or cyst. This doesn't happen very often, but frequently enough to make sure that an MRI of the spine is ordered in case of need.

Of course, variations in the pattern exist. People may experience hypersensitivity in the first intermetatarsal space if they have a herniated disc, so if they have a herniated disc and SS/PS, all the intermetatarsal spaces will be painful. This can frequently be identified by the pattern of the symptoms. As I mention elsewhere in this book, people with a herniated disc often have greater pain in either the back or the legs when sitting for a long time. Some find that their symptoms improve by sitting on a pillow or two. **I have also seen people with this pattern—greater tenderness in the first interspace and difficulty sitting—who responded well to treatment for Limb Length Discrepancy, as will be described in Chapter 12.** I have seen some people with nerve sensitivity in the third and fourth interspaces that was coming from spinal nerve compression, though that pattern is not as common.

It must be stressed that these findings are strongly suggestive but not one hundred percent diagnostic. They are, however, helpful in evaluating and following the role of SS/PS on neuropathic or other lower-extremity symptoms. How I use them on a *daily basis* will be clear to clinicians who read the stories in Sections 3 and 4 of this book.

Neuropathy or SS/PS? A recognized conundrum

Before the next sign is presented, I must set the stage by recognizing the difficulties inherent in differentiating symptoms of Peripheral Neuropathy from those of SS/PS. Differentiation often seems impossible. After all, an MRI or CT scan that shows Spinal Stenosis does not mean that neuropathy is *not* present or the cause of symptoms. Similarly, a nerve test or medical history that suggests neuropathy does not mean that SS/PS is not present or the cause of symptoms. In fact, many people have both of these conditions simultaneously, identified with nerve tests. Distinguishing between the two is a major dilemma.

The situation is made more complicated by the fact that standard nerve tests do not identify all forms of neuropathy. They can show neuropathy involving larger nerve fibers (*large-fiber neuropathy*) but not neuropathy involving the smaller nerve fibers (*small-fiber neuropathy*), so a negative nerve conduction study does not mean that there is no neuropathy present!

This problem has been somewhat mitigated in recent years with a new test called the "Intra-epidermal Nerve Fiber (IENF) Biopsy." This relatively painless test, pioneered in part at Johns Hopkins University in Baltimore, involves removing a small piece of skin with a punch biopsy. Special stains, combined with microscopic assessment, allow the counting and evaluation of small nerves and even autonomic nerves. This test has already been proven to have clinical value, and it has great potential for real breakthroughs in the understanding and treatment of neuropathy.

However, this test cannot rule out a contribution of SS/PS to the symptoms. I therefore consider this test only if my investigation and treatment does not provide relief or clarity.

In Chapter 7, I introduce Positional Testing, an original approach that can quickly relieve symptoms coming from spinal nerve compression and can thus help differentiate SS/PS from other conditions. This benefit, however, does not negate the value of clinicians understanding the physical findings reported in this chapter.

I want to emphasize that the section on PseudoStenosis is essential to understand, as PseudoStenosis must be considered when evaluating ALL PATIENTS with Spinal Stenosis.

Now, let me address the task of distinguishing SS/PS symptoms from those of Peripheral Neuropathy by introducing a helpful tool I have used for many years, the Loss of Protective Sensation pattern.

Clue 2: The Loss of Protective Sensation (LOPS) Pattern

Many patients with neuropathy have, or at least report, a reduced sensitivity in the toes, feet, or legs. One observation I have made is that *occasionally* people in whom Spinal Stenosis is present will report a long-term feeling of numbness, but physical examination will show that they do not have reduced sensitivity to either light touch or vibration. Others with SS/PS have a severe loss of sensation throughout the entire foot and much of the leg, even when symptoms are new. Based upon my experience, neither of these patterns would be expected with Diabetic Peripheral Neuropathy, the most common cause of neuropathy. It is valuable to check both light touch and vibration sensitivity in the physical exam, although in this chapter I primarily address the light touch.

Sensitivity to light touch can be measured with a device called a "Semmes-Weinstein Monofilament." In my 2003 *JAPMA* article (see the appendix) I present a "Loss of Protective Sensation (LOPS) scale" that can be used to establish the extent of loss of sensation as well as to track changes in loss of sensation with treatment of what may or may not be neuropathy. That scale, slightly modified, is presented in detail later in this chapter.

Most neuropathy is actually something called "Distal Symmetrical Polyneuropathy," or "DSP." "Distal" means "far away from the center of the body." In this case, it means that the neuropathy usually begins at the ends of the toes and works its way up. "Symmetrical" indicates that it is about the same on one side as on the other. In this case, "symmetrical" suggests similar abnormalities on both medial and lateral sides of the extremity, and equal effects on both left and right sides. Diabetic Neuropathy is usually both distal and symmetrical, involving many nerves—in other words, a polyneuropathy. (There are exceptions in diabetic patients involving individual nerves, but these are much less common.)

If patients have nerve compression, and specifically either Spinal Stenosis or PseudoStenosis, I find that the distal symmetrical pattern may or may not be present. In contrast to DSP, the loss of sensation may be worse in parts of the foot other than the toes, corresponding to specific nerves in the back. If sensation is better in the toes than in the arch or the legs, it most likely derives, at least in part, from nerve compression—most commonly SS/PS. I called this an **"atypical"** presentation, where the **loss of sensation is worse anywhere higher in the foot or leg than it is lower down in the foot**, such as in the tips of the toes. This is a strong sign of SS/ PS.

If the neuropathy is worse on the medial (big toe) side of the foot than on the lateral (baby toe) side, or if it is worse in one foot than in the other, it is not symmetrical and is therefore not a Distal Symmetrical Polyneuropathy.

Clinicians may take issue with me on this point based upon their own experience. They might agree that it makes sense for the pattern to be distal and symmetrical but claim that this may not happen in reality. I understand their opinion. **I believe that we disagree because they are diagnosing Peripheral Neuropathy in patients whom I would diagnose with having Spinal Stenosis or PseudoStenosis.** With all due respect, I maintain my position.

Such disagreements are the reason for my articles and lectures, and now this book and my website. I had already seen these asymmetrical or atypical patterns in over one hundred patients when I first published these observations back in 2003, and I have gone on to see the pattern in hundreds more in the following decade. While the research to document this in controlled studies has not yet been done, I hope that everyone, including physicians, podiatrists, and therapists, will at least consider this as a possibility, and will use the pattern clinically to **suspect** the presence of SS/PS.

Recording the Loss of Protective Sensation

The following protocol is *slightly* modified from the original presentation in the article entitled "Neurogenic Positional Pedal Neuritis: Common Pedal Manifestations of Spinal Stenosis" (*Journal of the American Podiatric Medical Association*, 2003).

I use a Loss of Protective Sensation (LOPS) scale of 0 to 10 to identify the severity of loss of protective sensation in the foot. I check this with a wheel that has three monofilaments. The 4.07 filament produces one gram of pressure, the 5.07 filament produces 10 grams of pressure, and the 6.45 filament produces 70 grams of pressure.

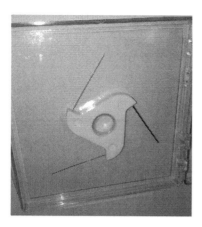

Picture 6.12. Semmes-Weinstein Monofilament wheel.

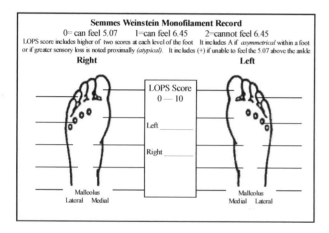

Picture 6.13. Semmes-Weinstein Monofilament record.

Each level is recorded on the diagram as one of the following:

0: Can feel the 5.07 filament

1: Cannot feel the 5.07 filament but can feel the 6.45

2: Cannot feel the 6.45 filament

I use five levels of checking on each foot, checking twice on each level, on the medial side and on the lateral side.

1. Bottom of toe
2. Ball of foot
3. Distal part of arch
4. Proximal part of arch
5. Malleolus

In the example shown in picture 6.14, the person cannot feel the 6.45 filament in the toes, the ball of the foot, or the distal arch. The patient can feel the 6.45 filament in the proximal arch but cannot feel the 5.07

filament. At the ankle, the 5.07 filament can also be felt. His LOPS score is therefore "7 (22210)" and is fairly simple both to record and to follow, whether it gets better with treatment or worse with time.

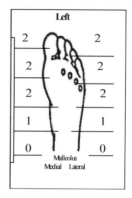

Picture 6.14. LOPS score "7 (22210)."

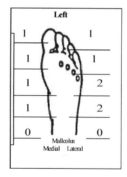

Picture 6.15. LOPS "6 A (11220)" or "6 A (M11220, L11110)."

More complicated to record but valuable to perceive is the case where the loss of sensation is either asymmetrical or atypical. The record shown in picture 6.15 demonstrates such a pattern. I would list it as a "6 A (11220)," as the LOPS is greater proximally than distally, and it is also different on the medial and lateral sides of the foot. (I could also list it as a "6 A [M11220, L11110]" to show the difference medially or laterally.) I perceive this as stemming not from a Distal Symmetrical Neuropathy, but from there being at least some nerve compression present contributing to the LOPS.

If the pattern is "A" (atypical or asymmetrical), recording it is more complicated—and maybe more than the patients need to know. I share this for clinicians.

As explained earlier, this LOPS scale has two major functions. It identifies the patterns that are suggestive of Peripheral Neuropathy or of SS/PS. It also allows a clinician to follow the improvement obtained in cases of loss of sensation arising from either condition, SS/PS or actual Peripheral Neuropathy.

> *Those paying strict attention will note that in the preceding sentence I claimed to see improvement in loss of sensation with Peripheral Neuropathy as well as with SS/PS. It is true. I find that some people with true Diabetic Neuropathy or other causes of Peripheral Neuropathy can often have their loss of sensation improved with appropriate treatment. This is addressed in Chapter 25.*

The Semmes-Weinstein Monofilament wheel that I use has three filaments, but we have only used two in this discussion. That is because, according to the guidelines presented by Medicare to document a loss of sensation that makes a diabetic eligible for Medicare neuropathy services, there must be a loss of sensation in the foot to the 10-gram (5.07) monofilament. Therefore, for patients and the podiatrists who care for them, that is not only a sign of risk, but also a criteria for getting essential care approved through Medicare. When I designed this protocol, that was my baseline for recording the presence or absence of neuropathy.

However, I also use the third (4.07) monofilament, which is not too much smaller than the 5.07. However, instead of applying 10 grams of pressure, it applies 1 gram of pressure—clearly much less. With absolutely normal sensation, one should be able to feel this filament. Those who cannot feel it do not qualify as having neuropathy that puts them at risk and are thus not eligible (based on that category) for certain treatments according to Medicare guidelines. It may, however, indicate that nerve dysfunction is beginning. It is a warning signal that may motivate individuals to take their diabetes management even more seriously. If the person can feel the 4.07 monofilament in all places, I record this as a "-5," which sounds worse but actually indicates totally normal sensation to light touch.

Biothesiometer and VPT

The following is a valuable test to use in evaluation of neuropathy, but I am not sure if there is value in differentiating neuropathy from SS/PS. I have seen many people who had improvement of this parameter with

treatment for SS/PS, but in truth I have not studied it enough to have confidence in using it for that purpose.

The test is Vibration Pressure Threshold sensitivity, or VPT. It is measured with a machine called a "Biothesiometer," which is basically an electronic and calibrated tuning fork. It identifies a reduction in sensitivity to vibration, which may be found with large-fiber neuropathy. Increased VPT is considered a risk factor for ulceration in patients with diabetes, with the number "25" having been established as the threshold number.

Picture 6.16 shows a Biothesiometer, along with the unit being used to test sensitivity at the first MPJ and at the tip of the first toe.

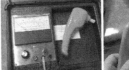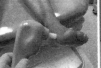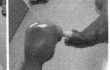

Picture 6.16. Testing with a Biothesiometer

I include this information not because of confidence that it may be used to differentiate SS/PS from neuropathy but because I believe it is of great value in evaluating diabetic patients. I also mention VPT several times in stories within this book.

Clue 3: The Extended-Leg Flexion Test

The third finding, the Extended-Leg Flexion Test, applies to the loss of sensation pattern as well as to the level of discomfort. I have had positive results with this a few dozen times over the last thirteen years, and I do not try this very frequently. It is, however, impressive when used. As background, know that when seated in a podiatry chair, the patient's legs are stretched out (extended), which may put a stretch on the spinal nerves, causing symptoms. Similar to when sleep position in bed is modified (Chapters 8 and 21), there may be an immediate improvement by bending the legs (flexing the knees), a position that mimics sitting in a recliner chair or lying down with a pillow under the knees. Individuals who report that their symptoms are constant, and present even while sitting in the podiatry chair, may have a quick (less than one minute) improvement in symptoms by flexing the knees as shown in Picture 6.18. This demonstrates that spine position has an effect on symptoms.

Similarly, if there is a loss of sensation that may be affected by spinal nerves, the same maneuver, flexing the knees and thus opening the spine, may immediately improve the sensation in the feet. This fact strongly supports that SS/PS is contributing to the numbness, and suggests to both patient and doctor the importance of using the gift of positional management. It is not a consistent pattern, but it is pretty impressive when it happens.

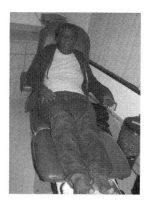

Picture 6.17. This patient is sitting with her legs extended in a podiatry chair. She had constant nerve pain, and loss of sensation was identified.

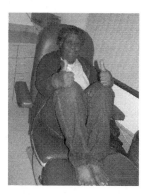

Picture 6.18. This patient is now sitting in a position of knee flexion, which flexes and opens the spine. She is giving me a "thumbs-up" to indicate the change in her nerve pain, as well as the immediate improvement in sensation.

Clue 4: The Professor Position

There are two additional maneuvers that are available to immediately examine the effect on the foot and leg symptoms caused by either Spinal Stenosis or PseudoStenosis. These were published in the *Journal of the American Podiatric Medical Association*, March 2013 issue. The title of the article—my seventh on Spinal Stenosis—is **"The professor position and the single stance flexion test may clarify the effect of lumbar spinal stenosis or pseudostenosis on lower-extremity symptoms."**

If a patient has pain in the feet or legs with standing or walking and obtains relief when leaning on a grocery cart or walker, it seems to make sense that the improvement comes from the reduction of weight on the body, which serves to reduce the pain. I have heard this repeatedly from therapists and doctors. These next two tests, however, support my differing approach and, I hope, will convince you to investigate that approach for yourself. To quote the article:

The first maneuver, shown in Picture 6.19, is the **Professor Position**. The patient is directed to stand erect until lower-extremity symptoms develop. The patient then places both hands behind his or her back, grabs one wrist with the other hand, and leans slightly forward. The patient stands and may walk in that position. If symptoms substantially reduce, it demonstrates that spine position contributes significantly to lower-extremity symptoms, in addition to or instead of weight bearing or dependent positioning. Holding the hands behind the back makes it easier for the patient to maintain that flexion position comfortably without putting muscle strain on the back.

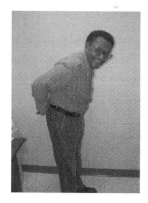

Picture 6.19 The Professor Position.

Clue 5: The Single Stance Flexion Test

The second maneuver, demonstrated in Picture 6.20, is the **Single Stance Flexion Test**. It is especially revealing in patients with asymmetrical symptoms. The patient stands erect in front of but not touching a counter or other source of support until lower-extremity symptoms develop. He or she leans forward, flexing the spine, and rests his or her hands on the counter. If that reduces or eliminates lower-extremity symptoms, the patient may perceive that it is the off-loading that provides relief. He or she then lifts the less symptomatic extremity off the ground, placing most of the body weight on the more symptomatic extremity. Maintaining relief in that position, and sometimes even bouncing up and down on that single extremity previously perceived as painful, demonstrates that spine position contributes greatly to the overall lower-extremity symptoms, in addition to or instead of weight bearing or dependent positioning.

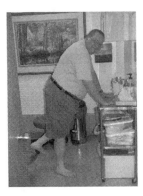

Picture 6.20 Single Stance Flexion Test.

Both of these maneuvers demonstrate that it is the **position of the lower back** that reduces the leg pain, not the removal of pressure on the leg or legs. If these maneuvers help, it is an indication that Positional Testing could be of great benefit!

The next three clues are consistent with Limb Length Discrepancy (LLDx), and they also require close physical examination. Limb Length Discrepancy is just one of many causes of PseudoStenosis, but by far the most common one. In that these findings are so important and can be clearly understood and routinely used by clinicians, I present them in detail in this chapter.

Clue 6: Asymmetric Equinus and Limb Length Discrepancy

Equinus is a condition in which there is inadequate dorsiflexion of the foot on the ankle. In other words, when pushed up, the foot does not get to a 90-degree (perpendicular) position. If equal on both feet, it is symmetrical and not reflective of a Limb Length Discrepancy. If asymmetrical, it MIGHT be caused by arthritis, a ruptured tendon, a stroke, or another neurologic problem. However, it is extremely common that asymmetric Equinus, involving tightness of the

Achilles tendon complex, is caused by a Limb Length Discrepancy. This has been reported in the literature.

It is not easy to measure exactly how much motion is present in the ankle, and doctors often disagree with the numbers. **However, it is fairly easy to note if one leg is tighter than the other,** or to check if the foot can go past the perpendicular (over 90 degrees), achieve a perpendicular position (90 degrees), or only achieve less than the perpendicular (less than 90 degrees). **In doing this test the knee must be <u>fully</u> extended, and the foot must be slightly inverted and held straight during the maneuver.**

Sometimes the asymmetry is apparent just by looking at the resting position of the two ankles.

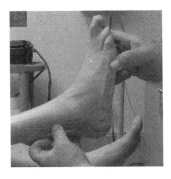

Picture 6.21. Measuring motion in the ankle with a tractograph. Exact measurements are not as important as is recognizing a difference between the two feet.

The following pictures utilize tape on the foot for clearer perception.

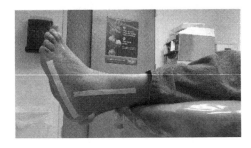

Picture 6.22. Resting, the foot is sitting at about 20 degrees short of perpendicular.

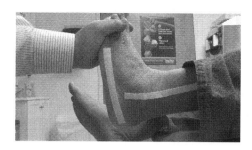

Picture 6.23. When the foot is held up, it gets to about a 90-degree angle (perpendicular).

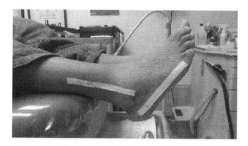

Picture 6.24. This foot is resting at a more plantar position, about 30 degrees short of perpendicular.

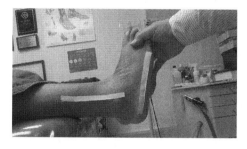

Picture 6.25. When the foot is held up, it is 10 degrees short of perpendicular, tighter than the left foot shown in picture 6.23.

These are subtle differences, which a clinician could appreciate if looking for them. Patients and their families often recognize the difference when I point it out to them.

There are two wonderful aspects of this finding:

• **As soon as it is identified on physical examination, a clinician should strongly suspect the presence of a Limb Length Discrepancy.** Other findings suggestive of a Limb Length Discrepancy are reviewed in detail in Chapter 12. However, this sign alone, if identified on clinical exam, should induce investigation of other possible clues, and should also prompt an aggressive Positional History to seek details of symptoms that might be related to PseudoStenosis.

• **Rapid resolution of Equinus is a great key to following the overall effectiveness of treating Limb Length Discrepancy.** If Limb Length Discrepancy is the cause of the asymmetric tightness, that tightness will disappear within 1–3 days of *consistently using a lift of the proper height.* This allows us to confirm, or at least strongly suspect, that an adequate amount of lift has been added. If the ankle motion is still more limited on the shorter leg at the follow-up visit, it usually means that there has *not been adequate lift, or there has not been adequate use of the lift.* I will then either add additional lift to the shoes or strap a lift to the foot to enforce compliance. (Of course, there could also be resolution of this if too much lift was used, either because of a mistake in evaluation, compliance issues, or the presence of a functional component to the Limb Length Discrepancy. Functional LLDx is addressed in Chapter 12.)

Since many people do not accurately report their compliance, this clue allows me to confirm or refute compliance. This is especially true for patients who initially report good relief of PseudoStenosis symptoms and have resolution of Equinus, but then note a return of symptoms. If the Equinus also returns, it is most common that there has been inadequate compliance, or that the lifts have flattened out, though it is also possible that the need for mechanical support has changed.

Clue 7: The *Invaluable* Iliac Crest Pain Resolution Sign and Limb Length Discrepancy

Measurement of Limb Length Discrepancy is usually done by one or more of three reported categories of methods: direct measurement, radiologic measurement, and indirect measurement.

Direct measurement involves use of a tape measure to measure distance between structures (such as umbilicus [belly button] to ankle-bone landmark) and then compare the two sides. While this method may have some clinical value, especially in the case of large discrepancy, I am among those who feel that it is not as dependable a method as the indirect method or the radiologic approaches mentioned below, especially for the slight differences that are so important.

Radiologic measurement has many possible methods, including performing a Scanogram, weight-bearing Long Leg Study, or weight bearing x-ray of the lower spine and pelvis with different levels of lift under the suspected short leg. This may be combined with lateral weight bearing x-rays of the feet. Each test investigates different structural components, and can provide useful information. However, the decision as to which technique to use may be based upon availability, insurance approval, and preference of the radiology department that is performing the tests.

I use radiologic testing less frequently than indirect measurement, as I often enjoy clinical success without it. However, it often has great clinical value. I order it most frequently if there is a lack of expected improvement after treating the discrepancy, or when I suspect a functional LLDx component—which I would suspect for one of two reasons: either an inconsistent appearance at different visits, or what appears to be a long-term significant LLDx without significant differences in the two extremities. I may also order radiologic testing if the clinical exam is not clear (such as in a very overweight person), or if there is a disagreement between professionals. This type of test also has value if enhanced detail is needed, such as when surgery is being considered for Limb Length Discrepancy or for joint replacement. The CT Scanogram is reported to be accurate, although literature and my experience suggest that there may still be a margin of error of 2 or 3 millimeters, and possibly much more. Further information about radiologic testing is presented in Chapter 14.

The **indirect measurement** technique is the one I use the most, and it is the one that provides wonderful and immediate information, including the **Iliac Crest Pain Resolution Sign**, which will be shared below. Indirect measurement involves the examiner palpating the Iliac Crest on both hips and placing lifts of known height under the shorter leg until structures of the hips of both sides become even.

This exam also allows evaluation for the presence of a functional Limb Length Discrepancy. If both the front of the hip bone (Anterior Superior Iliac Spine [ASIS]) and the back part (Posterior Superior Iliac Spine [PSIS]) are lower on the side of the shorter leg. the discrepancy is likely structural. If the ASIS is lower and the PSIS is higher on either side, a pelvic rotation is present. **This may be seen with either structural or functional Limb Length Discrepancy.**

It is essential to carefully monitor the position of the feet and legs when performing this examination. Individuals may subconsciously compensate for Limb Length Discrepancy in various ways, such as by slightly bending the knee of the short leg, by rotating or abducting the longer leg, or by plantar-flexing the ankle of the short leg. In that any of these could affect the level of the hips, it is important to ensure that the feet and legs are properly positioned during this examination.

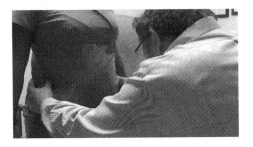

Picture 6.26. Palpation (touching and examining) of structures of the hip joint.

The Iliac Crest Pain Resolution Sign

This finding, which I have used for years, is not always present, but when it is, it is quite impressive. With palpation of the iliac crest (or perhaps the ASIS or the PSIS), one side, or occasionally both, is often quite sensitive; the sensitivity is reported usually as pain but occasionally, especially in children, as ticklishness. It is most common that the sensitive area is on the side of the longer leg if the LLDx is less than about ¼ inch, but it is common for one or both hips to be sensitive if the difference is about ¼ inch or more. The Iliac Crest is usually sensitive on the most dorsal aspect, centrally, but if not sensitive in that area I make sure to check both anteriorly and posteriorly.

That sensitivity often improves immediately after an appropriate lift is placed under the heel of the short leg. I don't know if this has ever been documented before. It is certainly not always present, and not everyone with a Limb Length Discrepancy has hip bone tenderness. However, when just a lift *immediately* eliminates that tenderness, both the patient and I are amazed. This finding, hip pain and immediate improvement with a lift, encourages patients to consider that an LLDx could be having a significant effect on their body and symptoms, something that they usually do not consider before my evaluation. I believe that this greatly encourages compliance. I refer to this as the **"Iliac Crest Pain Resolution Sign."** To the patients, I often refer to it as **"Happy Hips."**

Within a few days of proper use of a lift, this hip bone sensitivity often resolves. Sensitivity is then relieved not only when standing with a lift **but also when standing without a lift.** This is one of many examples in which there is dramatic improvement of clinical findings or symptoms with just 1–3 days of improvement of body misalignment.

It is important to note that there can be sensitivity in the Iliac Crest in the presence of a functional or structural LLDx, and it is commonly found if there is a combined (structural and functional) LLDx. This must be taken into account when deciding upon long-term need for a lift and on the need to reevaluate the amount of discrepancy present, as discussed in detail in Chapter 12.

Clue 8: Asymmetric Sensitive Pes Anerinus

This finding suggesting Limb Length Discrepancy is less common than the previous 2 listed. In truth, it is just one of many areas of biomechanical stress seen in the longer leg, that usually quickly resolves with proper treatment. The others, such as the sinus tarsi and the plantar aspect of the first metatarsal cuneiform joint, are presented in Chapters 12 & 19. I share this here because it is an area rarely checked in standard examination, and so easy for both clinician and patient to check and follow.

The Pes Anserinus is a spot just below the inside of the knee that is actually the combined tendon of three thigh muscles. Sensitivity in this area is quite often seen only in the longer leg of a patient with a Limb Length Discrepancy, though it could also be caused by local pathology such as a tendonitis or bursitis. It may be present in both legs if there is Flat Foot pathology or actual arthritis of the knees. The patient may not be aware of this being a sensitive area unless someone pushes on it, as the knee area may be painless. The sensitivity usually disappears quickly (1-3 days) with appropriate

mechanical control, often just a heel lift for the short leg or perhaps a heel lift combined with strapping in the presence of Flat Feet. If the area stays sensitive, I take that to mean that the mechanical stress in this area has not been compensated for. This area of sensitivity is not always present, but when it is, it makes an impression. It is an easy finding to both identify and follow, for both clinician and patient.

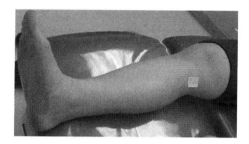

Picture 6.27 The location of the Pes Anserinus

I believe that the Pes Anserinus sensitivity is local inflammation caused by mechanical stress. Unlike the Iliac Crest, in which the sensitivity disappears immediately upon proper balancing, the Pes Anserinus stays sensitive even after appropriate strapping or balancing with a lift. In 1–3 days, the sensitivity is usually gone, but there is not an immediate change as there is with the Iliac Crest.

The Full Examination Form—Not Yet!

I have an intake form that has evolved over the years, a form that helps me follow a patient's history and physical examination that I find relevant to the challenges of SS/PS. Findings of this chapter are addressed on that form, but so are many of the findings that are presented in the upcoming chapters. This form is therefore included later in the book, in the appendix. Many of these findings represent changes that are consistent with PseudoStenosis, so Chapter 12 must be studied in detail in order to do a thorough physical examination for patients with possible SS/PS.

Positional Testing

The first part of positional management is taking a Positional History, which may be accompanied by the physical examination. These dual protocols, taken together, perform two important functions. First, they allow the suspicion of Spinal Stenosis or PseudoStenosis to arise, when neither may have been considered a possibility before. Second, they provide a baseline for both the symptoms and the physical signs that support such a diagnosis.

A Test and a Treatment

Once the diagnosis is suspected, testing and treatment are indicated. In this protocol for Spinal Stenosis (and at times, for PseudoStenosis), **testing and initial treatment are combined into what I label "Positional Testing."**

There are two things I'd like you, the patient, to bear in mind. First, filling out the LuSSSExt scale (Chapter 3) will give you a very good idea of your capabilities and symptoms, affording you much greater clarity as to the value—that is, the clinical improvement—of Positional Testing. After all, if you get only 50% better, using the Positional Testing techniques that you have learned is obviously worth cherishing and continuing. Without clarity about your baseline situation, you might be disappointed to see that some symptoms persist. Do not become discouraged or give up this life-changing route to improvement!

Additionally, I routinely use Positional Testing as my first line of treatment, unless I suspect (and can quickly treat) a PseudoStenosis condition. This condition will be more fully explained in Chapters 11 and 12, and is most common in people who have one leg that is longer than the other, feet that are different from each other, feet that are very flat with standing, very tight muscles, neurologic or muscular dysfunction, arthritis, or pain in the lower extremities. **I estimate that PseudoStenosis contributes to well over 50% of all Spinal Stenosis cases.** Nevertheless, I think it is often appropriate to start with Positional Testing, to confirm that spinal nerve compression is part of the problem and to get relief. If there is excellent but only temporary improvement, or if you suspect any of the abnormalities I've just listed, check out the PseudoStenosis chapters.

For treatment of PseudoStenosis, you may be able to treat yourself, or you may require the services of an excellent podiatrist, physical therapist, physiatrist, or orthopedist. But first, let us explore this common pattern and treat for likely Spinal Stenosis as a primary cause.

The Mainstay of Positional Testing

Sometimes, before explaining this, I ask patients to raise their right hand and promise not to hit Dr. Goldman. They almost always agree. Even those who do not promise do not actually hit me, thank G-d. There are some who resist, but I almost always get the cooperation I need, though it sometimes takes a couple of visits.

The mainstay of Positional Testing is the *temporary full-time use of an appropriate and properly set walker*.

Each of those italicized words is essential for you to understand. The *walker* must be the *appropriate* kind, *set at the right height*. The success rate is much higher if the walker is used *full time*, as explained below. Finally, please be assured that for the great majority of people, the full-time use is very *temporary*.

Why a walker? There are two distinct ways of opening up a spine that has Spinal Stenosis. One way is by surgery. The other way is by leaning forward. When you lean forward, the lumbosacral spine opens up, including both the central canal and the areas where the nerve leaves the spine. Whereas the narrowing of stenosis causes pressure, leaning forward widens the canal and relieves the pressure. This is why most people with stenosis walk better when pushing a grocery cart. As they lean on the cart, the areas of compression widen, and the symptoms in both the back and the legs improve.

But here is an original technique that makes all the difference in the world. I recommend, as the first-line treatment for Spinal Stenosis, or for any case in which Spinal Stenosis may be contributing to the symptoms, the full-time use of a walker. Even for people who can walk without a cane or walker, and who can even stand and walk for five or ten minutes without difficulty, I ask to initially use the walker, full time, for three days.

Why? I'm glad you asked!

A Positional Decompression

The answer can be summed up in two words, though those words do require explanation: *positional decompression*.

"Decompression" is the term that we use when speaking about eliminating the cause of compression in the body—usually compression on a nerve. A commonly recognized compression involves Carpal Tunnel Syndrome in the wrist. Nerve compression is also common with Spinal Stenosis, Tarsal Tunnel Syndrome, or even Morton's Neuroma in the foot. Decompression is standardly done surgically. Cutting the structure that puts compression on the nerve allows a normal blood supply to return, and it eliminates the pressure that leads to the inflammation that causes the symptoms. People often wake up after such a procedure with much less pain than they had before surgery, and they usually improve dramatically within just a few days.

This, then, is the goal of Positional Testing: to effect a positional decompression. Yet instead of cutting, we change the position of the body to relieve the pressure. By keeping that change in effect full time, or nearly full time, we allow a normal blood supply to return to the compressed area, and we thus eliminate the pressure that leads to the inflammation that causes the symptoms.

For this reason, the walker must be set low enough to cause the person to lean forward, creating enough flexion to open up the spine. The arms should be straight, and the flexion only enough to adequately open the spine, **but not so much that it is physically uncomfortable**.

This is quite different from the traditional physical therapy method that uses a walker, which calls for the arms to be flexed at about 30 degrees and for the patient to stand straight. While this position could be comfortable for patients with Spinal Stenosis, and while a walker can certainly help with balance and stability, this method does not result in the benefit that we seek.

Demonstration of Positions

Pictures 7.1–7.5 demonstrate the Positional Testing method of using the walker, the standard physical therapy method, and the far-from-optimal methods that people use to compensate.

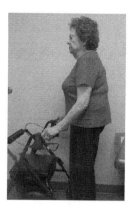

Picture 7.2. The more traditional position using a walker, which does not induce flexion.

In Picture 7.2, the walker is set at a more traditional position. The arms are bent, and the person is upright.

This does not open the spine. It does, however, provide balance and stability and therefore has some benefit for stenosis patients, though usually much less than the optimal positional setting provides.

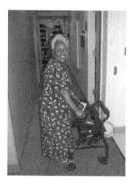

Picture 7.1. For Positional Testing, this is often the optimal position setting for walker use. The arms are straight, the walker is near the body, and there is a slight flexion of the spine. The shoulders are not elevated.

The exact height setting of the walker is a matter of a few minutes' testing and discussion between doctor and patient, as it must induce some flexion yet be comfortable for the patient.

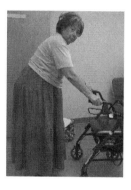

Picture 7.3. With the walker handle height high, the person instinctively seeks lumbar flexion by holding the walker far out in front of her.

In Picture 7.3, the walker height is at the traditional setting, but the patient, in order to achieve flexion, keeps the walker far in front of her and "chases after it" in an unstable manner. Occasionally, hyperextending the neck to look straight ahead may cause neck pain or arm discomfort.

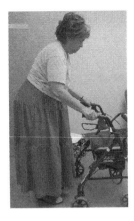

Picture 7.4. The person flexes her arms to achieve spine flexion, a position that is often hard to maintain.

In Picture 7.4, the walker height is at the traditional setting, but the patient achieves flexion of the spine by bending her arms extensively. This often causes the arms and the shoulders to become tired or uncomfortable with long walks, and sometimes leads to Shortness of Breath. (See Chapter 20 on Shortness of Breath.)

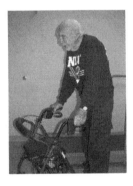

Picture 7.5. The walker height is slightly too high for proper Positional Testing, and the shoulders pop up, causing local shoulder, arm, or neck pain.

At times, individuals with other orthopedic problems need an unusual-appearing position to get improvement. The individual in picture 7.6 came in by wheelchair because of limited ability to walk even short distances. Because of Kyphosis, a curvature of the upper spine, he appears to be bending over excessively, but that is the fixed appearance of his upper spine. A low handle height was needed in order to have any lumbar flexion to open the lower spine. While it appears that he bends far too much, this position allowed him to resume walking, and within a few weeks, he could walk for up to three blocks without stopping.

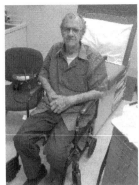 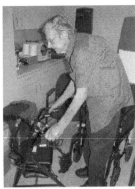

Picture 7.6. This individual came in by wheelchair. The curve of his upper spine makes it appear that he bends too far, but this position was comfortable and helpful. His arms are still bent at the elbow, but this was as straight as he could make them.

Understanding the Timing

People who improve with Positional Testing always do so within 1–3 days, tops. They may improve even more with time, but there must be at least good, rapid improvement. Otherwise, a reevaluation of diagnosis and treatment is called for.

In addition, the position must be comfortable immediately. It must at least be physically comfortable. Some people automatically resist because the position makes them lean forward, and they have spent a lifetime trying to stand straight even if it hurt. Accepting the slight forward lean is an emotional challenge for some patients. Helping them understand that it can provide quick relief of pain, and that it is usually only temporary, goes a long way in encouraging them to try this approach for a few days.

If the position is physically uncomfortable, it should not be used. Many people immediately feel much better, but not all do. The position should not, however, make the person feel physically worse. If it worsens symptoms, there must be a change in position.

StoryTime: Carol, 68, came in with a chief complaint of severe pain in her feet that had been bothering her for 10 years. She also had back and leg pain and could only walk for one to two blocks before she had to sit down. She'd undergone surgery for her left foot twice: one was a bunion surgery, and one was a major reconstruction surgery that was done by world-class surgeon. Though the results looked absolutely beautiful, Carol still had symptoms—and the same in both feet—so there was no improvement in overall discomfort. Before the major surgery, she'd used orthotics and ankle braces and had had months of physical therapy, all without results.

She had a positive Positional History. Pain in her feet and legs was worse with standing and walking and was relieved by sitting. She walked much better, without pain, when pushing a grocery cart. Symptoms were often worse at the checkout counter. My exam showed a positive First Interspace Fine Sign, the nerve hypersensitivity pattern suggestive of Spinal Stenosis.

Fortunately, Positional Testing provided relief. Within 3 days of using the walker properly, the pain was gone and she could walk much longer distances. Nerve sensitivity resolved as well. She used the walker extensively for a couple of weeks and then stopped. The improvement was maintained without the walker. Six months later, she only used the walker occasionally, if she was having a flare-up of foot or back pain.

Carol did need additional foot surgery, so I sent her back to the surgeon who'd done such a good job on her before. The fact that she had persistent symptoms did not mean that he hadn't done his work well. He had done a great job! It was just that, in this unusual situation, her pain was coming from her back—even though her foot deformities COULD have been causing similar symptoms.

The lesson? If there *might* be a Spinal Stenosis involvement, a brief trial of Positional Testing could go a long way.

The Prescription

When ordering a walker, it is necessary to specify the type and size and the height of the handles. Picture 7.7 is a copy of the prescription pad I use in the office. It is not rare to find that even with this clear prescription, the walker provided is not correct. This allows me to remind the provider that the patient needs to be provided with what I requested, which was specified in detail!

The Need for Compliance

After surgical decompression, patients often report improvement when they wake up from surgery, and they also experience a great deal of relief within a couple of days. The same is true with Positional Testing. Patients who have foot, leg, thigh, or back discomfort when standing usually report immediate and often complete relief when walking with an appropriately set walker. For most, the underlying ache (or burning, weakness, etc.) is usually much better and is often completely gone within a couple of days. In the physical exam, we see a dramatic change in nerve sensitivity (as explained in Chapter 6) in 1–3 days. In my practice, this change is used to corroborate the improvement that the patient reports.

If someone does not experience good improvement with (correct!) Positional Testing within 3 days, this method will not work. As will be explained later,

---

Name _____**Date**_____

Address _____

Standard Walker _____ Wheels in front, Skis in back

Rollator Walker _____ **3 wheel, include basket**

Junior Standard Bariatric _____ **4 wheel,** include basket, drop down seat

Handle height _____ **inches** (do not dispense if it is not correct)

    Diagnosis   _____ Spinal Stenosis   724.02

_____ Walking Difficulty 719.7   _____ Radiculopathy   724.4

_____ **Other** _____

____ Dispense as Written   _____D.P.M.

                                Stuart M Goldman D PM

Picture 7.7. Prescription for Walker.

there are a few reasons for failure, which need to be investigated. They will be discussed later in this chapter. **All the details of Positional Testing must be correct.**

StoryTime: Mary F was a woman in her late 70s who reported having pain in her legs and difficulty walking more than half a block at a time. Her history and exam suggested Spinal Stenosis. The exam also suggested that a walker height of 28 inches was optimal for her. Accordingly, I prescribed a walker of that height.

She came back the next week disappointed because her back and leg pain and her difficulty walking were all unchanged. No surprise: she'd been given a standard rollator walker whose lowest height was 32 inches! I rechecked, called the durable medical equipment dealer, and got it switched with a junior rollator walker. One week after using it, Mary returned with good news. All the back pain and leg pain had resolved, and she could walk for several blocks at a time. I cannot stress enough how often improvement only appears with an optimal walker height. While

---

Classification of Improvement

This may be a good place to add a clarification. Several times in this book I refer to "good-to-excellent improvement." The following categorization of improvement is as previously published in my 2008 article in the Journal of Family Practice on positional management of Spinal Stenosis. Improvement in symptoms occurs in 1–3 days when effective, but improvement in walking-distance ability can take longer if there is a need to overcome deconditioning caused by prior inactivity.

Excellent improvement is considered a 400% improvement in walking distance ability and a 75%–100% reduction in painful symptoms (measured using a visual pain scale). Good improvement includes a 250%–399% improvement in walking distance and a 50%–74% reduction in painful symptoms. This is what I expect to see quickly with either Positional Testing for Spinal Stenosis or PseudoStenosis, or Mechanical Testing for PseudoStenosis, if the intervention is going to work.

---

some people improve even when the walker is not set at the best height, many others improve wonderfully with just a slight improvement in position. I remind all to focus on walker height to induce a mild but comfortable flexion.

Mary F's interview can be enjoyed on our web set, WalkingWellAgain.com.

Be aware that **full-time improvement** of the spine's position is often necessary to obtain the full benefit of the treatment. And when I say "full-time," that's exactly what I mean! While I have had many patients who had excellent improvement with only partial compliance, I have also had a great many who did not. Often, a patient will come in and say, "Dr. Goldman, you're right. I am walking a lot better, and much farther—but my feet (or back or legs) still hurt." When I ask if they're using the walker full time, they respond that they either don't bother with the walker when at home ("Was that reeeealy necessary?") or else when they're *not* at home ("I'm too embarrassed to use it outside the house!"). When they try again, with full-time compliance, within a couple of days the pain disappears.

I admit that I have had many patients who did not use the walker at work, who just used it at night and on the weekends and still saw great improvement. I will take partial compliance over no compliance any day, and will recognize that it may still produce excellent results. To quote Voltaire, "The perfect is the enemy of the good." I appreciate that in order to accommodate or work around the responsibilities of daily living, a patient must sometimes compromise treatment.

For some patients, the best they can do is use the walker at night or when not at work, and full time over the weekend. Since I have explained that there must be good results within 1–3 days for there to be an expectation of success, **full compliance from Friday night to Monday morning is usually all that is necessary to achieve the hoped-for improvement.** In such circumstances, part-time use after that first 3-day period may be all that is needed to maintain improvement.

Rapid results may be enough to convince patients of the value of Positional Testing. After obtaining relief in a few days, patients may be more willing to request accommodations for using a walker at work,

About Hills and Irregular Surfaces

It is important to use the walker on flat surfaces. Walking either uphill or downhill with the walker can be very problematic and can even make the back or legs feel worse, short term or long term. Walking up hill with the walker may cause neck and shoulder pain. This is addressed below, and in Chapter 9. Try to avoid using the walker on hills.

*It is for some people important that the surface that is walked upon is smooth, and does not only **appear** smooth. There are certain shopping malls in which the floor tiles have depressions between them, and that makes the walker actually shake, which puts causes mechanical stress when a person walks while leaning on the walker. Having an irregular surface makes walking with a walker uncomfortable for some people. This is especially important to recognize during Positional Testing, as the person might not recognize the benefit of the walker because of the irregular surface.*

something they might have been too embarrassed to ask for if they were not convinced of its value.

Full-time use of the walker allows the nerves or structural tissues to be relieved of pressure, allowing healing. Patients often experience relief from symptoms that they have had for years, that they were told were untreatable, or that were of unknown cause. Of my successful Positional Testing patients, I believe that over 1000 had what they themselves described as "magnificent" improvement that was more effective than any previous treatment, including medications, injections, physical therapy, or even spinal surgery.

Moving Forward with Success

How active can you be with a walker? The answer is as individual as you are. You are like an athlete getting ready for the upcoming season, and you must use common sense. I can only provide guidelines.

If you have been inactive because of pain and weakness and have been unable to walk for more than a few minutes, then even without the Spinal Stenosis– or PseudoStenosis–induced pain, you may find that your legs, back, and body get tired quickly.

DO NOT BE DISCOURAGED! The road to recovery is not so very long, but you must have patience. Increase your activity level gradually and you will be rewarded. If you have been severely limited in the past, I advise that you walk many times a day, even if only in short bursts. Walk in your living room, or walk in the hallway of your apartment. Within a few days, you may be able to build up to taking a short walk every hour. After a few more days, if you feel that you are getting stronger, walk for several minutes, sit and rest, and then repeat.

Within a week or two, you may feel that you are ready to walk about in the outside world. Always use common sense. Try to walk in flat, safe, well-lit areas that provide convenient places to sit, especially if you are using a walker without a seat. A shopping mall is perfect for this, and it's a great place to get back into shape.

There is an exception to this approach. If you have been inactive because of pain and weakness, *but you have always been able to walk extensively at the supermarket when pushing a grocery cart*, then you have not slipped into as bad a physical condition as you might fear. Walking slowly in the supermarket PROBABLY corresponds to walking at about half-speed. Therefore, if you can walk in a store for forty minutes before sitting, with a proper walker set at the proper height you might be able to start by walking for up to twenty minutes. At a reasonable starting pace of two miles per hour, that twenty-minute walk would allow you to go two-thirds of a mile—about six blocks! This is far more than many people with stenosis even dream of walking. And it can be done for many people on day 1 or 2, once they have the necessary confidence.

Whatever your starting point, it is important to be realistic, use common sense, and increase your activity gradually.

Sometimes, patients who are just starting the recovery process, pain free for the first time in years, are eager to spend a day at the mall the first chance they get. The following day, they feel like marathon runners the morning after the first race, or as if they'd spent a couple of rounds in a boxing ring with Joe Frazier: sore all over and wondering which freight train had hit them. For some people, it takes several days to recover.

Although their spine and legs hold up, the rest of their bodies are just not ready for that particular challenge.

A month later that same stroll through the mall is like a walk in the park: comfortable and with no residual effects. It was the initial overdoing that carried a price. **So I must repeat: increase your efforts with common sense, understand where you are starting from, and be patient.**

Many of my patients who, before Positional Testing, could only walk one-half or even one-quarter of a block without having to stop, within a few months were able to walk two, three, or even four miles. Even after guiding such recoveries for over a decade, I am continually amazed at the amount of improvement that can be obtained. Remember that there may be the potential to walk as well as you did 10, 20, or even 30 years ago—but you have to build up to it gradually. Years of inactivity take their toll. You must give yourself a chance to get in shape again at a reasonable pace.

What If the Use of the Walker Is Uncomfortable?

If your lower back hurts more, or in a different way, when using the walker, the walker handles are most likely too low. DO NOT WAIT. Try raising the handles one inch at a time to reach a comfortable position. ONE INCH! I have had patients who responded to back discomfort by raising the handles several inches, whereupon they got no benefit at all and gave up on the whole process. When I saw these patients again, often for an unrelated reason, I figured out what went wrong and corrected the handle height, and the patient improved as initially anticipated. For this reason, only raise the walker one inch at a time when adjusting it for back discomfort. You can always raise it a second inch if it is still uncomfortable.

If your arms or shoulders are uncomfortable, it usually means that the handles of the walker are set too high. This sensation of discomfort usually does not occur immediately, like the discomfort in the back does if the walker handles are set too low. Rather, it occurs after you have walked for a considerable time and have flexed your arms or shoulders in order to be able to lean further. Lower the walker enough to make you lean forward slightly and comfortably, with your arms straight

and the walker close to you. If the symptoms still occur, lower the walker again.

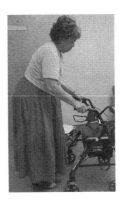

Picture 7.8. Flexion of the arms and shoulders in order to flex the spine.

If the walker does not go any lower, you need a different walker! It is not at all uncommon to need a lower walker. Many standard walkers only lower to 32 inches, a height that is often too high for people shorter than (about) 5'6". If you feel that this might be the case, go to a pharmacy or durable medical equipment dealer that sells walkers, and try the different heights to see how they feel. **As you now know from reading this chapter, the right height is often essential for success.** If you need a different walker, buy it! (As of August 2014, Medicare will pay for a new walker only once every five years. I have submitted information asking them to alter this policy. Wish me luck!)

More about Neck Pain

Neck symptoms can also be experienced by people who use bifocal glasses at the computer. In order to see the computer with the lower part of the lens, they hyperextend the neck. This problem can be solved by using reading glasses, with the refraction set for close distance only, when using the computer. Otherwise, severe pain can develop in the center of the lower neck.

I have also had many people with neck pain or headaches that resolved after treatment of PseudoStenosis issues, such as a flexible Flat Foot or a Limb Length Discrepancy. See Chapters 11, 12, and 19.

If your neck hurts, it might be because you are hyperextending it. This might depend on how much you have to lean forward to get relief. Some people must lean forward a great deal in order to relieve spine-mediated symptoms successfully. If they try to look directly forward into the distance, the position can cause neck hyperextension and pain. If you are one of these people, it is better to walk while looking at the ground perhaps 15 or 20 feet ahead of you. This reduces neck hyperextension and the pain it causes.

Should EVERYONE use the Walker as I Describe?

The answer is no! The great majority of people with SS/PS find immediate physical relief of symptoms from using the walker as described above. **Yet not everyone does.** *Some have arthritis or a herniated disc, both of which could make that position uncomfortable. Some are held back by the emotional distress they feel from leaning forward after spending a lifetime standing straight. In my own practice, I* **occasionally** *have patients who try the slight flexion position and reject it for either physical or emotional reasons.*

In addition, people without SS/PS who use the walker for arthritis or balance may prefer to stand straight with the arms bent, as is the classic approach.

Though I perceive great value in people with SS/PS using this approach, I realize that not everyone can use it, or even should. It is, however, of great potential benefit, so I believe that EVERYONE with suspected SS/PS should at least try it.

How Long Does Positional Testing Take?

Positional Testing is actually divided into two periods, one consisting of 3 days and the other of 10 days.

Within 3 days, it is time to reassess. If Positional Testing has not improved your symptoms, then you will not improve with further treatment unless changes are made. Perhaps the walker is not set at the right height, or perhaps you need some of the additional methods listed below. If you are no better within 3 days (of good compliance), study Chapter 9, "What If Positional Testing Did Not Help?"

If after 3 days you *have* had good improvement, the next step is to continue the Positional Testing regimen for a total of 10 days. Keep using the walker and the Adjunct Measures listed below. This will give the nerves a good blood supply with greatly reduced pressure, and a chance to fully recover. I believe that there is much less recurrence of symptoms if people complete the full-time, 10-day regimen.

This ten-day period, however, is the least firmly entrenched concept in my overall positional management approach. 7 days might be enough, while some people might be better able to get off the walker permanently if they keep up full-time Positional Testing for as many as 14 or 21 days. I admit that I don't know this time factor with precision. Research in a university setting could help establish such parameters in a way I have not. So far, this is only an educated guess on my part.

Introducing the Adjunct Measures

The following is a list of adjunct behavior modifications for Positional Testing. They are not always needed if you have seen great improvement by simply using the walker. If, however, you still have some discomfort or continue to be limited in your walking, standing, or sleeping, adding these behaviors can be just what the doctor ordered. They are explained in detail in the next

Adjunct Measures

1. Go down steps backward.
2. Modify your sleep position. Sleep with a pillow or two under your thighs and knees if you sleep on your back, and with a pillow between your thighs if you sleep on your side. If you must sleep on your stomach, put a pillow transversely, from side to side, under your lower stomach area.
3. Use a shower stool when showering.
4. Use a kitchen stool when doing work in the kitchen, and do as much work as possible in the kitchen sitting down.
5. Use the Professor Position when standing without a walker. This is achieved by putting your hands behind your back and leaning slightly forward, as if deep in thought.
6. Use the seat of the four-wheeled walker as a tray to carry objects such as food, laundry, or packages.

chapter, but for those who simply want to "get on with it," here are the recommended changes:

What Do I Do After Positional Testing Succeeds?

There is a third phase after Positional Testing called "Positional Therapy," which will transition you away from full-time walker use. This phase is detailed in Chapter 10.

Remember, even if using a walker and adopting the Adjunct Measures provides WONDERFUL relief, you should still consider the possibility that you have PseudoStenosis. If the relief is only temporary, you should definitely be evaluated for that. See Chapters 11 and 12, on PseudoStenosis.

What If Positional Testing Fails?

I repeat: those who improve with Positional Testing always do so within 3 days. If there is no improvement in my patient, I reevaluate for any of several possibilities. If you tried Positional Testing and Adjunct Measures but failed to obtain significant results, please review the possibilities outlined in Chapter 9.

The Grocery Cart Test

I was not sure where to put this section, and I finally chose to present it at the end of the chapter on Positional Testing. This is the first form of Positional Testing that I used in my practice. I used the "Grocery Cart Test" early on with many of my patients, to try to understand the effect of flexion on their symptoms and to help them understand the potential value of using a walker.

I still occasionally use the Grocery Cart Test. Some people are unwilling to try a walker because they fear it will affect their social standing. Some feel that it is too much of a concession to aging, a step closer to the grave. I believe that the opposite is true. Positional management affords you a great opportunity to improve your quality of life, and I believe that for some people it may also prolong the duration of life.

HOWEVER, I am not always persuasive enough. For people who are reluctant to use a walker temporarily, the Grocery Cart Test shows them just how much they can improve with wheeled support—without cost and without stigma.

The Grocery Cart Test

Choose a grocery store with numbered aisles, and a place to sit in the front. You will need to do this on two separate days. On each day you will follow the identical protocol, with one major difference. On the first day you will walk with no grocery cart, and on the second test day you will use a cart.

If you do not receive improvement with pushing a cart, and you are less than 5' 2" tall, you may try again, but with your arms resting side to side on the handle of the cart, to help you comfortably lean forward. Another option is to use a pediatric or junior walker, which we may lend you.

Enter the store. Rest on a chair for 5 minutes. Begin walking on Aisle #1. Record the time at which you start. Walk until you feel you begin to tire, and note where you are (which aisle) and what the time duration was. Continue walking until you feel you must stop or sit to get relief, and record the aisle and amount of time since you began. On the second test day, do the identical walk but pushing a grocery cart.

For consistency, **do not stop at all**, even to talk or to even look at any items, even when with a cart.

	Day 1 (no cart)	Day 2 (with cart)	Day 3 (if under 5'2", arms resting on cart or with walker)
Time (# of minutes) until tired			
Row at which you tire			
Time at which you feel you must stop or sit			
Row at which you feel you must stop or sit			

*The Grocery Cart Test may not work in mega stores like Sam's Club. The reason is that the carts there are larger and the handle height is much higher, at 46 inches rather than 42 inches. Several people have reported increased pain walking in mega stores compared to standard stores, which they attributed to **harder concrete**. What was actually happening was that the higher handle was not inducing the proper lumbar flexion needed to reduce SS/PS symptoms. Therefore, the Grocery Cart Test should not be done with a higher cart, unless the patient is at least (approximately) 5'10"!*

It is often necessary to take a formal Grocery Cart Test to see if the lumbosacral flexion truly improves the symptoms. **Many people with poor arterial circulation mistakenly feel that their lack of symptoms walking in a grocery store is due to using a grocery cart, when it is actually the frequent stops and starts of shopping that allow them to feel better when food shopping.** That is why the test requires walking without stopping, to compare UNINTERRUPTED walking capability with and without wheeled support.

The following paragraphs provide some supplemental insights that apply to use of the Grocery Cart Test. To understand the details, you need to consider PseudoStenosis. However, this test will tell you, with a great deal of confidence, whether you have either Spinal Stenosis or PseudoStenosis, and whether you can likely obtain at least good temporary help with Positional Testing.

Is there good improvement of symptoms with Positional Testing using a grocery cart, and worsening of symptoms at the checkout counter? If so, there is almost certainly a Spinal Stenosis or Pseudo-Stenosis component present. This is true for foot or leg pain, ankle arthritis, knee arthritis, hip arthritis, and of course, Low-Back Syndrome. Dramatic improvement of any of these symptoms when using a walker or a grocery cart strongly suggests that a large part of the problem is affected by spinal position. **If there is good improvement but no PseudoStenosis component that you detect (see Chapters 11 and 12), I recommend that you try full-time Positional Testing and all behaviors adjunct to Positional Testing.** The walker must be set at the right height and used as

much as possible, and the Adjunct Measures should be followed precisely. If this method proves helpful, the overall arthritic pain will be dramatically better within 1–3 days. **This can be true even if there is genuine arthritis.** Arthritis will still be present, but it may not hurt as much. If this works, transition to Positional Therapy as described in Chapter 10.

If there is good improvement, even if you decide that there might be a PseudoStenosis component, you can still seek and possibly obtain great short-term or even long-term relief by doing Positional Testing.

All patients with Spinal Stenosis should consider the possibility of PseudoStenosis. If this is present, the options include either addressing the PseudoStenosis component first, as I almost always do in my office, or obtaining relief with Positional Testing.

If there is no improvement or if there is poor improvement, still check for possible causes of Pseudo-Stenosis and have the PseudoStenosis addressed. If there is still only limited improvement, you can retry the Grocery Cart Test or other Positional Testing. It is possible that both mechanical treatment and other treatment for PseudoStenosis are necessary, as is Positional Testing for SS/PS.

If there is no improvement or if there is poor improvement, and there are no signs of PseudoStenosis, then you must seek additional help. This may include consulting a physiatrist, podiatrist, orthopedic surgeon, neurologist, vascular specialist, or rheumatologist. Discuss this next step with your primary care provider or with your podiatrist. Either may be able to give guidance as to which specialist would be best to see.

Thank You Drs. Goldsmith and Wiesel

*I have one final point regarding the Grocery Cart Test. The recognition of improved walking in Spinal Stenosis patients when using a grocery cart was published by Drs. GOLDSMITH and WIESEL in 1998, in an article in the **Journal of Clinical Rheumatology** entitled "Spinal stenosis: A straightforward approach to a complex problem." I am grateful to them for publishing this insight. It helped me begin on this long journey of exploration, which, in turn, has helped me help many thousands of patients.*

CHAPTER 8

Positional Testing Adjunctive Behaviors

For individuals suffering from Lumbar Spinal Stenosis or PseudoStenosis, the key to relief is opening the sections of the spine that have functioned in a narrow manner, causing nerve tissue to be compressed, inflamed, and painful. I've suggested Positional Testing as an excellent route to reach this end. However, there are many things besides the use of the walker that can help provide relief and that may actually be needed to effect the "positional decompression" we are aiming for in the first 10 crucial days. I listed them briefly in Chapter 7, "Positional Testing." Here they are again, presented in detail.

Modifying Use of Stairs

Descending stairs backward induces a change in the spine's position that maintains the spine in a comfortable, flexed position. When going down the stairs in the normal forward manner, it is very common to lean back slightly, in order to counteract the feeling of being about to fall forward. For many people who are afflicted with a variety of age-related conditions, stairs become an enemy, both because they are difficult to navigate and because they introduce a risk factor for falling.

If you lean backward to maintain stability while going down the stairs, you are performing the opposite function of the walker, which involves leaning **forward** to open the spine. Leaning backward can actually

narrow the spine. Many people find that going down steps makes the back, knees, legs, or feet ache, and that it generally aggravates their symptoms. They may feel unstable and have a sensation that they are about to fall. For many of these individuals, going down the stairs backward eliminates these problems.

Take a look at picture 8.1. When a person goes down backward, he leans **forward** the way he would with a walker, thus opening his spine. For most patients, this eliminates the compression seen with either Spinal Stenosis or PseudoStenosis. Simple but effective.

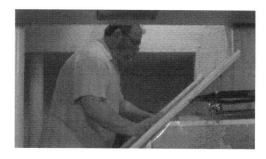

Picture 8.1. Going down the stairs backward opens the spine.

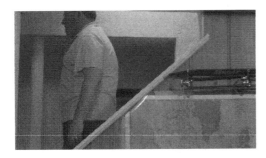

Picture 8.2. When going down the stairs forward, the person often leans backward slightly, which closes the spine and may increase pressure.

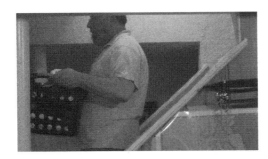

Picture 8.3. Going down the stairs forward carrying a basket, for example, causes one to lean backward even more.

In contrast, look at pictures 8.2 and 8.3. As shown in picture 8.2, a person goes down stairs standing straight or leaning slightly back—which closes the spine. As shown in picture 8.3, this condition is greatly aggravated when the individual is carrying a package or other object, such as a laundry basket, because carrying worsens the backward-leaning position.

Here are a few solutions:

1. Try to get someone else to carry your items downstairs. Asking others to do this might seem like an imposition, but it could spell the difference between your being able to use your basement and not. Relatives, friends, or even kids in the neighborhood can help. Remember, what might be poison for you—the simple act of going down steps carrying a basket—is effortless for them. Ask them, barter with them, or pay them—but get the help you need.

2. Use a pouch to carry things downstairs. A front pack, such as the kind hikers use, allows you to carry the items hands-free and leaning forward (while you go down the steps backward, of course).

3. Throw or push the stuff down the steps. This may sound a bit uncivilized, and you must be careful not to trip over anything that's lying on the ground. But if you are desperate it might be a reasonable solution.

Some of my patients were initially afraid that they would fall if they descended backward. No one has, to the best of my knowledge, but it is still a legitimate fear. Therefore, I offer three thoughts:

1. **Practice.** From the bottom of the stairs, go up one step forward, and then down one step backward. Go up two, and then down two. Up three, down three. This is far less frightening than starting with the entire staircase at once, and it builds confidence. When you are confident and comfortable tackling a small number of steps, you may progress to using this technique for the entire staircase.

2. **You MUST have a HANDRAIL for stability.** I believe that going down steps backward without a handrail is risky, and I do not recommend it. **If you are at all uncertain, have a second handrail put in for the other side of the steps.** This is not an expensive investment, and it might make you more secure and confident.

3. Of course there is always a risk of falling on stairs, no matter how they are navigated, so one must be careful and exercise good judgment. It is up to the person using the stairs to make the call. **If you are AT ALL unsure, see a physical therapist to practice with supervision and help.**

By the way, DO NOT FORGET TO HAVE A WALKER DOWNSTAIRS. This may be just for the 10 days of the full Positional Testing phase, or it may be long term, if the downstairs is an area where you carry things such as laundry that can place a strain on your lower back. Using the seat of the walker to move objects is a great way to prevent recurrence of your symptoms. Be open to realizing the benefit of the walker, and use it wherever and whenever it might be helpful.

I must give credit where credit is due. While virtually all other guidance on Positional Testing, Positional Therapy, and Adjunct Measures is original on my part, the idea of going down the stairs backward was provided to me by Ira Fedder, MD, a highly respected orthopedic spine surgeon in the Baltimore area. Thank you, Dr. Fedder!

Modifying Sleep Position

The position of the body affects spinal arthritis and compression of the nerves whether you are awake or asleep. Since we are trying to effect a spinal decompression, sleep position may need to be addressed as well.

Note that I said we MAY need to address the sleep position. Many people have no pain or discomfort at night or upon awakening, and they gain relief from all symptoms with only daytime modification, with no recurrence. For these people, no sleep modification is needed. **However, if you have back, leg, or foot pain at night OR when you first get up in the morning, or if you have recurrence after you stop using your walker, this set of modifications may help.**

The goal is to replicate in bed the position used during the day to make sure that the narrowing that is characteristic of SS/PS does not place abnormal pressure on sensitive areas of the spine. Since the narrowing of the spine can be relieved by changing the spine's position, we try to achieve this effect during sleep time too.

Sleeping in a recliner chair often provides the most comfortable position for patients with Spinal Stenosis. In fact, this is the only way that some people with SS/PS can sleep, and it is a great tool. However, two disadvantages spring to mind. The first is that changing positions in a recliner is not easy. Most adults naturally adjust their sleep positions at least a few times each night. This may have the advantages of keeping joints from stiffening up too much and being painful in the morning.

Also, as you may be aware, when someone is in a nursing home or hospital, the staff makes sure that the person switches positions occasionally in order to prevent the formation of **decubitus ulcers**. These ulcers form in areas of pressure, such as the heel of the foot or the low back, if the pressure is either too great or goes on for too long. Sleeping in a bed has the advantage of allowing a shift in position that may not be so easy to do in a recliner, thus preventing ulcers that could be caused by staying in the same position for too long.

A second disadvantage of using a recliner is that recliners are not built for two. You can share your sleep hours with a beloved person in a bed, if you are so blessed. If this is of value to you, try getting out of the recliner and back into bed. You may enjoy the benefits of the recliner position in bed by sleeping with a pillow or two under your thighs and knees while lying on your back. As will be explained, proper placement of the pillow is essential.

Many people, with the best of intentions—especially if they have some edema (swelling in the legs)—will raise their legs by putting a pillow underneath their feet or lower legs. While this does flex the spine a bit, it also seems to put a lot of strain on the nerves leaving the spine, and may worsen, rather than relieve, Spinal Stenosis symptoms.

Placing the pillow so that the knees flex eliminates that strain, and allows the spinal nerves to be relieved. I have had many patients who had comfortable sleep restored by using this simple maneuver. I repeat: the correct positioning of the pillow is crucial. Picture 8.4 demonstrates the recommended way of placing the pillow.

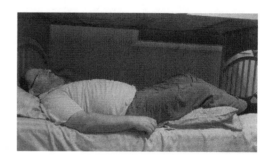

Picture 8.4. Pillows under the knees.

Remember, there is an advantage to being able to switch sleep positions. Therefore, if you have enough room in your bed, you can put the pillow UNDER THE SHEET so that it stays in place. Each time you shift to a side-sleeping position, you roll off the pillow. When you return to the back-sleeping position, the pillow is waiting for you. This handy trick has helped many people.

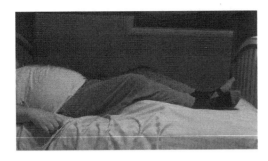

Picture 8.5. Pillows under the sheet.

For individuals seeking the positional decompression, I do not recommend putting the pillow under the feet. It is at times advised to do that to reduce swelling, but doing so may put tension on the nerves in the back of the legs and the back. This has caused much more discomfort for many of my patients. You can place a pillow under the knees and feet, as long as you have the knees bent!

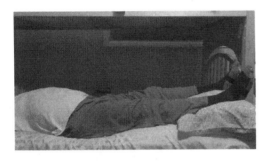

Picture 8.6. Caution: using pillows under the feet and lower legs can increase tension on the nerves in the lower back and thereby increase symptoms associated with spinal nerve irritation.

There may be a time when placing pillows under the feet is appropriate, such as after knee surgery, or if the doctor managing your heart condition wants to reduce swelling as much as possible. If this position is recommended and you have SS/PS nighttime symptoms, **check with your surgeon or therapist** to see if you can use the pillow under the feet to reduce swelling but also have a pillow under the knees to reduce spinal nerve irritation.

If you are a side sleeper, putting a pillow between the thighs is often helpful, too, as it changes the position of the nerves leaving the spine. If the pillow won't stay in position, you may find relief by using a long body pillow, demonstrated at the store section of WalkingWell Again.com. Alternatively, this problem can be solved by having a pouch sewn into the inner thigh of the pajama pants and inserting a small pillow into it that will maintain the separation between the thighs when you are lying on your side.

Two unrelated points: If you prefer sleeping on your side, be sure to use a thick pillow to support your head! Also, if you sleep on your side, keep in mind that some research suggests that sleeping on the left side may relieve heartburn symptoms, while sleeping on the right side may make them worse.

If you sleep on your stomach, put a pillow transversely, from side to side, under your lower stomach area, to open the spine. I have had some patients find relief of nighttime symptoms and achieve improved sleeping in this manner. However, if you find that you sleep well only on your stomach, you may have Sleep Apnea. Discuss this with your physician. Sleep Apnea is a very common condition, especially (but not only) in overweight people, in individuals with diabetes, and in individuals with large necks, many of whom snore badly. It is a condition that can cause major health problems, so do not ignore this possibility if you think it might apply to you.

Further information can be found in Chapters 21 (on nighttime symptoms) and Chapter 22 (on Sleep Apnea).

Using a Shower Stool When Showering

This is an obvious modification. If the goal is to minimize standing erect, that includes showering. For many people, this is only a temporary change during the initial days of Positional Testing, but it may make a difference. If you really want to do everything possible to eliminate the pressure on the nerves, this might be needed.

Modifying Kitchen Position

Use a kitchen stool, and do as much kitchen work as possible sitting down. Like use of the shower stool, this modification is simply to keep you from standing upright any more than you need to. When working in the kitchen you are often bending forward, bringing about some relief of the stenosis-induced symptoms. However, this relief of nerve compression may come at the cost of straining the muscles in your back to support yourself in that position. Many people find that a kitchen stool allows them to work at the proper height and remain pain free. In contrast to a shower stool, the height of the kitchen stool is important if you are trying to work at the counters, which are usually much higher than a kitchen table.

Try doing as much food preparation as you can while seated at the table. Use disposables whenever possible, eliminating the need for washing dishes at the sink. This expense may seem like a waste, but for the 10 days of Positional Testing it may have value, and the cost is really pretty small when you think about it. You could use the dishwasher—even for single items, if that is easier on your back.

In the kitchen, you may be tempted to compromise on some of your previous patterns, but the value of avoiding the wrong activity—especially during the Positional Testing phase, a time when you are trying to see how much better you can get with simple methods—may be tremendous. You must pay attention to see what works best for you, and what carries a price tag in terms of painful symptoms that are well worth avoiding.

The Professor Position

Use what I call the "Professor Position" when standing without a walker. This position is achieved by putting your hands behind your back and leaning slightly forward, as if deep in thought. (Think of Groucho Marx as Professor Wagstaff in "Horse Feathers.") This position flexes the spine without the person needing to lean on anything. This allows you to maintain a flexed position while standing, without straining the muscles in the back.

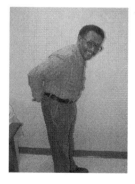

Picture 8.7. The Professor Position.

Although my aim is to have you use a walker as much as possible, or even all the time, during the initial Positional Testing phase, this is impossible for some

people for a variety of reasons, the most common being employment responsibilities. The second most common reason is ego: being unwilling to use the walker in certain social or professional settings. (I do NOT judge; I only observe.) For these individuals, being able to relieve SS-/PS-induced pressure by assuming the Professor Position whenever possible, or at least whenever needed, is of great benefit.

Picture 8.7 clearly shows the position and technique, although the amount of flexion needed is determined by the individual. Only bend as much as you need to in order to get relief.

Those who read about the Professor Position in Chapter 6 can now understand the expanded role of this maneuver. It can quickly corroborate the SS/PS role in symptoms of unknown cause. It can demonstrate the great potential of Positional Testing. Finally, it is an effective addition to therapy and allows those who cannot use Positional Testing full time to reduce pressure and inflammation on the nerves, with a therapeutic benefit all its own.

> **StoryTime:** Cheryl L, 61, came in because she'd been suffering with heel pain for a few weeks. She also reported severe knee pain and moderate back pain, both in bed and when walking, for many months. She'd had a fusion of her spine for scoliosis, which had provided moderate improvement.
>
> I resolved the heel pain with a strapping. Because the signs and symptoms pointed to Spinal Stenosis, I recommended Positional Testing and the Adjunct Measures. Wanting to avoid the use of a walker, she agreed to start with Adjunct Measures: the Professor Position when standing, a modified sleep position in bed, and going down the stairs backward.
>
> She never needed a walker. She found acceptable relief within a few days, just by using the Professor Position when necessary and by modifying her sleep position. She needed a grocery cart when shopping and limited her walking without the cart, but she was quite satisfied that her overall pain and sleep difficulties were resolved.
>
> The lesson? Sometimes only partial intervention is needed for relief. I will take partial compliance over no compliance any day, and I am sometimes pleasantly surprised. I make clear to patients that other

> *This section refers to an unusual use of the Professor Position: when walking downhill.*
>
> *Walking downhill* *can be difficult for patients with Spinal Stenosis, because of the need to lean slightly backward in order not to feel as if falling forward. That is why some people with Spinal Stenosis or PseudoStenosis find it easier to walk uphill (leaning forward) than downhill (leaning backward), even though gravity might suggest the opposite.*
>
> *This relates to the Professor Position.* *If going downhill, then taking the Professor Position and leaning forward might be hard to achieve or comfortably maintain. That can be corrected by simply turning around and resting for a few minutes while facing the uphill direction. Facing uphill, the Professor Position would be easier to maintain for as long as needed to relieve the SS/PS symptoms. Just don't forget which direction you were going!*

interventions may be needed, but it is reasonable to allow the patient to guide the order of intervention. In Cheryl's case, she avoided the walker, and had acceptable, although not perfect, results.

Two of Cheryl L's interviews are available on our web set, WalkingWellAgain.com.

Expanding Use of a Walker

Use the seat of the walker as a tray to transport objects such as food, laundry, or packages. After all, "full-time use of the walker" means full time! Even walking without the walker from the kitchen to the dining room, for example, is a break in compliance. Carrying food, laundry, or other packages may actually worsen symptoms, because leaning back in order to carry something in front may worsen the spine position.

For many people, proper positioning of the spine eliminates the need to sit and rest while walking. For them, using the seat as a tray to transport objects is the most essential advantage to using a four-wheeled rollator walker rather than a standard folding walker. During the initial Positional Testing phase, full-time walker use may spell the difference between complete and partial relief of nerve inflammation and secondary neuropathic symptoms such as burning, tingling, and aching. *Full time means full time!*

Having a walker on each floor that you commonly use of your home

It is obvious to me, but not necessarily to my patients, that a person experiencing problems that derive from the back should not lift heavy objects, especially up and down stairs. **The list of objectionable objects includes a walker—especially the heavier rollator walkers.** Since some people benefit from one-hundred-percent use but should not carry the walker up or down stairs, a solution is to have a walker on every floor. The walker for the secondary floors may be a cheaper folding walker (with wheels and sliders) unless you frequently need to transport things in the basement. Under that circumstance, a second four-wheeled rollator would be best.

> **StoryTime:** At the risk of sounding maudlin, I must tell you that I have an old friend who sent his father to see me from another city. The father spent a lot of time in his basement office, refused to get a second walker, and was dissatisfied with the results of Positional Testing. He admitted freely that he did not come close to full compliance and that he had much less pain when using the walker. An attorney with confidence in his own judgment, he decided to have spinal fusion instead and "just get back to normal." He did not survive the surgery. The price of the second walker was very high for him—far too high. Such a small change to make, and such a high price to pay.

Not everyone needs all these modifications

In this chapter, I present ways that the positional decompression can be maximized. However, to be honest, not everyone needs all of these modifications in behavior. If you are enjoying excellent results just from using the walker part time, that is cause for rejoicing! If, however, improvement over the first few days is not perfect, these modifications, all easy and inexpensive and safe, may be needed. Do not hesitate to add them to your healing regimen. They may be what allow you to begin Walking Well Again.

The Power of Combination Therapy

Proper use of the walker, especially when combined with these Adjunct Measures, has a very good chance of dramatically improving symptoms of Spinal Stenosis in a matter of a few days. But what if use of the walker does not improve symptoms, or what if the improvement is limited?

First, again, I recommend seeing a good podiatrist to check out the causes of PseudoStenosis.

Second, I recommend following up with a spine specialist. It is possible that you previously received care that did not provide long-term assistance, including anti-inflammatory medication, topical treatment such as a Lidoderm patch or a Flector patch, physical therapy, or epidural injections. Combined with Positional Testing, these therapeutic approaches might provide better results. For example, if epidural injection provided only moderate or temporary help, it is possible that combining these injections with use of the walker and these Adjunct Measures will provide better or longer-acting help. **Do not discount the effect of combining therapies if positional management alone does not provide the relief you seek.**

What If Positional Testing Did Not Help?

I have found that Positional Testing improves walking and reduces or eliminates symptoms in over 70% of people hampered by Spinal Stenosis. When effective, meaningful improvement is seen within 1–3 days. This leaves us with the question, what to do if Positional Testing *doesn't* work?

First we must define what we mean by "doesn't work." No, I am not splitting hairs. Remember our discussion of how vital it is to understand your symptoms well in order to appreciate the relief? The LuSSSExt scale introduced in Chapter 3 provides a clear presentation of what your symptoms were before Positional Testing. You may choose to repeat the scale. Perhaps it will clarify for you whether you are partially, though not all, better.

Are you a lot better, but still experiencing some annoying symptoms? Are you walking much better, but still experiencing pain in your feet, legs, or back? Are you walking much better, but find that you get out of breath or that your arms and shoulders tire? Are you better during the day but not in bed at night? Or are you not better at all? I will address the last question first.

Six Common Reasons

If you are not at all better, it is most likely due to one of the following six reasons.

1. The walker is not the right height.

2. There is a compliance issue. In other words, you did not use the walker and the Adjunct Measures the great majority of the time over the course of 3 days.

3. There is also a herniated disc or a spinal cyst or mass present. This (and some other pathology) can cause problems with flexion, so it makes the flexion of Positional Testing uncomfortable or ineffective.

4. There are severe anatomic changes that did not allow for elimination of nerve or structural inflammation with flexion.

5. There are moderate-to-severe PseudoStenosis issues.

6. The diagnosis of Lumbar Spinal Stenosis as the primary cause of symptoms is wrong, and another condition is the primary cause of the symptoms.

The Wrong Walker Height

Quite commonly, the handle height of the walker is not correct. It isn't always easy getting it exactly right. It requires judgment. Because of different body proportions, different arm lengths, and different pathologies, I cannot simply calculate the handle height based on the person's height. Rather, the height must be such that the back is leaning forward with the arms straight, all in a comfortable manner that relieves symptoms.

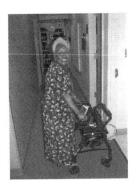

Picture 9.1. The correct walker handle height usually allows the person to lean slightly forward with the arms comfortably straight.

Reread Chapter 7 on Positional Testing if you have questions on how to achieve the proper height.

I have had many people—dozens!—who came in for a follow-up visit and reported only limited relief, but who did quite well after I adjusted the walker. Sometimes they had borrowed a walker, rather than purchasing what I'd prescribed, and it was the wrong height. Sometimes the durable medical equipment dealer had provided a walker that was set to the wrong height. In any case, setting the walker to induce the right amount of flexion is often necessary to obtain relief.

In fact, I have had many patients come to see me complaining of severe long-term symptoms, who had good relief when I simply adjusted the walker that they came in with. Thus, I repeat: the correct walker height is truly essential for many people.

If your arms or shoulders hurt when you walk with the help of your walker, it means the handles are too high. You are bending your arms and shoulders in order to achieve the appropriate height. In contrast, if your back hurts more with use of the walker, the handle height is most likely too low.

It is important to experiment with adjusting the handle height if you do not see comfortable improvement at the initial handle height. *Even I have occasionally recommended the wrong handle height, and have had to adjust the handle height to a different position at the follow-up visit.* Despite my having invented this approach

and having used it for fourteen years, I am not always right. **If I can occasionally be an inch or two off, so can you, as can your doctor or therapist.** Do not hesitate to experiment if you do not get the relief you seek.

Inadequate Compliance

The next possibility for why you did not improve may be inadequate compliance: using the walker less than what is needed to achieve the needed decompression. For example, if you used the walker less than 90% of the time for the first few days, there may not be adequate relief of pressure or inflammation in the nerves to bring about the sought-after improvement in your symptoms. I have had many cases where people presented that they walked much better but were still in pain. Then they admitted that they had not used the walker as directed. When fully compliant, many enjoyed real relief from pain that had NOT gotten better with limited walker use.

Sometimes failure in compliance is not the patient's fault. If there are two flights of stairs in a patient's home, he or she may not be able to have the walker both upstairs and downstairs. This person cannot (or should not) carry the walker up and down the stairs himself, and might not have someone to help with that task.

I would recommend that this person, as an experiment, simply stay home for a couple of days and use the walker full time. Another option, of course, is to have two walkers, one for upstairs and one for downstairs. If you do not own a car and use a cab or other car service, tip the driver if you need to, so that he'll bring the walker to and from the house for you.

A rollator walker may be too heavy and too bulky for an individual to lift. If you often use public transportation, a standard folding walker (with wheels in the front and slides in the back) may be a better choice. This walker is lighter—perhaps even light enough to be carried up and down the stairs, and it is easier to transport on a bus.

What if you work six or even seven days a week and cannot use a walker at work? Perhaps you need to arrange an extra day or two off from your job. That, of course, may be easier for me to say than for you to do. And yet, a day or two at home, fully compliant, might make all the difference.

Solving this dilemma is your responsibility. Enlist friends, family, or neighbors to help. You must look at your life critically and see how to comply with this protocol for at least 2–3 days to see if this approach will work for you.

A Herniated Disc or a Spinal Mass

At times, there is a herniated disc in addition to Spinal Stenosis. In such situations, the person may have a lot of pain when sitting as well as when lying down. **The same flexion that improves stenosis symptoms can actually aggravate symptoms caused by the disc**—symptoms that can include sciatica, local back pain, and pain radiating into the foot or leg. Pushing a grocery cart may actually aggravate back or lower-extremity symptoms. For such individuals, Positional Testing may be uncomfortable and is more likely to fail.

I have had some patients with a herniated disc who improved by doing a reverse of my Positional Testing (flexion) approach. Because sitting in a 90-degree position puts pressure on the disc, which irritates the nerve, any change that eliminates that pressure can allow the nerve inflammation to improve. I have directed such patients to try sitting on a pillow or two. Some noted immediate improvement. **If this position works, you should do so full time whenever sitting:** at home, at work, in a car. The sciatic pain may diminish within a day or two, but if this works I advise using the pillow as much as possible for 10 days. After the nerve irritation caused by the disc is quieted down, try Positional Testing with the walker, as the flexion needed to open up the spine may then be tolerated.

Another option for patients with both a symptomatic herniated disc and SS/PS is to combine traditional treatment with Positional Testing. Perhaps the herniated disc can be quieted by an epidural injection, by anti-inflammatories, or by medications that reduce nerve pain, such as antidepressants (Elavil, Desyrel, or Cymbalta) or anticonvulsants (Neurontin or Lyrica). Any method used to eliminate sensitivity from the herniated disc may then allow the use of Positional Testing.

Occasionally surgery is needed for a herniated disc, and this must be established through consultation with a spine specialist. While many affected patients improve with time, others experience persistent pain and the disc must be removed. Removing a disc is usually a far easier surgery to undergo than a spinal fusion, as it has quicker recovery and less morbidity. If the disc alone is removed, the person can then move on to using Positional Testing for Spinal Stenosis. I have had a few patients who saw success with this approach. The decision as to which surgery to perform must, of course, be made by the spine surgeon. However, such decisions are usually based on symptoms and disability and not just on the pathology present, so patients must be as clear as possible when explaining their symptoms and disability to the surgeon.

Lastly, sometimes a cyst or mass in the spinal canal area is causing pressure on the nerves that is not helped by manipulation of spine position. An MRI will identify this cause of spinal nerve compression that, as with a herniated disc, may require management by a spine surgeon.

Severe Stenosis or Post-operative Changes

Another reason for the failure of Positional Testing might be that, with Spinal Stenosis causing or contributing to the symptoms, there are anatomic changes that do not allow for elimination of nerve or structural inflammation with flexion. This appears to be more common if the stenosis is severe, or in the case of severe arthritic spurs or severe narrowing of the foramen (the windows that allow individual nerve roots to leave the spinal canal). It also appears more commonly in people with an unstable spine, in which there is actually a shift of one vertebra onto another. This condition is called "Spondylolisthesis," and it is sometimes only identified clearly with a modified (axial-loaded) MRI. More information on this condition can be found in Chapter 14, on radiology.

Patients who have already had spine surgery may have scarring around the nerves, a condition known as "perineural fibrosis." The presence of that scarring makes healing of the nerves more problematic. At the time of this writing, the year 2014, my understanding is that the prognosis of excellent pain relief is not good. I have found that such people often do have improved walking with a grocery cart or walker, but that the neuritic pain may not be well relieved by Positional Testing, injections, or even surgery. Such individuals need close supervision by a pain management specialist. They may improve with oral medication or with invasive pain management, such as an epidural stimulator or a morphine pump. I have very little follow-up with such approaches and do not have an opinion to share about them.

PseudoStenosis

While Positional Testing often provides excellent improvement in individuals with PseudoStenosis, there are times when it does not. The anatomic positional changes induced may not completely resolve with flexion, so the symptoms may remain. *Thus, if there is failure with Positional Testing, this is another reason to look closely for PseudoStenosis, described in Chapter 12.*

A Different Diagnosis . . . Completely

Finally, perhaps Lumbar Spinal Stenosis or nerve compression is not the primary cause of the symptoms. Stenosis mimics many different conditions. This means, of course, that many of those conditions may be mistaken for stenosis.

In my practice, I look primarily for conditions that can be successfully treated. Some of these conditions include PseudoStenosis, Diabetic or other Peripheral Neuropathy, CIDP or MGUS, Cervical Stenosis, NPH, arterial or venous insufficiency, myopathy, and others. I share information on some of these conditions near the end of Chapter 14.

If Positional Testing does not lead to improvement, I suggest you find a good podiatrist to examine you for possible PseudoStenosis, and a good neurologist or physiatrist to investigate other possible causes of your symptoms. Most conditions can be helped if the proper diagnosis is made, so find professionals who are willing to investigate.

This bears repeating. If you do not get the relief you need, there are professionals, including podiatrists, neurologists, physiatrists, pain management specialists, spine surgeons, rheumatologists, endocrinologists, physical therapists, and chiropractors, that you can consult. If you do not get better with the techniques I've shared, seek other help!

What if There was Partial Improvement?

What if there was incomplete improvement? In other words, you got better, but not all better. Here is a list of possible reasons, with explanation.

1. The walker is not set at the correct height.

2. A compliance issue prevented adequate decompression.

3. There is also a herniated disc present, which can cause pain and therefore problems with the flexion needed to open up a stenotic spine.

4. There are severe anatomic changes that do not allow for the elimination of nerve or structural inflammation with flexion.

5. PseudoStenosis-induced spine-position changes did not improve enough to resolve symptoms.

6. The diagnosis of SS/PS is correct, but there are other conditions contributing to the symptoms, which must be treated.

Those of you who are paying close attention will notice that reasons one through five are the same as those listed for patients who saw no improvement. To go from limited to excellent success, you may need to adjust the walker, improve your compliance, or address a herniated disc. You may have only limited improvement with this technique because of the severity of the spine changes, although I recommend experimenting with different walker heights and using all the tools of the Adjunct Measures (Chapter 8) before you accept incomplete improvement. You can also check my website (WalkingWellAgain.com) to see if there are new insights available.

The techniques reported here have approximately a 70% chance of good-to-excellent improvement with Spinal Stenosis in 1–3 days. Therefore, incomplete improvement may mean that some other spinal therapy is necessary. The patient should see a physiatrist for overall management.

It is common to have limited improvement for the sixth reason listed above—that other conditions contribute to the overall symptomatology. There are a great many conditions whose symptoms overlap, or that are exacerbated by Spinal Stenosis. **Chapters in Section 3 of this book address many of those individual conditions.** Others are detailed at the end of Chapter 14, on radiology.

If you have done the appropriate Positional Testing, used the Adjunct Measures, and obtained significant but only partial improvement of your symptoms, it is time to seek help in looking for other causes and treatments.

Positional Therapy

Wonderful. You've done Positional Testing—used the walker and perhaps the Adjunct Measures—and the results have been great. You are experiencing less back, leg, and foot pain. Maybe you have no pain at all. You're standing much better. You're walking much better and much farther than you have in a long time. Perhaps you're sleeping better, too. Now what? The answer: Positional Therapy.

Defining Positional Therapy

"Positional Therapy" is the term used to describe the transition from full-time walker use to the amount of use needed to maintain the improvement obtained with Positional Testing. In other words, this phase is only appropriate for those who have seen significant improvement of their symptoms through Positional Testing with the walker.

Remember: unless the patient sees good-to-excellent improvement within 3 days, there must be a re-evaluation of all the details included in the chapters on Positional Testing and its adjuncts—along, of course, with a consideration of the possibility of PseudoStenosis. If good compliance is not enough to bring about meaningful positive change, see Chapter 9, "What If Positional Testing Did Not Help?"

When seeing patients in my office, I guide the transition to Positional Therapy. In reality, however, the transition is largely controlled by the patient. While the Positional History and Positional Testing are both fairly consistent, Positional Therapy is *inconsistent* and tailored to the individual. I am not there with you, so I will do my best to help you with guidelines. Above all, common sense must prevail.

Five Factors Guiding Transition

1. What your original condition was
2. How much improvement you have experienced
3. How your body responds to reduced walker use
4. What your goals are
5. Whether or not you have PseudoStenosis

> *PseudoStenosis will be explained in Chapters 11 and 12. Even if you have great success with Positional Testing, it is important to consider PseudoStenosis, as controlling the cause increases the likelihood of maintaining the improvement obtained with Positional Testing without long-term use of a walker.*
>
> *The remainder of this chapter on Positional Therapy is directed to those who do not have PseudoStenosis, or those for whom treatment for PseudoStenosis has not provided adequate help, or those who, for any reason, are unable to treat the cause of PseudoStenosis.*

Positional Therapy can play itself out in various ways. Some people find that they can stop using the walker and all the Adjunct Measures and still remain symptom free. For others, as soon as they stop using the walker, the symptoms and walking limitation return. Many—perhaps the majority—fall somewhere in the middle, using the walker long term only for long walks, or if there is an occasional flare-up of symptoms. In this chapter I will not provide specific guidelines as I did elsewhere. Rather, I will describe concerns and present scenarios to help you use good judgment as you prepare for this phase.

There are some fortunate individuals who achieve total relief of all pain within a matter of days with Positional Testing and are quickly able to walk miles again with a walker. These are more likely to be younger people, people whose symptoms were not present over a long period of time, or those who are in overall better physical condition. In such individuals, there may not be any significant transition. Some simply stop using the walker, maintain their activity levels, and do not experience any recurrence at all!

More commonly, however, a Positional Therapy phase is necessary. This may be due to the fact that the affected anatomy is still present, capable of triggering symptoms when a certain threshold of activity level is reached. Positional Therapy may also be needed because of deconditioning (a reduction in strength or endurance), which requires a gradual increase in activity to allow for success in regaining one's former capabilities. If there has been a significant walking limitation for years, it is inevitable that a certain amount of deconditioning has occurred, weakening the muscles or the cardiovascular system. Strength must be recovered and rebuilt.

For this latter group, there is value in increasing activity levels *gradually*. A person who has not been able to walk more than half a block for years may be able to walk a few blocks after ten days, but not a few miles. I encourage patients to increase their walking gradually and to their tolerance. I repeat: I have had many patients who initially could not walk 1/2 a block, and who, in just a few months, built up their walking capacity until they could walk for two, three, or even four miles. I always encourage my patients to be patient and increase their activity gradually rather than all at once.

Three Qualifiers in Moving to Positional Therapy

1. The walker may not only help improve back or leg pain, endurance, and overall activity level, but it can also provide great balance support. **If you feel that your balance is at all a problem, then you should use either a walker or a cane.** Use of a cane has been shown to reduce the frequency of falls. Do not let pride get in the way. Using a cane when not relying on the walker can greatly reduce your chances of falling. Many falls occur at home. Make sure that all obstacles on the floor are removed. Check with your doctor to see if physical therapy or occupational therapy can be provided to help you with the challenges involved in **fall risks**!

It would be a tragedy if your painful symptoms were finally resolved and you were able to walk blocks or even miles again, only to end up falling and breaking a hip—all because you were reluctant to use a simple cane that could have prevented that fall. A broken hip can severely affect your life. Many people who undergo hip repair or replacement never return to their previous homes or activity level. How this would affect the people in your life is a story that you, and only you, can play out in your mind. **Please, do not go around without a walker or cane if you have balance problems!** Further information is in Chapter 23, on balance challenges.

Some patients who have eliminated all back and leg symptoms but still need a walker for balance, can raise the walker handle one or two inches. Of course, they need to watch out for a recurrence of SS/PS symptoms and should lower the walker handle height if spine-mediated symptoms return.

2. **If you are someone who has limited your walking to only a few minutes at a time over the last few years** because of discomfort in your feet, legs, or back, I'd like to reiterate the importance of raising your activity levels gradually. I have had a few patients who felt so good with the walker that they decided to go to the mall just a few days after receiving it. They tolerated hours in the mall but were in a great deal of pain afterward because of what my dear grandmother Goldie would have called "overdoing it."

It is essential to increase activity levels with moderation. For people who have previously been severely limited, I recommend taking advantage of short walks many times a day. If you live in an apartment building that has long corridors, start by walking them, to your tolerance level, once every hour. Little by little, increase the time you spend walking the halls. If you can traverse the length of a corridor one-and-a-half or two times, instead of walking for just a few minutes before you have to stop, you are making progress. By allowing progress to occur over a period of weeks, you are giving your muscles, bones, heart, and entire body a chance to improve at a pace they can sustain. This is especially important if you have been limited in your movement for a long period of time. Your body is eager to improve, but in order for the improvement to be safe, comfortable, and lasting, the process may need to be a slow one.

In contrast, if you have been limited to walking for only a few minutes at a time but were able to walk at the supermarket while pushing a shopping cart for a much longer period (half an hour or more), you will most likely be able to increase your activity levels much more quickly than a person who has not been routinely pushing a grocery cart. The reason is that pushing a cart while walking through the entire store constitutes a certain amount of exercise and has kept your muscles stronger than if you had not had that exercise. Therefore, though you initially expected to be able to walk only a few minutes at a time, you may find that you are able to walk many blocks within a few days, with a walker. The walker simply allows you to walk as well as you do when pushing a shopping cart.

3. **The question "How far can you walk without a walker?" is not quite as important as the question "How far can you walk *with* the walker?"** While a goal of Positional Therapy is to help individuals reduce or eliminate walker use, the walker may still be important for maintaining and even advancing your improvement. I would prefer that people continue using the walker part time for long walks of a few miles, rather than give up the walker and become reduced to walking only a few blocks at a stretch.

For this reason, it is of great value to monitor your walking capability. **Keep a walking diary,** and

compare how well you do with and without the walker. Perhaps, during the Positional Testing or Positional Therapy phase, you had built up to walking miles at a time with a walker, but when you stopped using the walker completely, you found that you could walk only a few blocks before the symptoms returned. If you keep track, you will recognize a pattern. You will then know that it is fine for you to go out and walk for a few blocks or for fifteen minutes without the walker, but that if you want to walk long distances (such as at a mall or art festival or with your grandchildren), you should take the walker along. Do not let pride get in the way of health and activity!

Even if you have total elimination of all symptoms when standing and when walking moderate distances after the 10 days of testing, you can still use the walker for long walks if you're trying to build up to long distances. For most people, how far they can walk is not something that can be answered after only 10 days. Many people whose mobility has been restricted for many years will have been subject to "deconditioning," the medical term indicating that the body's overall capacity for activity has been reduced. This may just be a fancy way of saying that they got out of shape, but it is nevertheless a real concern and needs to be respected and addressed. The way to address this is to increase your activity level gradually, with a realistic understanding of your starting condition and an equally realistic view of the ultimate goal.

Using the walker for long walks is often the needed key to walking well without pain, as well as to regaining physical strength. It may also be the key to fighting diabetes, fighting heart disease, keeping weight down, and staying fully engaged in life's opportunities.

StoryTime: Larry L was a 60-year-old gentleman who presented with difficulty standing and walking for many years. He could usually only walk a block or two before leg and back pain forced him to sit. As a result, he had become inactive and overweight.

Larry did full-time Positional Testing and had quick relief. He was soon walking two miles nonstop several times a week. After two weeks, he reduced walker use and only used it for long walks. He stayed much more active, lost a lot of weight, and reduced his use of the walker to only a few hours each week.

In his case, Positional Therapy involved using the walker whenever he took long walks, because taking long walks without the walker caused a recurrence of his symptoms. However, he is now frequently taking walks that he could not have conceived of taking for many years. A small price to pay for health.

Larry L's interview can be seen on our web set, WalkingWellAgain.com.

General Scenarios in Your Transition

I've drawn up several possible scenarios to help you understand the different possible paths ahead. You may find yourself described perfectly in one of them or you may fall somewhere between two of them, or you may be at the far end of either side of the spectrum. Please bear in mind that all of the scenarios assume that the patient has achieved good-to-excellent improvement with Positional Testing.

1. A patient who suffered pain and walking limitation for years uses a walker and builds up quickly to the point of walking longer distances without any negative symptoms. He stops using the walker, continues to be able to walk for miles, and has no recurrence. This individual does not need to use a walker unless there is either a recurrence of symptoms or an increased risk of falling.

2. A patient who suffered pain and walking limitation for years uses a walker and builds up slowly, because of years of deconditioning. Living in an apartment building and being unable to drive, the person has long stayed home, watching a lot of television. If the building has long indoor corridors, those are a great place to build up strength and stamina. One way to do so is taking a walk in the hallway every hour. The person should begin with a reasonable distance and time and should build up gradually. Over a span of weeks, what at first seemed like an accomplishment will likely become routine! Research strongly suggests that most seniors have the ability to regain strength and endurance if they increase their activity gradually. The hall, or any other available flat surface, can be a wonderful place to regain that strength!

3. A patient who for years suffered pain and walking limitation uses a walker and gets good improvement of discomfort, but still feels limited. After 10 days of full-time use, he may reduce using the walker in the house. After following his symptoms for the first couple of days, he should gradually increase unsupported walking time and keep track of the results. Once he is able to walk for 10 or 15 minutes in the home without the walker, it may be time to go outside without the walker for short walks, as long as there is no concern of increased fall risk. This person may need to continue using the walker for long walks in order to increase endurance and strength, even though short walks can be done without a walker or cane.

    IF you can take many short walks without the walker, use your judgment as to when to begin taking longer walks without it. Begin by doing so where there is a place to sit if you need to. Most shopping malls have many places to sit and rest, so those may be a good place to start.

    This may be a slow process, but be patient, and don't put yourself at risk for a setback by trying too long of a walk where there is no place to sit. Keep in mind as well that the Professor Position (Chapter 8) is there if you need it!

    You should periodically test your walking capability without the walker. If after some months you can cover miles with the walker and only blocks without it, continue to use the walker for long walks. It is important not to give up the effort to increase walking by putting away the walker if it truly is helpful. However, if walking-distance ability without a walker matches or nearly matches walking-distance ability with the walker, and your balance is fine, you may stop using it unless your symptoms return.

4. The following scenario is successful, but it may be disappointing. A patient who has done well with full-time walker use—that is, enjoys reduced pain and improved walking—experiences an immediate return of symptoms when walking without the walker. **This does happen in some people with more severe Spinal Stenosis or in those who have had back surgery.** It is possible that this person will

need to use a walker long term, or at least a majority of the time. *This could be a fairly clear picture.*

This is not a failure! Having someone who previously could only stand or walk for a few minutes before being disabled by pain and is finally able to walk blocks with a walker is a valued success and something to celebrate. Recall what I presented earlier in this chapter, that **how far you can walk without a walker is not as important as how far you can walk with it**! Increased mobility, exercise, and independence, coupled with less pain, is success! I hope you can appreciate the value of all of those changes.

HOWEVER, it is also possible that this person has PseudoStenosis and should be checked by an expert clinician.

In all of these scenarios (and the many that I did not detail), you will note that the patient is back in charge. During the Positional Testing phase, even if there is great and rapid improvement, I recommend good compliance for 10 days to reap the greatest benefit. I recommend that you use the walker the way I describe, even if you are already feeling better. In contrast, during the Positional Therapy phase, the patient is back at the helm. Listen to your body as you increase activity, and reduce your use of the walker accordingly. Just be sure to exercise your own good judgment.

What about the Adjunct Measures I've talked about? Do you still need to go down the stairs backward, use the pillow when you sleep, or stand in the Professor Position? Do you still require a stool in the shower and kitchen? **Don't ask me—ask yourself.** If the Adjunct Measures are comfortable and you'd like to continue using them, be my guest. If you feel you no longer need those measures, try living without them. The important thing is to **use your judgment**. Pay attention to symptoms and be ready to use common sense (which is not so very common, after all) to guide your actions.

Is It Better Forever?

There is a natural question that you may ask at this point: "Am I done with the walker forever? Will there be permanent improvement, or will there be a recurrence?" I must admit that I don't know. I often confess to my patients that while I may be the world expert on

this approach, I cannot predict the outcome for each individual patient. Even now, after fourteen years of use of the positional management approach, I cannot confidently predict who will be able to give up the walker completely and who will need to continue using it. I may have a reasonably good idea, but it's still only an educated guess.

I have had many patients who were able to stop using the walker for months and then had a flare-up. Maybe they lifted something the wrong way. Maybe they went to a mall and walked too long, for several hours instead of just one or two. Maybe they carried heavy packages while they were walking. For whatever reason, those old, familiar symptoms came back.

Don't worry. In almost all situations where a patient had a recurrence, a few days of full-time Positional Testing brought him back to where he wanted to be. The good news is that overcoming a flare-up that lasts for a couple of days usually takes far less time than overcoming a problem that has been in place for years.

The possibility of such flare-ups, with an occasional return of symptoms, is a reason why having a walker at home is important. Even if you are one of those fortunate people for whom there seems to be no residual need for a walker, it is possible that you will have a recurrence and will need the walker for just a couple of days to relieve your symptoms.

In my opinion, using a walker for just a few days is a pretty small price to pay to get relief. Consider your other options: You could take strong anti-inflammatory medication, which can have a negative effect on your stomach or blood pressure. You could take narcotic pain medications, which may cause constipation, breathing difficulty, and significant increase in risk for falls. Epidural injections carry a small risk of complication and often require an MRI, especially if it's been a couple of years since the prior spinal imaging. All of this risk, cost, and inconvenience can often be completely obviated simply by going back to the walker for a day or two and utilizing the Adjunct Measures. **Therefore, Positional Therapy includes the understanding that you may need to briefly go back to using the walker full time for a bit in the event of a recurrence of your old symptoms.**

Terminating use of the walker is a wonderful goal, but in my opinion it is far more important to get rid of the symptoms and to increase your walking distance as best as you can. I would much rather have you able to walk two or three miles at a stretch with a walker and without feeling pain afterward, than see you limited to walking only one, two, or three blocks without a walker. For many people, this means using the walker just a few times a week. Without the walker, these individuals would be far more limited.

Again, it is important that this transition be approached with common sense. Since I am not there to guide you, if you are not sure about how to proceed I hope you discuss the transition with someone you trust and who can understand the process.

The Value of a Second Walker

Please indulge me as I make this point with a personal story. My Aunt Laikee, who lives in Philadelphia, needed a walker, and she eventually reached the point where she could not walk without it. (She should live and be well; she is ninety years old, resides in an independent living facility, and is still fairly independent. Her body is aging, but her mind and judgment are both sharp as a tack.)

Knowing that many walkers eventually break with constant use, I bought her a second one. She resisted the idea, having a mindset from a generation that does not like waste or clutter. I insisted, and she allowed me to leave it in her apartment. No one mentioned it for a couple of years—until the first walker broke. She immediately went to Plan B and got out the preset walker waiting in her closet. She thanked me numerous times, knowing that even a day or two spent waiting for a new walker would have been a real hardship and would have held a risk of serious injury. At about one hundred dollars, it was a pretty inexpensive insurance policy.

If you do find that a walker provides great benefit, and especially if you need it for day-to-day functioning, please consider having a backup! You may find it an investment that repays itself many times over in terms of convenience and in terms of keeping those nasty symptoms permanently at bay.

Should You Use a Walker or Cane Long Term?

The final question of Positional Therapy is . . . . ..IS THERE A LONG-TERM NEED FOR A CANE OR WALKER? Here I must shift into a philosophical vein—albeit one with great practical implications.

How tragic it would be for someone who has lived with pain for years and has been limited by Spinal Stenosis to walking short distances, to finally have relief from the pain and regain ability to walk for blocks or miles again—only to fall and break a hip and lose everything gained. In that one fall, that person may lose the chance for an Indian summer, an opportunity to live actively and pain free in his or her senior years. Even more tragic—**in some instances the fall is caused not by poor balance but by pride**.

Refusing to use a walker or a cane when it is needed for stability because of poor balance is a bad, bad choice. Both walker and cane dramatically reduce the risk of falls for many people. If you are at risk for falls and you refrain from using the walker or cane, you put yourself at risk for tragedy.

If that fall happens and you lie helpless in bed, that disability will be made many times worse if it were coupled with the awareness that it might have been prevented by using the walker or cane. Your distress will be grievously compounded by the fact that, in cutting short your independence by an avoidable fall, you also ruined or disrupted the lives of those who love you. **If pride, ego, or vanity prevents you from using the support you really need, you are risking your future as well as the future of others in your life.**

There must be an honest evaluation regarding your risk for falling.

Of course, any instability could derive, wholly or in part, from the same problems that can cause PseudoStenosis, so you should be evaluated by a good podiatrist.

If after PseudoStenosis evaluation there is any question about your risk for falling, either in your own evaluation or in the opinion of those who know you well, I strongly recommend that you be referred to a physical therapist for balance training and for evaluation of your need for a walker or cane for long-term use. Your future and the happiness and future of your loved ones may depend upon your being honest with yourself regarding the need for a cane or a walker—and being strict with its use if it is determined that you do need it.

I'd choose quality of life over vanity any day. Wouldn't you?

CHAPTER 11

PseudoStenosis: Introduction and Overview

PseudoStenosis Introduced

In the next two chapters, I will introduce and explore an intriguing condition known as "PseudoStenosis." PseudoStenosis is a multifaceted syndrome that a great many suffering patients will be glad to learn about— and that clinicians also need to understand in order to provide their patients with the best possible diagnosis and treatment.

I am being literal in the use of the term *introduce*. PseudoStenosis is a concept I originally developed for my own use in 2008. I first presented it at the 2012 National Scientific Meeting of the American Podiatric Medical Association and later published it in an article in the *Journal of the American Podiatric Medical Association* in 2013. The importance and functionality of this categorization is a major impetus for this book.

This chapter explains the concept behind and the importance of PseudoStenosis. This material is valuable for patients and family members as background information, and, I believe, even more valuable for clinicians who want to evaluate and manage their patients' symptoms. This group of clinicians includes not only podiatrists, but also physical therapists, chiropractors, physiatrists, and neurologists, and especially spine surgeons. It should also be understood by internists, neurologists, rheumatologists, endocrinologists, geriatric specialists, general practitioners, nurse practitioners, and physician assistants, in order to enable them to encourage patients to seek help for their symptoms.

For anyone involved in the treatment of patients who may have Spinal Stenosis, these two chapters are as important as the one on Positional Testing.

Throughout much of this book, I refer to Spinal Stenosis/PseudoStenosis (SS/PS) as the potential unrecognized cause of symptoms. Often, the clinical presentation for both of these conditions is identical.

I believe that all patients with symptoms of Spinal Stenosis should be evaluated for PseudoStenosis as well. The reasons for this will, I hope, become clear to you by the end of these chapters.

PseudoStenosis can sometimes be treated by the patient alone, although he or she will often require professional help from a podiatrist or other clinician in order to experience long-term resolution. The important point to bear in mind is this: successful treatment of PseudoStenosis may eliminate both lower-back symptoms and symptoms in the lower extremities.

If suspected, PseudoStenosis is a condition that should be addressed aggressively, usually with mechanical, nonsurgical care. I call this care "Mechanical Testing," although it does at times include some non-mechanical care. As with Positional Testing for true Spinal Stenosis, I find that improvement occurs in just 1–3 days. Mechanical Testing, if successful, can almost always be usefully followed up with Mechanical Therapy, a permanent implementation of the changes temporarily brought about with Mechanical Testing.

PseudoStenosis Defined

The foot and leg symptoms of Spinal Stenosis occur because of spinal nerve compression. Stenosis, which means "narrowing," can exert pressure anywhere along the course of the nerves within the spinal canal. In Chapter 4, I review the different conditions that commonly cause stenosis.

"PseudoStenosis" is the term I chose to describe a condition in which the person has symptoms consistent with Spinal Stenosis, caused at least in part by anatomic changes or function in the lower extremities (and thus outside of the spine), which result in positional changes inside the spine.

Read that over. Anatomic or functional changes *outside* the spine result in positional changes *inside* the spine, which exert pressure or irritate nerves or local structures, causing stenosis symptoms. A person can have PseudoStenosis whether or not Spinal Stenosis is present.

Pressure from Within the Spine, Though the Cause Is Outside the Spine

Another way of explaining PseudoStenosis is to say that the spine or lower-extremity symptoms do not come from a primary spine problem, but are instead mediated through the spine.

To understand this concept, think about an electric carving knife, which moves back and forth on its own and can cut a roast on its own power with just a little pressure. For analogy's sake, assume that this is the effect of true, active Spinal Stenosis. By contrast, a regular carving knife placed with pressure on a roast does nothing unless there is a firm grip holding that knife and sawing it back and forth. In that situation, the energy comes from the hand and arm but is mediated through the knife. Similarly, in PseudoStenosis, the mechanical imbalance in the lower extremities causes the spine to malfunction in a way that puts pressure on the nerves; *that* causes the symptoms.

*Clinically, PseudoStenosis is a condition in which lower-extremity symptoms are brought on by irritation of the nerves, caused by narrowed structures putting pressure on those nerves, in which the body and spinal position induce that pressure, **and in which mechanical pathology in the lower extremities causes spinal structures to function in a narrowed manner.** This pathology may induce normal structures to cause compression as if they were anatomically narrowed, or it may exacerbate the effect of narrowed structures.*

Common causes of PseudoStenosis:

1. *Limb Length Discrepancy (LLDx)*
2. *A flexible Flat Foot, such as with Functional Hallux Limitus*
3. *A rigid or nearly rigid Flat Foot*
4. *Equinus, involving either a tight Achilles tendon in the back of the legs, or limited ankle joint movement for other reasons*
5. *An altered walking pattern caused by degenerative or other arthritis*
6. *An altered walking pattern caused by a stroke or other nerve or neuromuscular problem*
7. *An altered walking pattern caused by any lower-extremity pain great enough to make the patient walk differently*

With PseudoStenosis, the nerves in the back are irritated by physical means—pressure caused by spine structures. The only difference is that here, the spine pathology is affected by the foot and leg structures that cause the spine to function with a worsening of the narrowed areas. The symptoms are identical to those of Spinal Stenosis, because the mechanism—nerve compression aggravated by standing or walking (or sleep position)—is the same. Frequently, the MRI of the spine, even with axial loading, is negative, suggesting that the spine is not the culprit. And yet it *is* the culprit, or at least the mechanism for pain. The spine is the vehicle through which the pain is mediated, even if it is not the primary cause. Thus, many people that have back, foot, or leg pain deriving from spinal nerve compression actually experience these symptoms because of a spine imbalance caused by dysfunction in the lower extremities.

Spinal Stenosis and PseudoStenosis May Coexist

There are three possibilities that may be clinically present. A patient may have Spinal Stenosis, Pseudo-Stenosis, or both. It is by far the worst to have both: a potential clinical and personal disaster.

It is essential to grasp this concept, because it interferes with the usual way of understanding and testing symptoms. Suppose a person experiences symptoms (e.g., leg aches, burning, or tiredness) that are aggravated by walking and even standing, such as one would expect with Spinal Stenosis. An MRI is duly taken and indeed indicates the presence of Spinal Stenosis. One might then logically diagnose Spinal Stenosis as the cause of the patient's symptoms. An epidural injection might temporarily eliminate the symptoms by eliminating the inflammation of the nerves in the back. This outcome could be seen as confirmation of the Spinal Stenosis diagnosis. Periodic injections or even surgery would then seem justified to treat the symptoms. This is, I believe, the current standard of care.

However, if the symptoms are being mediated through the spine—meaning that nerves have been inflamed through mechanical pressure and irritation but are actually caused by lower-extremity problems that cause a spinal imbalance—**it is possible to achieve the same good, temporary results with injections.** In this case, there is actually nerve inflammation caused by pressure, which would improve with injections. If the spine dysfunction is caused or aggravated by lower-extremity dysfunction, though, the results of injections or even surgery would be temporary or incomplete. Even with aggressive and well-done surgery, in which one or more levels of the spine are fused, if a mechanical imbalance of the lower extremities persists, that imbalance could soon cause problems on a different level.

I strongly believe that failure to recognize this may result in the clinician providing medications, therapies, injections, and surgeries that are often doomed to failure or at least limited success, no matter how skillfully done. Failure to recognize PseudoStenosis is the reason that many Spinal Stenosis treatments fail.

This is essential. All clinicians treating either the back or the lower extremities should consider that there are three possibilities that may be clinically present. A patient may have Spinal Stenosis, PseudoStenosis, or both. It is much worse to have both, which makes for a clinical conundrum and often a personal disaster.

Even if existing Spinal Stenosis is treated with great skill and dedication and with the best of intentions, the PseudoStenosis factor may stand in the way of long-term success. I have unfortunately seen many patients who had undergone multiple spine surgeries and still suffered from persistent symptoms before having PseudoStenosis treated. Although, thankfully, many of these patients responded well to mechanical treatment of the feet and legs, they lost years of their lives to painful and ultimately unsuccessful spine management. Some, unfortunately, had severe arthritis or post-operative scarring involving the nerves, and they did not improve even when the PseudoStenosis cause was addressed. It is quite appropriate to treat PseudoStenosis even after failed spine surgery, but it is certainly better to treat it beforehand!

> *The 2011 guidelines of the American College of Physicians do not recommend spinal imaging for a diagnosis of Spinal Stenosis unless conservative care has failed and invasive treatment is considered, or unless there is clinically valid and significant doubt as to the diagnosis. A diagnosis of Spinal Stenosis may be made presumptively without spinal imaging.*
>
> *Similarly, a diagnosis of PseudoStenosis does not require a negative MRI. This diagnosis involves identification of symptoms (and perhaps physical signs) consistent with Spinal Stenosis, as well as identification of a lower-extremity problem that may cause PseudoStenosis—which is confirmed by relief of Spinal Stenosis symptoms through Mechanical Testing (the treatment of the lower-extremity pathology).*

StoryTime: Golether P was a middle-aged woman who came into my office early one morning with a chief complaint of severe back pain and leg pain, and burning pain in her feet. The symptoms had been present for about 9 months and were worsening. She reported an inability to walk or stand for more than a few minutes before the pain forced her to sit down. She had pain in her feet and legs at night in bed. A diabetic, she had been diagnosed with Diabetic Neuropathy as well as arthritis, both aggravated by obesity. My examination showed signs of PseudoStenosis, including a Limb Length Discrepancy and Flat Feet. We treated her with Mechanical Testing, as explained in Chapter 12. She was seen the following day and reported walking for a half hour the previous night with no pain, sleeping with no pain, and having only mild (20%) residual pain in the morning. She could stand and walk pain free.

This improvement occurred in just 1 day, with no medication.

Golether P's interviews on her first visit and on the following day are available at the website Walking WellAgain.com. Hear her story in her own words.

It is essential to understand that just as Spinal Stenosis symptoms usually improve within 1–3 days of Positional Testing, so too, do PseudoStenosis symptoms improve within 1–3 days of whatever management is needed for the lower-extremity cause.

The Risk of Having Both Spinal Stenosis and PseudoStenosis

I must emphasize as strongly as possible that PseudoStenosis can be a major factor in the pain process even when the person has actual Spinal Stenosis. To help you understand this, I will use a **"reverse example"** and then come back to PseudoStenosis. Please be patient.

Many people with foot, leg, or knee pathology suffer considerable added pain because they also have SS/PS. In other words, their bunion, Flat Foot, or knee arthritis hurts far more than would be expected from the pathology present. When I suspect this, I sometimes treat with Positional Testing, using the walker and Adjunct Measures described in Chapter 8. If Spinal Stenosis (or PseudoStenosis) is contributing to the symptoms, the pain may be dramatically reduced in a matter of a day or two. I have had patients with severe discomfort come in seeking foot surgery for quick relief—and after a few days with a walker for Positional Testing, declare in astonishment that they had no significant pain left at all.

Does that mean that there was no bunion, or no Flat Foot, or no arthritis? Of course not. It just means that the symptoms were much worse because of the hypersensitivity of the nerves in the back. This is actually a very common phenomenon.

StoryTime: A patient came in for surgical correction of a severely painful corn on a hammertoe. Normally, trimming a corn can provide weeks or even months of relief, but trimming this corn provided relief for only a few days. Suspecting Spinal Stenosis, I ordered an MRI that confirmed my suspicion. He received an epidural injection, and in addition to relief of pain previously attributed to neuropathy, he had relief of pain from the corn. He never had recurrence of severe pain. The corn was there; it just did not hurt very much! Surgery for the painful corn was never needed. (This occurred, I believe, in 1991, long before I ever thought of using Positional Testing for Spinal Stenosis.)

Using my "reverse example" above, if a patient comes in with a mild or moderate bunion that hurts a lot and interferes with his or her ability to wear shoes, and is given an injection that provides good but only temporary relief, the logical step might be to fix that bunion surgically. However, if an SS/PS component is suspected and treated successfully, the bunion, which has not been treated directly, may have relief of sensitivity, so that surgical treatment may not be indicated. However, successful treatment of SS/PS may also convert this from a painful bunion to a non-painful bunion, indicating that the obvious or most likely cause of pain was not the only or primary cause of pain.

Similarly, if a person comes in with classic symptoms of Spinal Stenosis that have had only moderate or temporary help with the classic treatment of therapy, medication, and epidural injections, the managing clinician not only should, but in my opinion *must*, investigate and treat for PseudoStenosis. If successful, the clinician will have converted a person with what seems to be painful Spinal Stenosis to a person who still has Spinal Stenosis—that is not causing pain.

It is essential to remember that PseudoStenosis in the presence of Spinal Stenosis is not an oxymoron. Many people have both Spinal Stenosis and PseudoStenosis. This is a very important phenomenon.

Clinician, if you treat symptomatic Spinal Stenosis with epidural injections while the lower-extremity cause of the imbalance is still present, the improvement will more likely be short-lived. For example, if you eliminated all inflammation of the spinal area and the patient walked around with only one shoe for a few days (the most obvious way to mimic a PseudoStenosis cause), what do you think would happen? The inflammation and symptoms would quite likely return. If the lower-extremity problem is not taken into consideration, you would reasonably conclude that the spine is the primary culprit, because the improvement was no more than temporary. Then you would probably decide that surgical treatment of the spine is a reasonable approach.

> *In individuals with PseudoStenosis, treatment of either the lower-extremity problem or the stenosis-induced symptoms with Positional Testing can provide a temporary, successful resolution of pain. Thus, the eventual road to long-term treatment may be guided by the path that is taken. **This is essential and life changing.***

SS and PS: A Potential Disaster!

Oftentimes, spine surgeries fail. Many people first undergo a laminectomy (decompression), a procedure that opens up the spine by removing bone and thick, soft tissue. After affording the patient some temporary relief, it eventually fails, and the person goes on to have a spinal fusion. Some patients have fusion on one or more levels of the spine but still experience a recurrence of painful symptoms and limitations. This is something that might be expected if they walked around with only one shoe after surgery. The lower-extremity structure affecting the back function is, in my opinion, a common contributing factor to failed spinal surgery and other treatment. I believe it is also frequently the cause of surgery being necessary in the first place! If the lower-extremity mechanical problems would be addressed, a great many patients with Low-Back Syndrome would be absolutely fine. They would not need any back treatment at all, let alone surgery.

I want to make my position absolutely clear. Even if there are Spinal Stenosis changes present on the MRI, the causes of PseudoStenosis must be evaluated for any patient with Spinal Stenosis symptoms. **Failure to**

address the lower-extremity problems may doom the spine treatment to failure.

This paragraph may be the most controversial of this book. I believe that any clinician treating the feet and legs must *always* be aware of the possible effect of spinal nerve compression on lower-extremity symptoms. I also believe, just as firmly, that any clinician treating the spine (especially spine surgeons!) should *always* keep in mind the possible effect of lower-extremity biomechanics on spine pathology.

Doing so might prevent a great many surgical failures; equally important—a great many surgeries could be prevented in the first place. Having tunnel vision—treating one part of the body without considering the whole anatomic system involved—is an all-too-common phenomenon, one that may be exacerbated in the training of specialists. I hope this book will play a small role in reducing this particular problem.

> *A final reminder: The classification of PseudoStenosis, which I find to be so essential in managing patients with lower-extremity symptoms that could be consistent with Spinal Stenosis, is original on my part and not found elsewhere in the literature. Keep in mind that this is not part of standard medical practice, nor has it been supported by broad medical research.*

This chapter has introduced and explained the concept of PseudoStenosis, and has outlined the reason that understanding it is of paramount importance for those treating both the lower extremities and the spine. The next chapter will address individual causes of PseudoStenosis, practical means of deciding whether it may be present and is affecting the overall symptoms, and treatment methods.

For the Clinician and the Very Curious: About the Name "PseudoStenosis"

As I chose the term "PseudoStenosis," I was aware of the prior use of the name for another condition in which non-stenosis conditions in the spine cause similar symptoms. When preparing to publish an article, I consulted Dr. Charles Hennekens, the author of Epidemiology in Medicine, a text on medical research. He is the internationally lauded researcher who discovered the major role of aspirin in heart disease, and he is identified as the third-most quoted author in medical research in the world. I was greatly privileged to coauthor an article on Spinal Stenosis with him in 2008. He advised me to use the term "PseudoStenosis" but to explain how my use differs from the one in the prior article published thirty years earlier, which I did. I will now add three clarifications.

1. *My version of PseudoStenosis could be called "PseudoStenosis LEI," standing for "Lower-Extremity Induced."*

2. *Another way of classifying Spinal Stenosis could be dividing it into three categories: Primary SS, in which the symptoms are caused by actual stenosis in the spine; Secondary SS, in which lower-extremity dysfunction induces spine dysfunction and symptoms—i.e., PseudoStenosis; and Tertiary SS, in which both structural Spinal Stenosis and PseudoStenosis are present.*

3. *Because the spine pathology that was reported in the 1983 pseudostenosis article (Postacchini F. "Lumbar spinal stenosis and pseudostenosis." Italian Journal of Orthopedics and Traumatology) does not generally give rise to stenosis symptoms, I believe it is possible that the premise of that article was mistaken. Perhaps symptoms were induced by the lower-extremity dysfunction as I've presented in this chapter, and the unusual findings in the spine were incidental or only partially responsible for the symptoms. It is my goal that lower-extremity causes as factors in Spinal Stenosis symptoms become routinely considered, and that was certainly not the case back then.*

CHAPTER 12

PseudoStenosis: Practical Evaluation and Management

Since this chapter is so extensive, I have divided it into 7 sections, 12 A-G. I hope the divisions help make the material in this long chapter less overwhelming.

Diving into Details of PseudoStenosis

Some people read every book from cover to cover. To skim, skip, or otherwise give less than their full attention to every printed word is unthinkable.

And then there are those who tend to focus on the sections that apply to their own particular situation and gloss over the rest. Or those who choose to leapfrog over a chapter here and there in the interest of getting to the end more quickly. For those who decided to give the previous chapter a miss, here is a brief overview of the phenomenon that I have dubbed "PseudoStenosis."

"PseudoStenosis" refers to a clinical presentation in which symptoms of Spinal Stenosis, either in the spine or in the lower extremities, occur because biomechanical dysfunction in the lower extremities induces spinal dysfunction. Spinal Stenosis may or may not also be present. Lower-extremity symptoms and nerve sensitivity are **mediated** through the spine, even if they are not caused by spine pathology. This confusion of symptoms is, in my opinion, a common reason for the lack of long-term success with standard treatment commonly used in treating Spinal Stenosis.

Treatment of the lower extremities, usually begun with what I label "Mechanical Testing," may eliminate the symptoms of Spinal Stenosis. As is the case with Positional Testing, the effectiveness of Mechanical Testing usually becomes apparent within just 1–3 days.

I suspect that the causes of PseudoStenosis are often the causes of actual Spinal Stenosis, but I do not have data to back that up. For further details about the nature of PseudoStenosis, please see the preceding chapter. The present chapter deals with suspecting and identifying the problem and describing possible treatment approaches for each cause.

The Seven Common Causes of PseudoStenosis

Some of the common causes of PseudoStenosis are listed in the box below.

1. *Limb Length Discrepancy (LLDx)*
2. *A flexible Flat Foot, such as with Functional Hallux Limitus*
3. *A rigid or nearly rigid Flat Foot*
4. *Equinus, involving a tight Achilles tendon in the back of the legs or limited ankle joint movement for other reasons*
5. *An altered walking pattern caused by degenerative or other arthritis*
6. *An altered walking pattern caused by a stroke or other nerve or neuromuscular problem*
7. *An altered walking pattern caused by any lower-extremity pain great enough to make the patient walk differently*

For Patients and Their Families: A Brief Guide

Sections on each of the common causes of PseudoStenosis are generally divided into three basic parts: **recognition** of the presence of a condition (such as Limb Length Discrepancy), **investigation** as to whether it may be causing PseudoStenosis issues, followed by **treatment** of the problem. If the proper treatment is given for the true problem or problems, we can expect quick improvement of PseudoStenosis and the many symptoms it may cause. How quick? Just as with Positional Testing for Spinal Stenosis, only 1–3 days.

A lot of information is included to make the condition clear, and to share with clinicians my perspective on evaluation and treatment. This is thus a complicated chapter. **If the reading becomes tedious, you may certainly skim the sections, find the cause of Pseudo-Stenosis that may contribute to your problems, and proceed to the guidance on treatment.**

If you know you have a Limb Length Discrepancy, you may choose to just address that as guided and see if treatment helps. If you know you have Flat Feet, you may read the section on that condition and seek to understand evaluation and treatment. The same is true for all of the other conditions. **However, with ALL conditions, you must consider the possible presence and role of Limb Length Discrepancy, because it is such a common problem and because it can affect all others.**

Patients and family primarily need to take two main points from this chapter:

- An awareness that any of these conditions can cause PseudoStenosis and thus any symptom that might present as Spinal Stenosis, affecting any of the conditions presented in Section 3 of this book.

- Direction about how to consider these conditions, and about how to seek treatment for the pathology that might be having such an effect on quality of life.

Limb Length Discrepancy (LLDx): Suspect it and Detect it

The most common cause of PseudoStenosis is Limb Length Discrepancy. This condition is something that, when present, can often be quickly and safely treated at home. It is common to see wonderful results in a matter of a day or two. I will therefore go into great detail to help you recognize and understand this common condition, and I will hope that the information does not overwhelm you. There will not be a test afterward! Just read this section and extract the information that may apply to your situation.

"Limb Length Discrepancy" refers to a situation in which one leg is longer that the other. The discrepancy may be structural (where one leg is actually longer than the other) or functional (where, because of a problem higher up—primarily in the pelvis or low back—one leg functions *as though* it were shorter than the other, even though the actual length is the same). It may also be **combined**, meaning that both factors, structural and functional, are present.

How Common Is Limb Length Discrepancy, and How Much Discrepancy Is Important?

One oft-quoted study* reported that 32% of 600 military recruits had a 1/5- to 3/5-inch (5–15 millimeters) difference between the lengths of their legs. In that there was no perceived correlation comparing low-back pain in those with and without that much LLDx, the study presented that this discrepancy is a variation of normal that is not clinically significant.

I strongly disagree with this conclusion, for multiple reasons, two of which I share. *First, I observe that even mild LLDx of 2 or 3 millimeters can have a profound effect on symptoms. Second, these were healthy young men whose bodies were strong enough to compensate for the differences, and who had not yet experienced the wear and tear of life. They were men who did not yet have arthritis or spine problems in addition to the Limb Length Discrepancy. The imbalance that was present had not known the cumulative destructive effect of millions of steps taken over a lifetime of walking and working.*

*Thirty-three years of practical experience with senior citizens tells me otherwise. My practice has had so many patients who appeared to have small **1/4-inch, 1/8-inch, or even 1/16-inch discrepancies**, who were treated with lifts and had excellent relief of symptoms. Not just symptoms that had been bothering them for days or weeks, but symptoms that had been present for years. Follow-up months or even years later showed a maintained improvement, with no other intervention.*

Therefore, I believe with all my heart that even small Limb Length Discrepancies should be addressed if there are any symptoms, often before any other treatment is tried. *There is nothing quicker, cheaper, or safer. And it is often the last treatment that you will ever need.*

Who is right? Those who suggest that the discrepancy must be over 3/8 (or even 3/5) of an inch to be a problem, or those who say that smaller differences can have a big effect? I report to you that I have had success with hundreds of patients with just a small lift that relieved long-term symptoms in a day or two, so you know how I vote. What is important in this situation, however, is YOUR SYMPTOMS. If this is a suspected cause of problems, treat even for small differences, and see how you do. The proof is in the pudding!

*Hellsing, A. L. 1988. "Leg length inequality: A prospective study of young men during their military service." Upsala Journal of Medical Sciences 93 (3): 245–253.

A Limb Length Discrepancy may have been present since youth, or it may have developed later. It may be the result of an injury, a surgery such as fracture repair or knee or hip replacement, or an auto accident. It may come from a stroke or an ankle injury causing arthritis and limitation of motion. There are many potential causes, but the result is the same: the person is walking and standing differently enough to cause a change in spine function, which may result in spinal nerve compression and the accompanying symptoms. Even subtle changes may bring on symptoms.

An important point to note, especially in dealing with senior citizens, is that a long-term LLDx may not have caused symptoms throughout the earlier years but can cause symptoms later in life.

For those people who think that a subtle difference of 1/8 or even 3/16 of an inch can't make a difference in a person's gait, I suggest that you walk around for a few minutes with two different shoes on, one a little thicker than the other. Or just fold up a few napkins and put them under the heel of the removable insert of a sneaker. Within minutes, you will most likely be aware that "something" is wrong. That is what people live with when they have a Limb Length Discrepancy. While some individuals, especially if young and strong, subconsciously adjust to the difference and experience no symptoms, for many others the condition is very unpleasant, or worse. **Their symptoms may be severe enough to cause disability, including back pain, leg or foot pain, or symptoms identical to Spinal Stenosis, which may in turn interfere with standing, walking, sleeping, sitting, working, and overall quality of life.** The situation is often aggravated by the fact that even a small Limb Length Discrepancy can lead to significant arthritic changes in many parts of the body.

An environmental Limb Length Discrepancy may occur when someone walks extensively on the side of a road or where the walking surface is uneven. Other causes include wearing two different types of shoes, walking with a cast or removable cast that is higher than the shoe, or even wearing down one shoe more than the other while using a cast or crutches, and then using the now uneven pair of shoes when restored to normal footwear. Once aware of these possible causes, an alert person may solve the problem himself.

Environmental Limb Length Discrepancy may also occur when a person or the clinician tries to solve one problem but causes another. The patient may wear an in-shoe ankle brace to treat foot or ankle arthritis, and that brace may be thicker than the insert in the other shoe. I have had a few patients who removed the insert from their shoe to make room for a bunion or hammertoe, but only did it on one side. In those cases, efforts unwittingly created an environmental Limb Length Discrepancy.

Tragically, I have had several patients for whom this condition was the unrecognized cause of symptoms that forced them to go out on disability. Years of inability to support themselves and their families, of living on disability or welfare—all because of a minor difference in leg length that **caused *or prevented resolution* of a major set of symptoms.** The tiny difference had an impact that changed their very lives. "For want of a nail, a shoe was lost; for want of a shoe, a horse was lost; for want of a horse, a message was lost; for want of a message, a battle was lost; for want of a battle, a kingdom was lost."

*The message here is that a seemingly inconsequential, "MINOR" Limb Length Discrepancy can change a life. The severity of symptoms and the amount of damage caused is not necessarily related to the amount of discrepancy. Even a small difference can have profound effect. **"Mild" does not mean "Minor".***

Never underestimate the effect that a Limb Length Discrepancy can have on the body.

Clues Suggesting LLDx That You May Already Know

How can you know (or strongly suspect) that you have a Limb Length Discrepancy? There are several clues, which you may already be aware of:

1. If your feet need two different shoe sizes, or if one shoe usually fits more tightly than the other

2. If your two feet, ankles, or knees are physically different from each other

3. If you need to have your pant legs modified by a tailor to get a good fit, or if one pant leg frequently becomes more frayed than the other

4. If you know—or at least recognize, now that the question has been raised—that you frequently shift from side to side when standing (or if you find that standing is harder than walking)

5. If you have an abnormal walking pattern or if the wear pattern is different on your two shoes

Clues Found in Patterns in Standing and Walking

Before examining for physical signs suggesting LLDx, we should focus on clues in standing and walking. **Often, a person with a Limb Length Discrepancy shifts from side to side when standing, either consciously or unconsciously.** When I ask them about this, they frequently acknowledge it to be true, although sometimes they have to think for a minute before answering. **People with Limb Length Discrepancy often find it difficult to stand.** Some have to "shake a leg" periodically, trying to shake symptoms out of their leg. **For many, it is harder to stand than to walk. They often, especially in later years, report balance problems.** These patterns usually improve IMMEDIATELY with the proper treatment.

Individuals with LLDx also sometimes have a "funny" walk. Sometimes they have difficulty walking in a straight line. There may be **vaulting,** where the body is higher when lifted by one leg than when by the other. The arm swing may be uneven. There may be tilting of the head. They may walk and stand with one foot turning out more than the other, or with one knee slightly bent. They may commonly place one or even both hands on a hip when standing, or frequently seek to lean against a counter or even a wall. All of these patterns may be found with LLDx.

Physical Signs and Examination for LLDx

Using a direct examination to check for LLDx is sometimes, though not always, a straightforward matter. Findings are more apparent if the discrepancy is large, say, over 3/16 of an inch, about 5 millimeters. You may require help from a friend, or you might need a podiatrist or other clinician. But you can begin the process yourself. The first thing to decide is if you want to examine from the top down or from the bottom up.

Examining from the Head Down

If you are examining from the head down, you will need a tall mirror. Stand in front of it, and see if your shoulders are the same height. You may have looked at yourself in a mirror thousands of times and never checked for or noticed that difference. Notice it now. If there is a discrepancy in the two shoulder heights, you most likely have a Limb Length Discrepancy, scoliosis, or both. **In fact, it is clear that Limb Length Discrepancy can *cause* scoliosis.** The two often go hand in hand. If you are not sure, ask someone else to check you, either from the front or from behind.

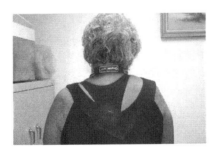

Picture 12.1. Difference in shoulder height from behind, and tilting of the head, suggesting LLDx, scoliosis, or both.

Note: This is a clue suggesting the need to evaluate. The longer leg may be on the side of either the lower or the higher shoulder.

Secondary Scoliosis

If the shoulder is higher on the side of the hip that is lower, it suggests a secondary scoliosis caused by a Limb Length Discrepancy. I have at times seen the following situation: the higher shoulder was caused by secondary scoliosis, but the higher shoulder becomes lower and even with the other shoulder when I put the

lift in the shorter side. Reread that, and consider this example. The left leg is longer. The left hip is higher. The left shoulder is lower. The left shoulder may immediately become the same height as the right shoulder after an appropriate lift is placed in the right shoe. **This is a flexible scoliosis caused by Limb Length Discrepancy that straightens out after the cause is corrected.**

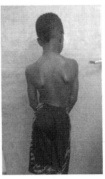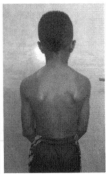

Picture 12.2.

Initially, the left hip was much higher and the left shoulder lower in this young man with scoliosis shown in Picture 12.2. After compensation for Limb Length Discrepancy, improvement in spine position was immediately noted.

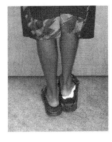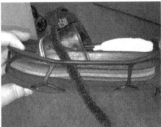

Picture 12.3. Building up his shorter leg by using an Evenup, spacers, and felt added to the heel of his sandal immediately allowed this patient to stand and walk with better balance, and to produce the changes seen in picture 12.2 above.

The person pictured in picture 12.2 and 12.3 has an extreme example of a *secondary scoliosis* that can be caused by a Limb Length Discrepancy, with the curve developing to keep the head as vertical as possible, not leaning toward the shorter leg. In contrast to a fixed (rigid) scoliosis, a flexible scoliosis can often be corrected quickly by compensating for the Limb Length Discrepancy. Once the need to compensate in order to try to keep the head and upper torso straight is gone, the individual may no longer curve the spine.

Head Tilt and Neck or Shoulder Pain

I have seen patients with Limb Length Discrepancy who consistently or frequently stood with the head tilted a little to the side, whose head and shoulders evened out as soon as the proper lift was put in. When this intervention works, it is so obvious and often so rapid as to be unbelievable. **I have also had dozens of people report improved neck pain and often shoulder pain when the Limb Length Discrepancy was addressed.** Not enough to be confident about certain success, but I thought I would mention it.

Sometimes one can suspect LLDx if clothing or even a belt consistently sits unevenly on an individual in the hip area. This may be made easier to detect if the person wears a shirt with stripes!

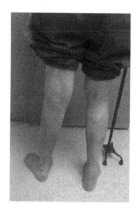

Picture 12.5. The longer foot turns out to the side, away from the midportion of the body. The longer leg has a foot that is flatter and a knee that bends in more, an increased "Q-angle" (the angle between the thigh bone and the tibia). The knee on the shorter side is straight.

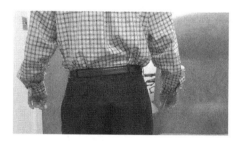

Picture 12.4. The angle of the belt appears higher on the right side, the side of the longer leg and higher hip.

Checking the Knees

If you are checking the lower extremities, there are a couple of clues in the knees and a great many in the feet that suggest a Limb Length Discrepancy.

There are specific patterns of the knees that suggest LLDx. First, the knee of the longer leg may, especially in a long-standing LLDx, develop arthritic changes, which cause the knee to bend inwards. One knee—on the shorter limb—is straight when you check from in front or from behind, but the other knee has an inward angle that is seen with arthritis.

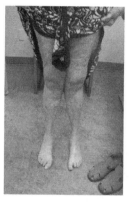

Picture 12.6. One or both knees has an increased Q angle when the knees are together or near together and the feet are not close together.

Another sign of an LLDx is the asymmetric sensitive Pes Anserinus, and was presented in Chapter 6. The Pes Anserinus is a spot just below the inside of the knee that is actually the combined tendon of three thigh muscles, where they insert into the bone. Sensitivity in this area is quite often seen only in the longer leg of a patient with a Limb Length Discrepancy, though it could also be caused by local pathology such as a tendonitis or bursitis. Sensitivity in this area may be present in both legs if there is Flat Foot pathology or actual arthritis of the knees. The patient may not be aware of this being a sensitive area unless someone pushes on it, as the knee area may be painless. The sensitivity usually disappears quickly with appropriate mechanical control, often just a heel lift for the short leg or perhaps a heel lift combined with strapping in the presence of Flat Feet. If the area stays sensitive, I take that to mean that the mechanical stress in this area has not been compensated for. This area of sensitivity is not always present, but when it is, it makes an impression. It is an easy finding to both identify and follow, for both clinician and patient.

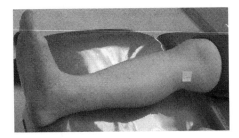

Picture 12.7 Location of insertion of Pes Anserinus-

Another pattern is a deformity called "Genu Recurvatum," in which the knee curves backwards when the person is standing with the knee fully extended. Not a common condition, I find that it is more common in a shorter leg, more frequently if the discrepancy is about 5 mm or more.

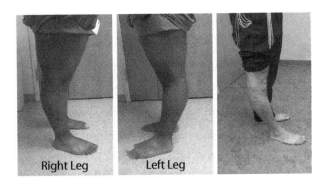

Right Leg   Left Leg

Picture 12.8. Genu Recurvatum.

One may also compare the knees' positions when the patient is lying down. If the knees are bent and the feet are placed parallel, both knees should be equally elevated. If they are not, this suggests the presence of a discrepancy. This will not be visible if the discrepancy is small.

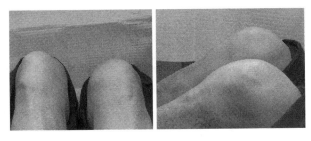

Picture 12.9. From the front and from the side, it is apparent that the knees are at different heights.

Checking the Feet

Frequently, someone paying close attention from behind can see a difference in the legs of a person with LLDx even when the person is standing or walking in shoes. One shoe, usually the shoe of the foot of the longer leg if there is a structural Limb Length Discrepancy, is turned (angled) farther away from the center of the body.

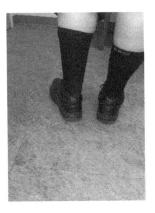

Picture 12.10. When walking or standing, one shoe, *usually* that of the foot of the longer leg if there is a structural Length Discrepancy,may be turned farther away from the center of the body.

If you are looking at the feet with the shoes off, there are some clues you can see yourself, but for others you will need the help of an observant friend. Let us start off with what is often for me the first clue, a difference in the feet when in a sitting position. To check this, you must be sitting up in a straight position and not leaning. Your back must be flat against the back of a chair with your legs extended straight forward. Your helper should look at the bottom of the heels and see if one is higher than the other. You will need to check several times, shifting against the back of the chair to make sure. If there's a difference, there's most likely LLDx—either functional or structural.

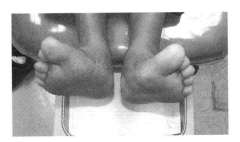

Picture 12.11. Heel difference in position.

Do not overreact to this appearance. This imbalance may reflect a structural or functional Limb Length Discrepancy, or it may just be the way the person is sitting! One must measure, which I do indirectly as will be described below, before concluding if there is a discrepancy—and before concluding how big the discrepancy is and which leg is longer! These are clues, but please be patient!

Foot Asymmetry

A valuable sign suggesting Limb Length Discrepancy is an asymmetry between the feet. Though LLDx is not the *only* cause, such asymmetry is most common in patients with LLDx, especially one that is of long duration. Common but not universal findings follow. **Less frequently, the opposite is true, and a shorter leg will have a flatter foot or worse bunion or it will turn out more. That atypical presentation is sometimes seen with a functional, rather than structural, LLDx, or when there are other structural problems in addition to LLDx.** The following patterns are far more common.

> *These changes are most commonly seen with a* **structural Limb Length Discrepancy. If, however, there is a chronic functional Limb Length Discrepancy caused by a primary problem in the pelvic area or lower spine, the shorter leg may turn out, and its foot may be flatter and have a greater bunion and more pronation problems.**
>
> *Much less commonly, these changes may also occur if there is a structural orthopedic deformity of the hip or knee, which may be either present from birth or caused by an injury, even if there is no LLDx.*
>
> *If you have a question about this, get evaluated by a professional, and consider seeking radiologic evaluation, as discussed both below and in Chapter 14.*

In addition to these signs, a Limb Length Discrepancy can also cause a variety of arthritic problems in the back, hips, knees, ankles, and feet. For further information, please see Chapter 19.

> *Longer leg may have some or all of the following symptoms:*
>
> 1. *A more Flat Foot that may become arthritic and develop tendon problems*
> 2. *A foot that turns out to the side (away from the body) more when standing*
> 3. *A larger bunion*
> 4. *A callus in the center of the ball of the foot*
> 5. *Hammertoes*
> 6. *Swelling along the inside of the ankle if there is tendonitis*
> 7. *Greater nerve sensitivity, even if the discrepancy is only 1/16 of an inch (See section on the First Interspace Fine Sign in Chapter 6.)*
> 8. *An increased "Q-angle" of the knee with soft tissue swelling, involving tendonitis and bursitis*
> 9. *Increased sensitivity of the Pes Anserinus, just below the inside of the knee.*
> 10. *Increased arthritis of the knee*
> 11. *Arthritis of the hip (although more common on the short leg)*

> *Shorter leg may have some or all of the following symptoms:*
>
> 1. *A less Flat Foot (although it may still be flat)*
> 2. *A foot that is likely to be straighter when the person stands or walks*
> 3. *A callus or pain on the ball of the foot, behind the baby toe (at the fifth metatarsal base)*
> 4. *Hammertoes and, occasionally, dislocated second or third metatarsal phalangeal joints*
> 5. *Greater tightness of the Achilles tendon (as will be explained in detail)*
> 6. *Limited motion or altered position of the knee or hip, or Genu Recurvatum (backward curve) of the knee (if the leg is shorter by more than about 1/4 of an inch)*
> 7. *Greater nerve sensitivity, if the leg is over 1/4 of an inch shorter (See section on the First Interspace Fine Sign in Chapter 6.)*
> 8. *Greater wearing-out of the outside of the heel of the shoe on the short side*
> 9. *Increased arthritis of the knee, but without the large medial bulge of the increased "Q-angle"*
> 10. *Arthritis of the hip (although not uncommon in the long leg)*

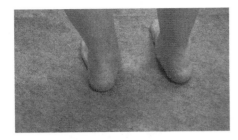

Picture 12.12. Feet are different: foot arch appearance may be very different or only slightly different. This may be noticed both when standing and when sitting.

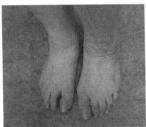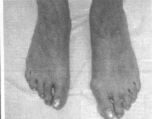

Picture 12.13. Asymmetric Bunions.

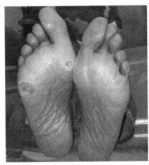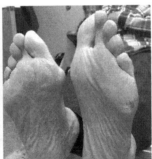

Picture 12.14. The right (shorter leg) foot (on the left of the picture) has bad calluses on the ball of the foot behind the first and fifth toes. The far right picture shows a callus under the fifth metatarsal, a callus that is common in the shorter leg.

I have seen many people who had an isolated hammertoe of the second toe in the shorter leg. Many of them had an extremely painful metatarsal phalangeal joint on the bottom of the foot, and some even had a dislocated metatarsal phalangeal joint. Therefore, even though it is more common to have the callus behind the baby toe, be aware that full or partial dislocation of the second MPJ may also be present in the shorter leg.

Differences in Shoes or Orthotics

In that the foot of the shorter leg often inverts more, there is a difference in the shoe wear. Specifically, the

heel of the shoe often wears down more on the outside of the shoe of the shorter leg.

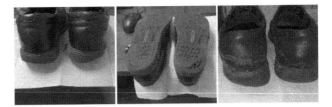

Picture 12.15. Shoe wear is often greater on the outside of the heel of the shorter leg, or the inside of the heel of the longer leg.

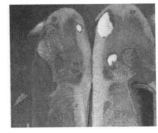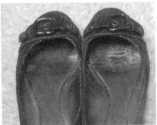

Picture 12.16. There may also be difference in the wear pattern of the inside of the shoes or the orthotics. Greatest wear is seen in the area that a foot is more likely to develop a callus. Such asymmetry is a strong indication of a Limb Length Discrepancy

The preceding signs are those which can be observed by even casual observation. An upcoming sign, asymmetric Equinus, requires more focused attention, and was presented in greater detail in the section for clinicians in Chapter 6. In the section "Measuring LLDx," there will be information on the Iliac Crest Pain Resolution Sign. First we briefly address an important set of findings, physical examination of nerve involvement.

Physical Examination for Nerve Involvement in Limb Length Discrepancy

Nerve abnormalities are addressed in both Chapter 6, on physical examination, and Chapter 15, on Peripheral Neuropathy. The nerve hypersensitivity pattern commonly seen with both Spinal Stenosis and PseudoStenosis is the **First Interspace Fine Sign**, which is frequently seen along with tenderness upon palpation of the tibial and femoral nerves.

Significant asymmetry of nerve sensitivity suggests Limb Length Discrepancy. Less frequently, it may be caused by another asymmetric cause of PseudoStenosis. This is an absolutely essential clue to investigate.

Asymmetry in **Loss of Protective Sensation patterns** also suggests the possibility of PseudoStenosis secondary to Limb Length Discrepancy, although that pattern is not consistent. **Details from Chapters 6 and 15 must be considered.**

Asymmetric Equinus

The structurally shorter leg usually has a tighter Achilles tendon (or tendon complex). I believe this is caused by a **subconscious effort of the body to keep the torso even**; it attempts to functionally lengthen the shorter leg. When examined, the Achilles complex actually feels tighter when the foot is pushed up as high as it can go—and it goes up less.

It is not easy to measure exactly how much motion is present in the ankle, and doctors often disagree with the numbers. **However, it is fairly easy to note if one leg feels tighter than the other,** and to see if the foot can go past the perpendicular (over 90 degrees), achieve a perpendicular position (90 degrees), or only achieve less than 90 degrees. **To get a feel for the tightness of the tendon, the knee must be *fully* extended and the foot must be slightly inverted and held straight during this maneuver.** Sometimes, the asymmetry is apparent just by looking at the resting position of the two ankles.

Picture 12.17 shows the measuring of motion in the ankle with a tractograph. Exact measurements are not as important as recognizing a difference between the two feet. The following pictures demonstrate examination with tape on the foot for enhanced perception.

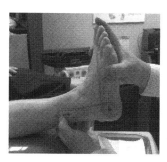

Picture 12.17. Measuring with a tractograph. Having the exact numbers is not nearly as important as is simply recognizing the difference and following up after treatment.

Picture 12.18 shows a foot that, with the knee fully extended and the foot slightly inverted, gets to approximately 90 degrees (perpendicular) when the motion is tested.

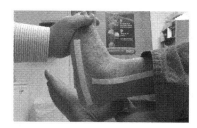

Picture 12.18. With the foot held up, it gets to about a 90-degree angle (perpendicular).

Picture 12.19 shows a foot that can only be moved to 10 degrees short of the perpendicular.

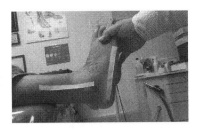

Picture 12.19. With the foot held up, it is 10 degrees short of perpendicular, tighter than the left foot.

These are subtle differences that a clinician should be able to appreciate, but only if specifically looking for them. Patients and their families often recognize the difference when I point it out to them.

The Importance of Quick Resolution of Equinus

Here is an original observation that is one of the keys of managing a Limb Length Discrepancy. I say original, but perhaps it is not unique. Perhaps other people have observed and used it. Perhaps it has even been published, although I do not recall seeing it. In

> *At the beginning of this chapter, I referred to a disagreement among various authors as to how much Limb Length Discrepancy is necessary to cause problems.*
>
> *I believe that this asymmetric tightness represents a subconscious effort by an individual to compensate for the discrepancy; the person tries to lengthen the shorter leg by pushing down with the Achilles tendon.*
>
> *This seems to support the position of those who feel that a small difference is important. After all, the body would not try to compensate for a discrepancy that was not having any potential negative effect. It only compensates for something that is perceived as "wrong."*
>
> *Any discrepancy that is enough to cause an asymmetric tightness is also enough to induce changes in function that can cause symptoms. Even 1/16 of an inch, about 2 millimeters!*
>
> *Therefore, identifying this asymmetry can automatically direct a clinician to investigate symptoms that **might** occur from a Limb Length Discrepancy.*

any case, **this is a great key to following the overall effectiveness of treating Limb Length Discrepancy**.

If Limb Length Discrepancy is the cause of the asymmetric tightness, that tightness will disappear within 1–3 days of consistently using a lift of adequate height. This allows us to confirm, or at least strongly suspect, that an adequate amount of lift has been added. **If the ankle motion is still tight on the shorter leg at the follow-up visit, it usually means that there has not been adequate lift or there has not been adequate use of the lift.** I will then either add additional lift to the shoes, or I will strap a lift to the foot to enforce compliance. (Of course, there could also be resolution of this if too much lift was used, either because of a mistake in evaluation, compliance issues, or the presence of a functional component to the Limb Length Discrepancy.)

Individuals with a Limb Length Discrepancy may subconsciously stand differently to compensate for the problem. Sometimes the LLDx is apparent at the heel when standing, but usually it is not.

StoryTime: One day, I was examining a woman who presented in many ways as if she had PseudoStenosis from a short leg. She experienced back pain within a few minutes of standing. When I had her stand for the examination, I was surprised that her shoulders and hip bones were even. However, as I looked at her from behind I saw that the heel of the short leg was just a bit off the ground. As she stood in place and tired, her heel dropped, and her shoulder and hip on that side became lower. She had been compensating by lifting herself higher on the short leg, and she was unaware of it. In a totally subconscious move, her body was trying to compensate for the Limb Length Discrepancy. Once the leg got tired, her back went into an uneven position and began to hurt. Use of a lift for the short leg immediately eliminated all of her symptoms.

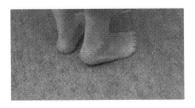

Picture 12.20. Pushing up higher on the short leg to compensate for Limb Length Discrepancy.

If Asymmetry of Equinus is not from LLDx

Other conditions besides Limb Length Discrepancy can cause limited ankle motion. This restriction could be caused by an ankle injury, arthritis, or a nerve problem, including stroke, nerve injury after knee surgery, or dysfunction of a nerve in the low back. This ankle with reduced upward motion may then act as a longer leg. This problem with ankle motion/tendon tightness does not usually resolve with the proper lift. Such patients often have difficulty standing and feel that they are falling backward. Help for these individuals may be obtained by putting an **adequate lift in both shoes**. Further information is presented in the section on Equinus in this chapter, in Chapter 19, on arthritis, and in Chapter 21, on nighttime symptoms.

Measuring Limb Length Discrepancy

This seems a good place to talk about something still controversial: evaluation and measurement of Limb Length Discrepancy. These details are presented in Chapters 6 and 15, so I will mention them briefly and then move on to the invaluable Iliac Crest Pain Resolution Sign.

Measurement can be made by three reported categories of methods: direct measurement, radiologic measurement, and indirect measurement.

Direct measurement involves use of a tape measure to measure distance between structures (such as umbilicus [belly button] to anklebone landmark) and then compare measurements of the two sides. While this method has clinical value, especially in cases of large discrepancy, I am among those who feel that it is not as dependable a method as the indirect method or the radiologic approaches mentioned below, especially for the slight differences that I feel are so important.

Radiologic measurement techniques investigating the leg length include performing a (non weight bearing) Scanogram, a weight-bearing Long Leg Study (Teleroentgenogram), or weight bearing x rays of the lumbosacral spine and pelvis, with different level heel lifts to ascertain the benefit of the lifts on the spine. The decision as to which technique to use is guided by clinical details but may also be based upon availability, insurance approval, and preference of the radiology department.

I use radiologic testing much less frequently than indirect measurement, as I often enjoy clinical success without it. I order testing primarily if I do not get the expected clinical success, if there is suspicion that a functional LLDx is clouding the clinical appearance, if the clinical exam is not clear (as in a very overweight person), if there is a disagreement between professionals regarding the status, or if it is necessary to provide corroboration to the patient or family regarding the presence of the discrepancy. It must be conceded that there is a margin of error in performing and interpreting the tests that may exceed 2 or 3 millimeters.

Further discussion on the different forms of radiologic testing, the advantage of individual tests in different clinical situations, and the limit of accuracy of the tests is provided in Chapter 14, which deals primarily with radiology issues.

StoryTime: Mary was a 67-year-old woman who presented for chronic foot pain that was worse with standing or walking for more than a few minutes and that had been present for many years. Orthotics previously provided were comfortable, but they did not provide relief. She had arthritic pain in her low back and knees as well. All symptoms began after an auto accident 9 years earlier. Treatment by podiatrists, chiropractors, and orthopedists, and by extensive physical therapy, was not effective.

She had right-sided Equinus and a heel that was higher appearing when not weight bearing. Her left Iliac Crest was higher. She had a positive First Interspace Fine Sign on both feet, but it was worse on the right. That pattern, of being more sensitive in the short leg, is unusual, but I find it more frequent if the LLDx is at least ¼ inch. Her longer left leg had a flatter foot. Both Iliac Crests were sensitive; the higher left side was more painful. It took a ⅜-inch lift under the right heel to make the hips even and pain free. I provided several ⅜-inch lifts, and I also ordered a CT Scanogram.

At the next visit, I got mixed messages. The patient had near 100% relief of foot, knee, and back pain, and was standing and walking better than she had in years. She had elimination of all nerve sensitivity, Equinus, and hip sensitivity. However, a CT Scanogram suggested a 7-millimeter discrepancy, and I had provided ⅜ of an inch, just over 9.5 millimeters. I decided I did not want to overtreat, and provided ¼-inch lifts, 6.3 millimeters.

At the next visit, she had slid backward. She had a moderate return of symptoms, as well as Equinus, nerve sensitivity, and hip sensitivity. Deciding to treat based upon my findings rather than the exact radiology report, I again provided ⅜-inch lifts for full-time use. She had relief of symptoms within a day. Follow-up evaluation three weeks later showed elimination of Equinus and sensitivity along the hips and nerves. Indirect examination again showed need for ⅜-inch lifts to make the hips exactly even.

There are many lessons to this story, but I focus here on radiology. Just as the findings of spinal imaging are only a guide to treatment, so too are radiologic findings only part of the puzzle, though often a very valuable and helpful piece. I recommend radiologic testing, but not complete dependence upon it.

> ### For the clinician and the very curious
> *Examination of the hips may offer insight as to whether part of the problem is a functional LLDx, caused by pelvic rotation or low-back misalignment. In a functional LLDx, the foot of the short leg may be flatter and turned out more. In addition, the ASIS (Anterior Superior Iliac Spine) may feel higher on what appears to be the longer leg, but the PSIS (Posterior Superior Iliac Spine) may be higher on the shorter leg. If the discrepancy is merely structural, both the ASIS and PSIS will be lower on the side of the shorter leg.*

The **indirect measurement** technique involves placing lifts of known heights under the shorter leg until structures of the hips of both sides become even. This exam also allows evaluation for the presence of a functional Limb Length Discrepancy as described below. After other clues cause one to suspect LLDx, this indirect measurement is an essential step to confirm and measure the discrepancy present. This provides a starting place from which to begin treatment. I believe that

> ### For Everyone—
> ### Patients, Family, and Clinicians:
> ### Structural, Functional, or Combined?
> *As we discuss evaluation and treatment, it is necessary to reinforce the idea that the LLDx may be structural (caused by actual shortening of the leg), functional (caused by pelvic or lower-back misalignment), or a combination of the two.*
>
> *If there is a functional component, at the second or third visit the appearance of the discrepancy may be different from its appearance at the initial visit. Quite often, the amount of discrepancy appears smaller after successful treatment of the spine, the LLDx, or the other causes of PseudoStenosis. Such treatment may include strapping, lifts, inserts, braces, physical therapy, spinal manipulation, and epidural injections. **It is important to recheck LLDx after any treatment that may affect the spine.***
>
> ***There are times one must be especially cautious in diagnosing a structural Limb Length Discrepancy.** If a person has recently injured his back, it may be misaligned, causing a functional LLDx. It is appropriate to consider and even experiment with treating perceived LLDx, but it is important to wait until the acute misalignment is resolved before firmly diagnosing the presence, nature, and extent of LLDx. If there is a question, consider radiologic testing.*

clinicians should routinely use this technique when evaluating and treating LLDx.

Keep in mind that the amount identified may include both structural and functional LLDx, so one may not diagnose with finality the amount of discrepancy present with this exam. It is a starting point from which to begin treatment. **It is essential to repeat the examination at follow-up visits to confirm that the findings are consistent and to identify if the amount of the apparent discrepancy has changed. Repetition is essential, as the functional LLDx component may resolve with successful treatment.**

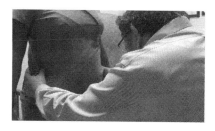

Picture 12.21. Exam of hip symmetry shows palpation (touching and examining) of structures of the hip joint. Indirect measurement is an essential step in evaluating the presence and extent of Limb Length Discrepancy.

The Invaluable Iliac Crest Pain Resolution Sign

This finding, which I have used for years, is not always present—but when it is, it is quite impressive. With firm palpation of the Iliac Crest as shown above, one side, or occasionally both, is often quite sensitive. The sensitivity is usually reported as pain but occasionally, especially in children, as ticklishness. It is more often found that the sensitive area is on the side of the longer leg if the LLDx is less than about ¼ inch, but it may be found with either hip if the discrepancy is over that amount. **That sensitivity usually improves immediately when an appropriate lift is placed under the heel of the short leg.** I don't know if this has ever been documented before. It is certainly not always present, as not everyone with a Limb Length Discrepancy has hip bone tenderness. However, when just a lift *immediately* eliminates that tenderness, both the patient and I are amazed. It is very encouraging, and, I believe, it greatly encourages compliance. I refer to this as the **"Iliac Crest Pain Resolution Sign."**

Often, after using an appropriate lift consistently for a few days, the sensitivity resolves so that the hip bone is not sensitive even when the person is not standing on a lift. Similar to the resolution of asymmetric Equinus and the First Interspace Fine Sign presented in Chapter 6, I regard this as a confirmation that we have identified a problem and have taken steps to address it. At that time it is appropriate to repeat indirect measurement to reevaluate the amount of LLDx that is clinically present, as described above.

I do have an alternate name for this sign that I sometimes use with patients. When the hip is so sensitive and improves immediately with a proper lift, I

note that the patient has a "Happy Hip." On follow-up visits I recheck when the lift is in shoes and again when the shoes are off. If there is no sensitivity, I refer to this as "Happy Hips." The patient almost always agrees.

Great clues to use and be guided by

The value of these three clues (asymmetric Equinus, asymmetric First Interspace Fine Sign, and Iliac Crest Pain Resolution Sign) will be clear as one addresses the many clinical problems presented in later chapters of this book. The presence of any of these three causes me to suspect LLDx as a contributing factor to PseudoStenosis-induced symptoms.

*I have occasionally treated patients with only one or even none of these clues who still had improvement of spine-related symptoms by treating the discrepancy. Therefore, these must be considered valuable clues, **but not findings that must all be present to consider this diagnosis.***

If there is a mixture, I become suspicious and more cautious. An example could be a person with greater nerve sensitivity on the left side who also had greater Equinus on the left rather than the right, as would be expected. If the three clues do not line up as expected, I stress to the patient that there may be a functional component, and that it is even more important than normal to build up slowly and to be checked a few times.

Limb Length Discrepancy: Correct it, or at Least Treat it

Treatment Tips: 13 Points

We have now addressed the causes for suspicion and methods for evaluation of Limb Length Discrepancy. **Let us move on to treatment.** How do I treat for Limb Length Discrepancy in my office—and what guidance can I give *you*?

The idea of using a lift, either in the shoe or built into the shoe, is as old as old can be. If there is a discrepancy of ⅜ of an inch or more, it has most likely been recognized and addressed in the past. Most likely, but not necessarily. I have had patients who had the discrepancy recognized but were told it was not important to address. In addition, I have had others who recalled that for years they used a lift but simply stopped on their own.

Frequently, some of the improvement that comes with treating the Limb Length Discrepancy is noticed immediately. Just as you would notice a problem right away if you were walking with only one shoe on, with proper balancing you may notice improvement—though not necessarily all the improvement that you will eventually get—immediately. **As with all Spinal Stenosis or PseudoStenosis treatments, there should be excellent overall improvement within 1–3 days.**

StoryTime: Marie D was a 62-year-old woman with insulin-dependent diabetes who presented for treatment of a rash. She reported that she'd had nerve pain in her legs for 5 long years—pain that did not respond to oral medicines. She had even taken a nerve test, which had not shown any pathology.

Marie had frequent back pain, leg pain, and foot pain, which was always much worse with standing or walking. She was able to walk much more comfortably when pushing a grocery cart. My exam showed a Limb Length Discrepancy, along with the supportive signs of asymmetric Equinus, a positive First Interspace Fine Sign, and a positive Iliac Crest Pain Resolution Sign. **One lift and one day later, all of the foot and leg pain, previously attributed for years to neuropathy, was gone.** Her follow-up interview is available on WalkingWell Again.com.

The lesson? By treating the cause of PseudoStenosis, in this case a Limb Length Discrepancy, five years of nerve pain can disappear in a single day!

Goals of Treatment

I perceive three basic goals of treatment when attempting to compensate for the Limb Length Discrepancy.

- Rebalance the spine position enough to eliminate the spine dysfunction that causes either local back pain or pressure on the nerves, which in turn causes the symptoms in the lower extremities.

- Eliminate the effect of the imbalance on the mechanical function of the lower extremities. Both the shorter leg and the longer leg have abnormal mechanical stress that can cause deformity and disability in the feet, ankles, knees, and hips. **These deformities have been touched upon in this chapter but are more thoroughly detailed in Chapter 19.** Proper treatment relieves the mechanical stress causing arthritic symptoms, which lead to development of degenerative arthritis changes and may also affect balance, as is addressed in Chapter 23. This benefit is often appreciated short term, but it may also be of ultimate long-term value.

- Allow successful mechanical control of the feet and legs with orthotics or braces. The mechanical stress of LLDx is a factor that often makes people unable to benefit from, or at times even tolerate, their orthotics or custom-built ankle braces. Proper balancing often allows the orthotics or braces to become more comfortable and effective.

First Do No Harm: Cautions with Treatment

The first precept of medicine is "Primum non nocere," a Latin phrase that means "*First* do no harm." We want the treatment performed in a manner that will accomplish the most possible good with the least chance of harm. There are different ways to cause harm by using too much lift.

1. **Too much change might be uncomfortable for a body that has compensated long term for this problem.** If the lift is uncomfortable, you might feel that this approach is a failure and then stop using it, when all it needs is to be done judiciously.

    Story Time: Ben came in for a painful ingrown nail. Exam showed Equinus on the left foot, a positive First Interspace Fine Sign on the right foot, and a positive Iliac Crest Pain Resolution Sign, with the optimal lift seeming to be 3/16 of an inch. He had gone to a chiropractor for many years for frequent adjustments for an aching and weak back, although he did not describe the back as actually "painful."

    I strapped him with a 3/16-inch lift and looked forward to the next visit. Whoops! He went to the chiropractor and got adjusted the next day, and had a lot more pain. The chiropractor evaluated him and felt there was absolutely no discrepancy. I advised him to remove the strap and lift and sent him for a CT Scanogram, which reported a 5-millimeter discrepancy, 3/16 of an inch, just as my exam had suggested. I gave him several lifts of 1/16-inch thickness and had him increase the lift slightly every couple of days, to try to avoid the need for periodic spine adjustment. He did somewhat but not all better, and only felt comfortable with 1/8 inch, not the full 3/16 inch that was the discrepancy suggested both by my exam and by the CT Scanogram.

    The lessons? In Ben's case, there had to be a gradual adjustment to the amount of lift needed to compensate for the discrepancy. **If an increase in symptoms suggests an overcorrection, patients and clinicians should be patient.** Start with a lower lift, and only gradually increase the height of the lift used, to try to achieve the goal of optimal compensation. Ben simply did not tolerate what I felt was the appropriate full correction. **The amount used should only be the amount that is comfortable.**

The second lesson of this story is that it is possible for there to be a disagreement between professionals. I have often disagreed with findings and treatment plans noted by excellent professionals. I am often proved right by successful treatment, **but I have also been proved wrong enough times to keep my ego in check.** If there is a disagreement in the perceived findings or diagnosis, go for a third opinion, or have a test that can shed some light on the matter. In this case, I was appreciative to have the CT Scanogram support my findings, even though, as must be repeated, the radiologic evaluations are helpful but not necessarily exact.

2. **Very often the amount of discrepancy originally perceived is not correct. A person who has a *structural* discrepancy often also has a *functional* discrepancy,** so that the amount perceived initially is exaggerated. Someone might appear to have a ½-inch discrepancy at the first visit, but only appear to have half of that—a ¼-inch discrepancy—after a few days of treatment, as the body begins to walk more normally. Thus, the discrepancy is much milder than originally thought. Adding ½ of an inch might actually aggravate the spine!

StoryTime: Betty was a 58-year-old woman who presented with chronic pain (burning and aching) with her feet for many years, despite anti-inflammatory medication, therapy, and a few pairs of orthotics. Indirect examination suggested a ⁵⁄₁₆-inch LLDx. She had an asymmetric Equinus, a positive First Interspace Fine Sign that was worse in the longer left leg, but only mild mechanical changes with the feet. In addition, areas that are often sensitive with mechanical foot problems caused by Flat Feet were not sensitive. This is explained in Chapter 19.

Looking for a home run, I provided her with ⁵⁄₁₆-inch (8-millimeter) lifts. Here we developed a temporary love/hate relationship. Within 2 days ALL of her long-term foot pain was gone. However, the lift exacerbated the long-term but previously only mild back pain she had. I told her to stop using lifts and follow up in a week. I also ordered a CT Scanogram.

The pain in her feet returned in a few days, so she went back to using the lift. Yes, foot pain was again relieved, but back pain returned. I should not have been shocked. Her CT Scanogram showed a 4-millimeter LLDx, not the 8-millimeter one that my initial exam had suggested. I gave her ⅛-inch (3-millimeter) lifts. They were well tolerated, and she maintained improvement of the foot pain without worsening of her back symptoms. Indirect measurement at a follow-up examination suggested that ⅛ inch was the appropriate amount.

The lessons? I have at times over-treated the LLDx, and the patient paid the price with new symptoms. In Betty's case, there was a combined LLDx, both structural and functional. In cases like this, **STOP using the lifts if new symptoms develop.** Follow-up examination is essential. **You should not give up on the potential for treating LLDx because of initial failure.** If in doubt, reevaluate, and consider radiologic testing.

> *For everyone—patients, family, and clinicians*
>
> *In my office practice, the great majority of people do well without complication when I treat them for LLDx. Throughout Section 3 of this book, you will read about many of them. However, not all do. I share these stories not to discourage patients or professionals from aggressively investigating and treating LLDx, but to reinforce that treatment is a process that may require at least a few visits.*
>
> ***Do not be discouraged if the first try is not perfect! And be willing to put in a lot of thought if all of the clues do not point in the same direction.***
>
> *In addition, not everyone with a Limb Length Discrepancy requires treatment. While I lean toward treatment if there are any symptoms, or even areas of sensitivity that reflect either nerve or arthritic imbalance, they are not always present. **Especially in older adults who are functioning well,** I may identify the LLDx, inform the patient, and discuss future treatment that should be considered if any symptoms develop. **First, do no harm!***

When to Use the Two Different Protocols

There are two conflicting protocols that may be used to treat LLDx. One is to identify the perceived difference and immediately compensate for it. For example, if you suspect a ½-inch LLDx, you immediately treat with ½ of an inch. This approach may hit a home run, but it also may cause the kind of problems described above and end the experiment. The second way is to start out with less than the perceived difference and slowly increase the lift height.

I am more aggressive in my office than I would recommend patients or less experienced clinicians to be. Experience counts, but that does not mean I am always right, so I caution patients that we may need to change the lift. I stress that it is okay if the use of the lift feels a little funny or different, but that it should not be used if it causes any increased discomfort.

One can be more confident of there being a true structural LLDx (rather than just a functional LLDx) with a few clues described below.

- If the two feet or legs show significant structural differences as described earlier in this chapter (If this is the case, the structural LLDx will usually have been present for years. Structural differences rarely occur quickly.)

- If there is severe asymmetric Equinus present

- If the person acknowledges that changes in symptoms occurred after a surgery such as a joint replacement or an orthopedic injury such as for a fracture (This scenario suggests two possibilities. One is that the LLDx was more recently formed. The other possibility is that the physical challenges after the surgery or injury made it harder for the individual to compensate for a long term LLDx. More in Chapter 19.)

In such cases, I am more aggressive with lift height, and may use the total or near-total amount that is suggested by indirect measurement and the Iliac Crest Pain Resolution Sign.

If there is not such clear support for a structural LLDx, I use a more conservative approach, starting with a lesser amount, often half of what is perceived, and increasing gradually. For example, if I perceive a 5 mm discrepancy, but there are no structural differences and there is no history of probable cause, I may begin with only a 3 mm lift and have the patient add 1 more mm every 2 days, until he either experiences relief of symptoms or finds that the lift is uncomfortable. I also request that patients return to the office, usually within 7 days, so I can recheck the apparent discrepancy.

Sometimes patients do not add the lifts on their own as directed, and they simply return for me to adjust the lift height. Clinicians should be aware that active cooperation is not always what we would hope for, and they should be prepared to completely direct the lift height during office visits with some patients.

The second approach I described is more appropriate for patients and families to use and for clinicians to consider. Start conservatively, using less than the perceived difference, and increase gradually, every couple of days. Below, in the section entitled "Self-treatment for Limb Length Discrepancy," I present information on lifts available via the Internet that can be easily acquired by both patient and clinician.

Can a Limb Length Discrepancy Disappear or Change Sides?

The answer is yes! Sometimes, because of any Spinal Stenosis or PseudoStenosis treatment, a person begins walking better, his low-back joints work more normally, and the appearance of a Limb Length Discrepancy completely disappears. **In that circumstance, it was a functional rather than a structural difference.** For this reason, there is value in the patient being rechecked after using the lift and periodically after that, to make sure that what seemed initially to be a Limb Length Discrepancy is still present. The perceived LLDx may have just been a functional discrepancy, secondary to spine misalignment.

As is explained later in this chapter, any cause of significant foot or ankle pain may cause the patient to walk differently to avoid pain, and may thus affect the function of the back, causing PseudoStenosis. It may also cause a functional Limb Length Discrepancy. Thus, treating the cause of pain and rechecking at the next appointment is appropriate.

Need for Consistency in Use

Initially, use a lift full time to achieve and maintain optimal improvement. Just as use of the lift can provide immediate improvement of symptoms, even occasional standing or walking without the lift can affect the mechanical function and secondary nerve inflammation. Having the lift at all times is often essential for success.

If I am not confident of the patient's compliance, I often test for success first by attaching the lift to the foot. The lift may be added just to the heel or it may be extended farther forward. This allows accommodation of painful areas, and also may prevent the foot from being forced forward as if in a high-heeled shoe. **I have had many patients who initially reported no or limited improvement of symptoms, who reported excellent improvement when a lift was strapped to their foot.** It was obvious to me that poor compliance had prevented them from improving, and that having the lift attached to their foot removed the challenge of compliance from them.

Just as it is most effective in the initial phase of Positional Testing for Spinal Stenosis to use the walker full time for at least a few days, it is most effective to use a lift at all times during the initial trial to have the greatest likelihood of successful improvement of symptoms caused or maintained by the Limb Length Discrepancy. In either case, walking a small amount of time without the correction may prevent the inflamed or irritated tissues from healing. Once inflamed tissues improve, strict compliance may not be quite as important for many people. The first days, however, are essential. **Poor compliance may prevent the improvement that could be obtained with good compliance, leading all to believe that the LLDx treatment was not of value.** This can result in a lifetime of continued problems.

In addition, once good success is enjoyed with just a few days of good compliance, patients are encouraged to maintain the success with long-term compliance. Once symptoms are improved, patients usually become willing to do whatever is needed to maintain their improvement.

StoryTime: This is a fun story, as well as one with an absolutely ESSENTIAL lesson. A woman came to me presenting with a toenail problem. She also acknowledged a long-term problem with lower-back pain, which I suspected was due to her Limb Length Discrepancy. My exam also showed asymmetric Equinus and a positive asymmetric First Interspace Fine Sign.

I gave her lifts to use for her shoes, but she reported at the next visit several days later that she had received no help and was flatly not interested in the other recommendations that I offered. The Equinus and nerve sensitivity were as unchanged as her symptoms.

When she returned for a follow-up for an unrelated issue months later, I again brought up the PseudoStenosis and Spinal Stenosis options, including orthotics. During that discussion, she noted that, as a "country girl," orthotics were not an option, since she rarely wore shoes in the house and spent most of her time there. AHA! No shoes, so she had not used the lift much on the first try! I treated her with a lift again, but this time strapped it to her foot in a Low Dye strap. She returned a few days later and reported that her back pain had disappeared. The exam showed elimination of the unilateral Equinus and elimination of the nerve sensitivity that had been present at each of her prior visits.

Seeing such dramatic improvement, she became motivated. She agreed to wear the lift as much as possible, in both her shoes and her bedroom slippers. She maintained her improvement long term. In her case, the secret was to maximize compliance, especially for the first few days. After that, she wore shoes full time—country girl or not. A small price to pay to eliminate chronic back pain!

Treating with Lifts

I provide my patients with lifts to wear **at all times**. That means I provide a lift for the shoe they are wearing, and a few more to use in other shoes. I do not expect them to remember to switch the lift from shoe to shoe, so this is the optimal way—to start off with lifts in all shoes. This includes sneakers, dress shoes, crocs, bedroom slippers, and anything else they may wear in the upcoming week.

I use vinyl lifts, or thin 1 millimeter plastic lifts, or piano felt that has an adhesive side to build up the inside of the shoe on the shorter side. Depending upon my confidence, especially if the apparent discrepancy exceeds about 6 millimeters, **I sometimes start with less than the full amount, and provide additional thin lifts,** so that additions may be made by the patient at home.

The Order of Professional Treatment is an Art

Medical treatment is a combination of both science and art. Multiple symptoms are often present simultaneously, and many physical abnormalities may be present or suspected. Knowing which to treat first, or how many to treat first, is definitely an art. At home, you are limited in your options, whereas in the office a provider will have many choices.

If a person comes in and gives me a blank check (for time, not money!) and understands that investigating treatments one at a time may afford the best insight, then I may treat one condition and then add another treatment 2 or 3 days later. Within a few visits during the course of a couple of weeks, we would discover what interventions work and should be used.

That blank check of time and cooperation is not always present. Perhaps the patient is skeptical. Perhaps he or she lives far away, or has high co-pays and limited finances. I may then get more aggressive and do multiple treatments on the first visit. This is especially true if the person came in for something simple (such as an ingrown nail), and I did an exam and history that suggested to me that I could help him overcome long-term and life-changing disability. Under those circumstances, I may choose to do many things to bring the patient and family on board. Once he experiences significant improvement, he usually becomes willing to work with me on evaluating which interventions are needed long term.

If multiple conditions or multiple types of symptoms are present, a clinician employs his best judgment and a little guessing as he tries to unravel a mystery. Patients, be patient, and allow the process to take place. In many cases, your patience will be well repaid.

At times I will attach the felt (with adhesive) to an insert that came with the shoe, or to an orthotic, as well as provide extra lifts so that the person can put them in the other shoes.

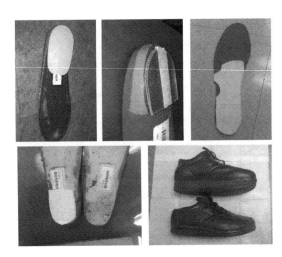

Picture 12.22. Lifts added to the bottom of the orthotic or to the shoe insert, or built into the shoe.

If I suspect (for any reason) that the patient may not be compliant, or if the patient was previously not compliant and did not improve as expected, I will attach the lift to the bottom of the foot. This may be done with taping, or with a wrap called an "Unna boot." Details on strapping and Unna boots may be found in the appendix.

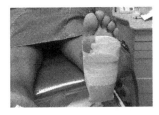

Picture 12.23. The foot has been strapped to induce the pronation control that that can be obtained with a custom built orthotic, and can include a lift or other modifications.

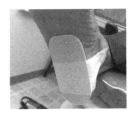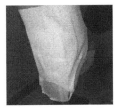

Picture 12.24 When only a lift is needed, I strap a (durable and waterproof) vinyl lift with a waterproof strap. This allows the patient to shower, and enhances compliance.

Should Lifts be Permanent or Temporary Additions to Inserts?

Clinicians directing treatment need to decide if the lifts should be temporary and removable additions to the shoes or inserts, or if they should be permanent additions.

I believe that the decision should be based primarily upon confidence of the long-term need. Supporting factors include the following:

- Lifts that quickly resolve a long-term problem

- Maintained consistent appearance of LLDx after the clinical symptoms resolve

- Asymmetric structural changes suggesting long-term structural discrepancy

- Awareness of an incident such as a fracture or joint replacement surgery that contributes to the discrepancy

- Radiologic evidence that confirms the structural discrepancy

Insofar as structural discrepancy often is joined by functional discrepancy, there is value in following the patient's progress and appearance before adding a permanent lift to shoes or inserts. **Patients should also be cautioned to return for reevaluation if any of the symptoms of PseudoStenosis or arthritis ever worsen.**

Here is yet another reminder of the need for consistency. If a patient uses lifts, the lifts should be *in all shoes and sneakers*. They should even be placed in bedroom slippers. Otherwise, an hour of walking in the house without compensation may cause recurrence of symptoms that would suggest that this intervention is not effective. Facilitate strict compliance!

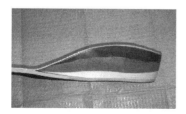

Picture 12.25. A tapered lift is built into the orthotic.

Self-treatment for Limb Length Discrepancy

Limb Length Discrepancy is a condition that patients can often treat at home. Experiment by adding a lift to the shoe of the shorter leg, and wear shoes with a lift as much as possible, following direction in this section. Pay attention to your symptoms and activity capability.

How do you get the lifts? Obviously, a clinician who treats this condition will have lifts in the office. But if you, the patient, want to treat this on your own, you need lifts with the correct dimensions.

Availability and Selection of Lifts

There are basically three types of lifts. The first, the kind available in almost any pharmacy, is a soft material that is used primarily for shock absorption. Packaging does not list the height of the lift. These lifts do not come in graduated heights, and of course getting the right height is *essential*. Therefore, these lifts will not be optimal for most people treating LLDx.

Fortunately, on-line providers sell other types of lifts that take care of this problem. One type is a solid lift that is an established thickness, while the other type can be modified to be multiple thicknesses, as is described below. In my office I usually both types, but also at times use different layers of felt and sometimes make gradual adjustments. **For patients investigating their long-term need, being able to experiment, by making subtle adjustments in height, can help them discover what is most helpful**.

The lift that allows individuals to do the same is a lift made of clear plastic layers that are each just one millimeter thick. It's functional height is 12 millimeters thick, about 1/2 of an inch. **It is a little more expensive than other lifts, but the possibility of gradual minor modification will be valuable for many people.**

Recall what I said a few pages ago, about the conservative approach to achieving the right height. In the *"experimentation phase"*, start with only about half of the perceived difference and then build up gradually, increasing the height just 1 or 2 millimeters every couple of days. Because improvement occurs so quickly, patients may increase the height quickly. **Just be sure to stop or to reduce the height if you feel new discomfort, and to make sure that you add the same amount of lift to ALL your shoes that you are using during this phase.**

This plastic layered lift has other advantages. It can easily be trimmed, so that users can get multiple lifts from one unit if the amount of elevation needed is small. For example, if you need 4 millimeters of lift, you could get three functional lifts from this one lift, that is 12 mm thick. In addition, the thin plastic layers are quite durable. Finally, being plastic, it can be used in water, and can be glued on to a sandal or thong, to maximize time of correction. These are important factors.

Once the proper height is determined, you should prepare for the "long-term use phase". **For most people, the lifts should be used their entire lives, and should be in all shoes.** Durable vinyl lifts come in various heights, such as 3, 5, 7, 9 and 12 millimeter, and can last for years. If necessary for optimal height, you may glue a 1 MM layer to the bottom of a vinyl lift. The lifts are very inexpensive, most of which are currently less than 10 dollars each.

Let me make sure that this information is clear. The most important factor for the success of a heel lift is the height, which is measured in millimeters (MM) or in fractions of inches. This is not only important, but essential. **One or two millimeters too little can prevent**

Ordering Lifts Through my Affiliate

I will have a "Store" section on my website (Walking WellAgain.com) in which my books as well as other products that I feel are helpful can be purchased. I will have links to what I perceive as appropriate lifts in that section. Patients can also order them directly toll free by phone at (844) 433-5538 (844-Heel-LFT).

*There is, in addition **a sock that is modified to accept a heel lift so that the person can wear it with sandals and even barefoot.** Many people can benefit from using this sock and lift when taking a shower, or walking around the house, and even at the beach. Access to these modified socks will also be available at WalkingWellAgain.com, or by the toll free number 844-Heel-LFT.*

*In that appropriate use of lifts is so important, I will include a section on WalkingWellAgain.com with further innovative ways of using the lifts, and **I invite any patient or professional who uses lifts in an innovative way to share it with others through the website.***

success, while one or two millimeters too much could cause new discomfort. It is therefore essential to pay attention to the exact amount used and to use it full time for the period of time needed to see improvement, which is usually just 1–3 days.

The second-most important factor is durability. A lift of the exactly correct height that provides great improvement will fail if it compresses with time. Therefore, after identifying the proper height needed, it is essential to have appropriate lifts for all shoes and to select lifts that will stand the test of time, and to replace them when necessary.

About full length lifts

In addition to standard heel lifts, there are lifts that fit the entire length of the shoe. The advantage of such lifts is that they do not shift the foot forward, which might make you feel less balanced or might put pressure on the front part of the foot. **This is usually only a concern if the lift needed is large, over ⅜ of an inch.** It may be combined by having part of the lift go the full length, and part being just in the heel. In that this lift can also be trimmed, it may also be modified to reduce pressure on painful areas.

There are, however, two potential disadvantages of the full-length lift. First, if your shoe is at all tight, or if you have hammertoes, using a lift along the full length might make the shoe much tighter in front and cause increased pain and curling of toes. That problem can be adjusted for by trimming the lift so that it ends at the sulcus, the part of the foot behind the toes. It can also be negated by wearing extra-depth shoes, the kind that compensate for hammertoes and other forefoot problems by having extra room in the toe box of the shoe. If this is of concern, it is best to adjust for this problem with a good podiatrist, orthopedic surgeon, or pedorthist.

The other problem relates to Equinus, the tightness of the ankle discussed extensively earlier in this chapter. Recall that temporary use of the appropriate heel lift will usually cause the tight Achilles tendon complex to loosen up, and the Equinus to disappear, within a day or two. However, if while the Equinus is present, you use a full-length lift, either on the inside of the shoe such as the lifts we are discussing or built into the shoe, the tightness could make the calf very uncomfortable or cause you to feel imbalanced and tilting backward. In contrast, if the proper amount of heel lift is initially used full time, Equinus usually resolves quickly. Afterward, a full-length lift might be well tolerated. Keep this challenge in mind as you choose the lifts.

In What Shoes can Lifts be Used?

Obviously, it is easiest to use lifts in closed shoes that have a removable insert, such as those that most sneakers and many men's dress shoes now have. Simply put the lift under the insert and it will then stay in place. Having the insert on top of the lift also pads the edge of the insert so that the insert has an effect but is not necessarily even felt.

Fortunately, many flats for women now come with removable inserts, so that a lift can be inserted underneath them. Less easily accessible, there are bedroom

---

About Taking Showers

It is well known that the bathroom can be a dangerous place, with some sources reporting hundreds of thousands of emergency room visits each year caused by falls occurring in the bathroom. While getting into the shower or bath can be problematic, it is reported that falls are far more frequent when getting back out.

I consider those with Limb Length Discrepancy to be at much higher risk, not only because of their balance problems, but because standing in a shower may tire them out. Remember, with an LLDx, standing is often harder than walking. When it is time to leave the shower, a person with an LLDx may be much more strained and at greater risk of fall.

The solution? Wear a lift in the shower. This may be achieved either by using a pair of waterproof shoes with a removable insert under which you can slip a waterproof lift, or by gluing or even taping a waterproof lift to the back of a sandal. You could also use a sock with a pouch for the lift. Of course it is important to wear something that is secure and not slippery.

Use your judgment as to what works best for you. If you think this MIGHT be a problem, consider this as one more tool to try to make the bathroom a safer place.

---

slippers and sandals for casual wear, and even water shoes that you can use in the shower, with removable inserts. If you cannot find them locally, look online. I will try to have links to such shoes, bedroom slippers, and sandals on the WalkingWellAgain.com store section.

Another option would be for you to use double-sided tape or superglue to affix a lift to the heel of a shoe without an insert, or one with an open back. These methods can help you keep an insert in place in a shoe in which it would otherwise shift and no longer be comfortable or effective. Patients, help yourselves be compliant by being creative and proactive!

Be strict about your compliance. If you have a significant Limb Length Discrepancy, you should use a lift as much of the time as possible. If you are going to try to be one hundred percent compliant, you must exercise good judgment!

If the Discrepancy is Large

If the perceived discrepancy seems large enough to require a lift greater than ⅜ inch (10 millimeters), you have two options. First, you can go to a podiatrist or to an orthopedic shoe store that sells extra-depth shoes. These shoes can accommodate a much thicker lift than a regular shoe. If you do need lifts of ⅜ of an inch or more, you can put the lift not just under the heel, but also under spots farther forward, so as not to cause increased pressure in the bottom of the forefoot. You may extend it, at least in part, to just behind the toes, so as not to cramp the toes, especially if you have hammertoes.

Some extra-depth shoes have multiple layers of inserts inside them. In addition to using lifts, one may simply remove some of the layers in the shoe of the longer leg. The shoe may feel looser, but it may be well tolerated. In addition, sometimes the foot of the longer leg is actually bigger or wider, so that can be considered in shoe selection. Discuss this with your doctor, or perhaps with the pedorthist at the shoe store.

Another option for those needing greater lift on one side is to purchase an Evenup. Available through WalkingWellAgain.com, this device attaches by straps to a shoe to provide a thicker sole. It may provide additional height of either 1 centimeter (⅖ inch) or 2 centimeters

(⅕ inch). Promoted to help prevent problems for people with casts or cast boots, I also use it to provide immediate balance assistance for people with large Limb Length Discrepancies.

If you experience good improvement with this device, adding a sole lift to your shoes becomes a logical next step. This can be done by a pedorthotist, who may modify new or existing shoes.

That brings us back to a point mentioned above, which must be reinforced. **In patients who have a discrepancy of ⅜ inch to ½ inch or more, the tightness of the Achilles tendon can be severe.** It may be so severe that adding a lift to the entire sole of the shoe or using an Evenup makes the leg feel like it is pulled backward and makes the wearer feel like he or she is being pushed backward.

What is the solution? Temporary use of a lift, either strapped on or used FULL TIME, can reduce or eliminate the Equinus. Tightness improves in just 1–3 days. Afterward, the same sole lift or Evenup could be very comfortable. More is presented in Chapter 19.

Following the Improvement with Five Findings

Here is an essential clinical question: since measuring for lifts is an inexact science, how can we determine if enough lift has been added to compensate for the discrepancy? My method usually involves following five findings.

1. Look for **symptomatic relief**. If you experience resolution of symptoms, it is cause for celebration, and it may be that no more lift is needed. It's simple, but simple is not bad. It is, however, important to follow up with the physical signs and symptoms at least a few times, to make sure that an appropriate lift height is used long term.

2. Check for nerve hypersensitivity (**First Interspace Fine Sign**), as described in Chapter 6. Keep in mind that nerve sensitivity usually resolves in just 1–3 days, but the loss of sensation from SS/PS often takes at least 10–14 days to achieve optimal improvement.

3. Follow the **unilateral Equinus**. As you may recall, this means that the Achilles tendon of the shorter leg is tighter than that of the longer leg. If the muscle that was much tighter on the shorter leg achieves the same amount of dorsiflexion, then

adequate lift has been added. This usually occurs in just a day or two. In contrast, I have had several patients who continued to have symptoms, sensitive nerves, and a tight leg muscle, but saw all three of these presentations resolve within a couple of days by adding additional lift to the shoe (or switching to full-time use of the lift).

4. Perform the **essential repetition of the indirect measurement of LLDx**, which should be repeated on follow-up examinations. This step should include following up on both the hip imbalance and sensitivity. If there is a structural Limb Length Discrepancy, the examination will still show that one hip bone is higher than the other. *This is essential to check, as many people have a functional LLDx that disappears or improves with treatment.* In addition, recall that the Iliac Crest Pain Resolution Sign identifies hip sensitivity that improves immediately with use of an adequate lift for the short leg. Usually, after using the proper amount of lift consistently, the hip sensitivity is gone at the follow-up visit, even when the person stands without a lift, even when the hip height discrepancy is still clear. The tenderness that might have been severe before treatment is usually completely gone.

StoryTime: Virginia was a 50-year-old woman who presented with long-term numbness and pain in her left foot, ankle, and leg, plus aching in her back, which was aggravated by standing and walking. Examination showed that she had Flat Feet on both sides, a little worse on the left, which by indirect measurement appeared to be a longer leg by about ³⁄₁₆ of an inch. She had pain in the sinus tarsi and the plantar arch, and a positive First Interspace Fine Sign, all also worse in the left foot. Treating both the Flat Feet and the Limb Length Discrepancy, I applied a Low Dye strap to both feet and included a ⅛-inch lift for the shorter right leg.

At the next visit she was much better, but not all better. She shifted much less and found standing easier, and estimated relief of approximately 75% of her pain. She still had a mild Equinus only of the right leg, a mild positive First Interspace Fine Sign of the left foot only, and mild residual hip sensitivity of the left side only. There was elimination of the tenderness in the sinus tarsi and arch of the foot, suggesting that the strap had provided enough support to eliminate the discomfort caused by the Flat Feet.

Suspecting that I had not used enough lift, I gave her several $\frac{1}{16}$-inch lifts to use in each of her right shoes, including her bedroom slippers. Several days later she returned, reporting elimination of all discomfort in her back and leg. The three signs of Equinus, nerve sensitivity, and hip sensitivity were all totally relieved as well.

I have stressed that if these signs do not improve or do not resolve completely, it is often because of inadequate compliance or inadequate lift. Since the lift was strapped to her foot, I knew that compliance was not the issue. The additional lift added was small, only $\frac{1}{16}$ inch, less than 2 millimeters, but it was the amount needed to adequately compensate for the LLDx. Follow-up is needed, with strict attention to the details described in this story.

5. The fifth finding is not as consistent, and is more applicable to Chapter 19. That chapter deals with the arthritic presentations of LLDx, not the neurologic presentations or compensations as this chapter does. I presented earlier in this chapter as well as in Chapter 6 **the Asymmetric Sensitive Pes Anserinus,** the spot where three tendons insert just below the inner side of the knee. This is not as consistent of a finding as the other four mentioned above. In addition, the Pes Anserinus is just one of many places where the biomechanical stress of LLDx and pronation can cause local inflammation. Other common places include the Sinus Tarsi, the Posterior Tibial Tendon, and a joint on the bottom of the foot, the first metatarsal cuneiform joints, as is explained in detail in Chapter 19. I routinely check these spots after treatment for LLDx, if they were sensitive beforehand. Commonly, tenderness in sensitive spots in the longer leg disappears completely after use of the proper lift for the shorter leg. If tenderness does not disappear, it may mean that I need greater compliance or greater lift, but it also might mean that I need other treatment such as strapping or orthotics to control the pronation. This finding is therefore not as specific to following LLDx treatment, but often very helpful.

To Clinicians who take LLDx seriously:

First of all, my compliments. Being willing to be open to a totally new approach is hard for successful and experienced clinicians. This is especially true when that new approach might negate the need for some of the services they provide. To any specialist who makes evaluation and treatment of LLDx part of the initial protocol, my hat's off to you.

I want to caution you about the need for being aggressive with the use of the lifts. It is NOT ENOUGH to provide a lift and discharge. Either enough lifts should be provided for multiple shoes for the first few "test" days, or the person must specifically agree to use the lift all of the time and switch it from shoe to shoe, even in the house, or the lift must be strapped to the foot. There should be rapid follow up to follow the signs of PseudoStenosis associated with LLDx. Less than this aggressive approach will result in failures due to either poor compliance, or improper lift height. All of the magic that can occur is premised upon strict use of a proper lift for a few days, and it is essential that everything possible be done to ensure that compliance.

I keep a large supply of vinyl lifts in the office, in packs of 4. My profit on them is quite low, and they end up taking room and effort. They are, however, great for the bottom line, if resolution of pain and restoration of activity is how you measure your practice success. Just remember that whether you strap with a lift as an initial test, or you provide durable lifts, or if patients order them on line, it is essential to confirm the potential benefit by a few days of strict use of the proper size lift, and to help patients succeed long term by guiding to the proper, durable lifts that most patients will need forever.

Limb Length Discrepancy: Final Thoughts, until Chapter 19

Children, Limb Length Discrepancy, and Growing Pains

Kids make up only about ten percent of my practice, so their stories are only a small portion of those in this book. I want to take a "time out" to focus on them.

The arthritis and other disabilities all too common in adulthood do not develop in a vacuum; most often they develop because of poor mechanical function caused by the same problems that cause PseudoStenosis. Arthritis caused by poor mechanical function is the focus of Chapter 19. Here I want to stress the importance of evaluation and management of LLDx in children, since their symptoms are usually not caused by obvious arthritic changes.

Many children suffer from what are labeled "growing pains." WebMD.com defines growing pains as "cramping, achy muscle pains" that children feel in their legs, with symptoms often occurring in the late afternoon or evening, or during sleep, causing the child to wake up. Other than activity, there is no cause suggested on that website.

Since the early 1980s, I have been among those who recommend stretching exercises as treatment for this leg discomfort. In addition, it is common knowledge in the podiatry community that children with flexible Flat Feet and growing pains usually have good improvement with orthotics, with surgery being necessary less frequently. I continue to use stretching for tight muscles and orthotics for Flat Feet, as described in detail in this book.

However, I find that a great many children have growing pains because of a mild (but not minor!) Limb Length Discrepancy. Identifying and treating a discrepancy as small as $\frac{1}{16}$ of an inch, just under 2 millimeters, by using the tools presented in this chapter, often provides quick and persistent relief. This should be the first avenue of investigation.

I now repeat something that is easy and essential to follow. Remember the Iliac Crest Pain Resolution Sign, presented in Chapter 6 and reviewed in this chapter? Most frequently, children do not report that sensitivity as pain, but as ticklishness. When they stand, one or both hips are sensitive. With the proper lift, the ticklishness disappears immediately. (Just be sure not to over-treat. Use only the minimal amount of lift needed to make the hips coplanar and eliminate sensitivity, and follow cautions explained in this chapter.) After a few days of *full-time* use of a lift of the right size, the ticklishness is gone, even when the child stands without the lift. Often, the growing pains are gone too. For many children—and adults as well—using both orthotics and a heel lift is best.

Does Limb Length Discrepancy Run in Families?

I have had many families in which multiple children, as well as parents and grandparents, had symptoms and/or deformities caused by LLDx. It is therefore a pattern that I keep in mind as I evaluate individuals. However, a definitive answer to this question can only be answered by large medical studies.

* * * * *

Now that you appreciate the subtleties of confronting Limb Length Discrepancy, I will share two more stories that stress the need to pay attention to details, appreciate the patient's history, and use thoughtful clinical judgment.

StoryTime: Jane J was a 70-year-old woman who presented with a 4½-year history of progressing foot, leg, and back pain. She could at times walk up to a block before being forced to sit because of pain, but often standing or walking for even one minute was too much. She had been awakened by foot and leg pain every night for years. The whole process began after she was in an automobile accident in which her left heel bone (calcaneus) was badly fractured. Within a few months she had fusion of the joints in the back of the foot, which successfully relieved the severe arthritic heel pain. Months later, when she began walking, the pain in her back, leg, and throughout the bottom of her foot became progressively worse. She had two epidural injections for the spine pain and suspected nerve pain, but one provided only a few hours of relief, and the other provided less than one day of help. She declined the spine surgery recommended and lived with chronic pain and severe restriction in activity.

Fast-forward four years. My examination suggested a structurally short right leg. She had Equinus greater on the right, far greater nerve sensitivity on the left, a higher and extremely painful left Iliac Crest, which improved with a ³⁄₁₆-inch lift under

Reasons that LLDx Might be Undertreated

I strongly believe that Limb Length Discrepancy is undertreated because of four factors that this book can help overcome, and because of two factors that will likely present an ongoing challenge. The four are as follows:

1. *Lack of awareness of the wide range of symptoms LLDx can cause*
2. *Lack of awareness that LLDx as small as 1/16th of an inch, which is less than 2 millimeters, can cause significant symptoms*
3. *Lack of awareness of the tools that can facilitate suspicion and then identification of LLDx*
4. *Lack of awareness of the details needed for successful treatment*

One factor that will likely present an ongoing problem is that there is an inconsistency of presentation when a functional component to LLDx is present. The clinical appearance of the LLDx often changes. This could undermine the confidence of any treating clinician, as inconsistent findings would make it hard to make clear recommendations. This problem may be magnified by the reality that the time constraints of a busy medical practice may not include the opportunity to treat and recheck quickly, something I find so helpful. Even a clinician sensitive to the importance of LLDx might find it challenging to make the time to follow this condition with confidence, because of the change in appearance that may be present with an unresolved functional LLDx. I believe that success will require a greater awareness on the part of patients, combined with the conscious decision within the medical establishment to make management of this pervasive condition a priority.

The second factor is the lack of a radiology protocol to definitively guide management. Testing (as explained in Chapter 14) is often quite helpful, but the management decisions should be guided by detail oriented cooperation by patient and clinician, an ongoing challenge.

the right heel. She had acute tenderness along the tarsal tunnel area, making me suspect entrapment of that nerve, which I treated with a topical diclof-enac anti-inflammatory gel. I strapped both feet and included a ⅛-inch lift for the left foot and a ⁵⁄₁₆-inch lift under the right heel.

Five days later, Jane returned to the office a different person. From the second night after her initial visit, she was able to sleep without interruption. She had 100% relief of chronic back pain, almost 100% relief of leg pain, and over 70% relief of left foot pain. The day before, she had gone to a mall and had walked extensively without limitation, and she reported that the foot pain was mild to moderate but did not interfere at all with activities. Examination showed that the asymmetric Equinus was resolved. Hip sensitivity was completely resolved, even when she was standing without a lift. The left hip was still higher, suggesting a structural LLDx. The nerve sensitivity of her left leg was resolved,

although she was still somewhat sensitive at the tarsal tunnel area, which I felt was responsible for the limited symptoms she still had within her left foot. A single steroid injection for Tarsal Tunnel Syndrome resolved the residual foot pain.

Jane J's interview from her second and third visits may be found on WalkingWellAgain.com.

The lessons? I have had many patients in whom a fracture was the cause of development of a short leg causing LLDx. **In this case, the fusion of the rear-foot resulted in a slightly longer leg,** a situation that cascaded into a full-blown case of Pseudo-Stenosis, which caused years of back, leg, and foot pain that made it so hard to walk, stand, and sleep. **A CT Scanogram would have been negative, as the problem was below the ankle joint.** Based on Jane's history, I would have suspected the left to be

---

Self-Care for Patients: Essentials of Treatment for Limb Length Discrepancy

1. *Start with less than the perceived difference, especially if the perceived difference is ³⁄₁₆ of an inch or more. One may be more aggressive with lifts if there is structural difference between the feet, or if an injury or surgery caused the LLDx.*

2. *Use the lift full time, inside and outside of the house, even in bedroom slippers.*

3. *The lift should immediately be relatively comfortable. If it is uncomfortable, do not use it.*

4. *If symptoms do not improve within 2 days, you may add additional lift.*

5. *If Equinus of the shorter leg does not improve within 2 days, add additional lift.*

6. *Recheck within a few days, and again within a few weeks, and again periodically, to ensure that the discrepancy is still present. Remember that it is important to be sure that you are not dealing with, at least in part, a functional Limb Length Discrepancy. Even if still comfortable, the lift may be removed if the apparent difference between the limb lengths resolves. **Long-term unneeded use of a lift can cause problems.** If you have any question, discuss the issue with a podiatrist, physical therapist, physiatrist, chiropractor, or orthopedic surgeon, preferably one who is familiar with the ideas in this book. If unsure, seek radiologic examination such as a CT Scanogram or Long Leg Study, or X-ray of the spine with various lifts.*

7. *You may need an extra-depth shoe, an external shoe modification, or an Evenup, if the discrepancy is over 3/8 of an inch.*

8. *If you have Flat Feet or one Flat Foot, you also may need an orthotic or a brace. Check with a medical professional such as a podiatrist or orthopedist regarding the options.*

9. *Modifying your old orthotics may be helpful. If it is not, seek evaluation for possible new orthotics or brace.*

10. *If you have only partial improvement, you may also need Positional Testing for Spinal Stenosis, or you may need to receive care for other causes of PseudoStenosis.*

11. *If you have persistent pain from other areas of arthritis, see an appropriate specialist. **Keep in mind that treatment that previously failed may become more effective once the Limb Length Discrepancy is properly addressed.***

12. *If a functional discrepancy is suspected, it is best to work with a clinician!*

shorter, but this was not true. Fortunately, all physical findings suggested a short right leg, and she responded well. In my opinion, all other treatment would have been doomed to failure.

StoryTime: Bayla was a 65-year-old woman with chronic left hip pain. Therefore, this story might be better for Chapter 19, but for the purpose of focusing on managing LLDx, I include it here.

She had improvement of chronic foot and ankle pain with custom orthotics, but she still had hip pain. Exam suggested a ³/₁₆-inch discrepancy with the left being shorter, but she did not have the classic findings of asymmetric Equinus or asymmetric nerve sensitivity. In fact, she had a moderate bilateral nerve sensitivity. I added a ⅛-inch lift to her left orthotic, and she reported moderate improvement. She still had some hip pain, and the findings were not classic, so I removed the lifts and ordered a CT Scanogram.

The results reported that there was an LLDx of 0.0 millimeters. No difference! However, without the lift, her left hip had gotten worse. As we talked further, she reported having had scoliosis since she was a child. Feeling that this was a fixed functional LLDx, I provided her with the full amount of lift, which again moderately reduced her left hip pain, but I referred her to a physiatrist for further evaluation and overall management.

The lesson? In her case, findings were not classic, and this appears to have been a functional, rather than structural, LLDx. The lift was moderately helpful, but it was not the long-term answer.

I present a great many cases throughout this book in which there is wonderful and complete resolution of long-term symptoms. **I believe it essential to also include stories in which the treatment I tried provided limited or even no help, and the patient required other specialists for overall management.** This is one of those cases.

For Clinicians: My Strongest Encouragement

For clinicians, I present a final summary, a story, and a baseball analogy about LLDx, now that you have *so much* background. As strongly as possible, I encourage all of you to make LLDx awareness a part of your clinical routine.

I pick up LLDx in just a few minutes with new patients or with return patients with new problems, or, to be honest, if I did not look quite thoroughly enough at the prior visits. **Let's get that in print. We all see things on follow-up visits that we missed earlier.** In addition, we search for new observations if new symptoms require a new evaluation.

I am directed to look for a Limb Length Discrepancy by ANY of the shared clues:

- Asymmetry of feet, including Equinus
- Uneven heel position when sitting
- Shoulder asymmetry when sitting or standing
- Positive Positional History
- Symptoms of Spinal Stenosis or of any of the conditions listed in Section 3 of this book
- History of sciatica, Ilio Tibial Band Syndrome, Meralgia Paresthetica, or herniated disc
- History of degenerative arthritis of spine or lower extremities
- History of major fracture or any major joint surgery
- Lower-extremity symptoms of neuropathy or poor circulation
- Pain in the back or legs when standing, walking, lying down, sitting, or upon arising
- History of neck or shoulder pain
- Recalcitrant spine or lower-extremity symptoms of any cause

I do a QUICK check for the signs. I check for Equinus to assess if the shorter-appearing leg is the tighter one. I check the First Interspace Fine Sign. If bilaterally symmetrical, it is usually not just LLDx causing problems, but if primarily on one side, it might be! I check if the longer-appearing leg is more tender, as is most common in mild discrepancies of about ¼ inch or less. If the discrepancy is over ¼ inch, greater nerve hypersensitivity is more common in the longer leg, but also may be found in the shorter leg. I check for structural differences between the feet, ankles, and knees. I check the Pes Anserinus, and also check for other areas of biomechanical stress, which will be addressed in Chapter 19. I have patients stand, and I then check hip symmetry. If the hip bone is tender, that often resolves immediately with the proper lift, that amazing Iliac Crest Pain Resolution Sign. I rebalance with lifts until hips are symmetric, although I may treat with less than that amount, as has been described. Once this process is mastered, it can take only five or ten minutes minutes. The result is frequently invaluable information, and often, an amazed patient.

I encourage ALL CLINICIANS who treat any of the conditions addressed in this book to make LLDx awareness part of your routine. Not just podiatrists. Primary care providers, including internists, family practitioners, nurse practitioners, and physician assistants, can also check this. Specialists, including physical therapists, physiatrists, rheumatologists, orthopedists, spine surgeons, vascular surgeons, neurologists, and sleep specialists, should consider this diagnosis and quick exam. Since so many conditions are caused or exacerbated by this

Home Run or Strikeout at the First At-bat

Treating LLDx is often an essential part of successful treatment for any of the conditions mentioned in this book. When indicated, I almost always include mechanical treatment for LLDx (and at times, Flat Feet) as part of my initial intervention, and most often wait a few days before adding other treatment such as medications, injections, Positional Testing, or physical therapy.

If the patient is not significantly better in a few days, I may have struck out, but it was only my first at bat! As long as I have been clear on the possibility that other treatments should be added, I will (usually) get additional at bats.

If, however, there is good success, then the patient and I have hit a home run. We've achieved success without the other treatments such as injections, medicine, surgery, and even physical therapy, treatments that many people prefer to avoid. Success leads to the ability to provide long-term resolution of a chronic problem with mechanical treatment that is safe and often inexpensive, what I consider to be a grand slam.

In baseball, it is accepted that home run hitters will strike out occasionally as they strive for the long ball. Similarly, I find that most patients are willing to be patient and to try simple and safe treatment first before adding medicines, injections, casting, or therapy, and to delay other treatments to see if the initial treatment provides improvement.

incredibly common problem, it should be on everyone's radar. **If you suspect or even consider LLDx but do not feel comfortable checking for it yourself, or if you want to have a more thorough exam regarding PseudoStenosis, please refer the patient to an appropriate clinician. The results can be life changing.**

Story Time: This one is an unbelievable story, which the patient's caregiver tells on WalkingWellAgain.com. Corey H was a middle-aged man with a severe mental disability, who was brought to me to have his thick fungus nails trimmed. He was non-communicative, neither speaking nor responding to any verbal efforts on my part. His caregiver had a relationship with him and was able to direct him. She had been taking care of him for over five years. Obviously, he did not complain of any other symptoms. His caregiver reported that he could walk adequately for the very limited distances that were part of his daily life. He had, however, for the past several years, a problem of rubbing and scratching his feet throughout the day. He had been evaluated by a dermatologist, who had provided topical creams, none of which had provided relief.

My exam suggested a Limb Length Discrepancy of about ⅜ inch, a tight Achilles tendon on the short side, and a positive First Interspace Fine Sign on the longer leg. **These findings suggested possible PseudoStenosis from a Limb Length Discrepancy, which, among other things, could cause neuritic pain in the feet or legs.** I provided ¼-inch lifts for the shoes for the shorter leg along with appropriate discussions, and wished them good luck.

Three months later the patient was brought back to the office for trimming of thick fungus toenails. The caregiver had a new story. By the first day after his first visit, all rubbing and scratching had stopped, and it had not resumed during the entire three months! My exam showed no nerve sensitivity, and the tightness of the Achilles on the shorter leg had resolved. He still appeared to have a Limb Length Discrepancy, but both the secondary signs and the symptoms had resolved. All improvement was maintained at the next (six- and nine-month) visits.

The lesson? A podiatrist, or anyone else examining feet, should look for signs consistent with Pseudo-Stenosis, especially Limb Length Discrepancy, and if found, should immediately suspect that it may be causing problems. There should then be a doubling of effort to take a complete Positional History, combined with questioning the possibility of all the other conditions addressed in this book. I cannot tell you how many times this clinical exam and a quick Positional History clued me in to find conditions that patients had not bothered to mention, or as with this young man, could not explain.

The six other causes of PseudoStenosis are less common than LLDx. Flexible Flat Feet and #7, a lower extremity pain conition that alters a person gait, are usually seen at least a few times each week in my office, while the others are less common.

Keep in mind that success with any of the other causes of PseudoStenosis often requires addressing the LLDx.

Is a Mild Discrepancy a Minor Discrepancy?

For years, when patients asked me if the surgery I was going to perform was major or minor, and I always replied that there is no such thing in the world as a minor surgery . . . if it's being done on me.

I believe the same is true with Limb Length Discrepancies. While a larger LLDx is more likely to cause visible changes, even a mild LLDx may cause a lifetime of problems. I emphasize now, as I did at the beginning of this chapter, that I have had hundreds of patients who had wonderful improvement with only a 1/16- or 1/8-inch lift, approximately 2 or 3 millimeters. It is essential to understand that mild does not mean minor!

Patient Information Handout on Heel Lifts and Limb Length Discrepancy

I believe that you have a Limb Length Discrepancy that may be causing you problems. I am providing you with heel lifts for you to use in shoes or add to your orthotics.

Basic information you need to know

1. *Success requires that, at least initially, you use the lift as much as possible. It should be in all your shoes, those worn both inside and outside of the house. Do not go barefoot. You may even attach a vinyl lift to a flip flop or croc for taking a shower.*

2. *If this will be helpful, there will be improvement of symptoms within 1–3 days.*

3. *If the lift causes worsening of your condition, stop using it! If it feels a little funny, or you note the difference but it is not uncomfortable, you may continue to use it.*

4. *There are two types of LLDx. With a structural LLDx, one leg is actually longer than the other leg. With a functional LLDx, spine or pelvic imbalance provides the appearance and at times induces the symptoms of a Limb Length Discrepancy. You may have both structural and functional discrepancies at the same time. It is necessary to follow up to make sure that the clinical appearance does not change. It is therefore essential that you have a follow-up appointment. At times the appearance may change, and the amount of discrepancy may seem less, or occasionally more, than that seen at the first visit. We will reevaluate you at the next visit.*

5. *If clinically necessary, we may order radiologic testing to further investigate this LLDx.*

6. *There is sometimes value in beginning with a lift less than the amount of LLDx seen, and increasing gradually. _____ If improvement is limited, increase a small amount after 2 days*

7. *It appears that your shorter leg is the ____left ____right, and the discrepancy is, in MM:*
   ___1 ___2 ___3 ___4 ___5 ___6 ___7 ___8 ___9 ___10   Other_____

8. *The initial lift height we are starting you with is in MM:*
   ___1 ___2 ___3 ___4 ___5 ___6 ___7 ___8 ___9 ___10   Other_____

9. *If this provides valuable assistance, you may need to use lifts long term (forever).*

Inexpensive excellent lifts can be purchased on line through the store section at WalkingWellAgain.com or directly by calling 866 Heel-Lft.

Pes Planus—Flexible Flat Feet

The role of the Flat Foot in lower-back pain has been recognized for decades, and has been written about by giants in the fields of both podiatry and biomechanics. Drs. Howard Dananberg, Douglas Richie, Richard Blake, Paul Scherer, Kevin Kirby, Steven Subotnick, Sheldon Langer, and Justin Wernick are just a few of the many great clinicians and authors who have shared great clinical insights about biomechanics and orthotics over the past decades.

Readers should know that my advice on how to treat Flat Feet biomechanically is not original. My contributions are limited to connecting this problem to the concepts of PseudoStenosis and to promoting the idea of coupling the Flat Foot treatment with other successful approaches presented in this book.

Readers should also know that evaluation and treatment of Flat Feet is a deep subject, and I only scratch the surface in this section and in Chapter 19.

Flat Foot, also known as "Pes Planus," is a deformity in which the arch of the foot collapses, has collapsed, or never developed properly, with the bottom of the arch coming into complete or near complete contact with the ground. This may greatly affect the function of the foot and leg, and it may also affect the knees, hips, and spine, as will be presented in this chapter and in Chapter 19.

This foot type, also described as a "pronated foot type," is in most cases flexible but may also be rigid. This is an important point to remember, as the treatment approaches for different types may be different.

"Pronation" refers to motion in three planes: DORSIFLEXION (when the joints of the foot move upward), EVERSION (when the outside of the foot comes up), and ABDUCTION (when the joints and structure of the foot turn outward, away from the midline of the body).

What you need to know is that a pronated foot is flatter than it should be. If it is flexible, the foot looks like it has more of an arch when the person is sitting. I have had many patients who denied having a Flat Foot by pointing out a beautiful arch . . . that disappeared with standing.

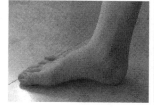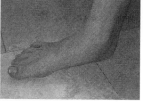

Picture 12.26. A moderately flexible Flat Foot. Looks more normal with sitting; flattens with standing.

Functional Hallux Limitus

One distinct feature often associated with a Flat Foot is a condition called "Functional Hallux Limitus," or "FHL." The person with FHL has good motion of the big toe joint when not standing, but limited motion and altered function when standing or walking.

This is in contrast to a structural Hallux Limitus, a condition in which there is arthritis and limited motion of the big toe joint. In FHL—at least early in the disease process—the person has good motion of the big toe joint when not bearing weight.

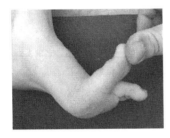

Picture 12.27. Normal motion of the big toe joint.

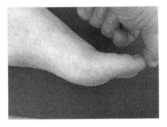

Picture 12.28. Limited motion of the big toe joint.

With FHL, it may be noticeable that the big toe has an unusual, or at least distinctive, shape. The end bone of the big toe (the distal phalanx) turns upward. This may be seen both when the person is sitting and when he is standing, and is called "Hallux Extensus Interphalangeus."

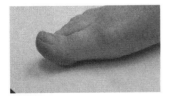

Picture 12.29. Hallux Extensus Interphalangeus.

This foot type is often seen with significant pronation (flattening) and often affects the overall posture.

It may be associated with Kyphosis, a mild or worse hunching of the thoracic spine, which is below the neck.

> *Functional Hallux Limitus has (for decades) been identified as being associated with chronic or frequent low-back pain, neck pain, TMJ (jaw pain), and even migraine headaches.*
>
> *Whenever I see a patient with FHL, I question the patient regarding the above-mentioned symptoms. If the symptoms are present, I test for whether the FHL and the symptoms are related, by testing the effect of mechanical control, either by strapping the feet or by applying Unna boots, both of which are described extensively in the appendix. This Mechanical Testing, like Positional Testing, usually provides relief within 1–3 days. If you suspect this problem, walk—or run—to a good biomechanically aware podiatrist.*

Strapping as a Mechanical Test

Once the condition of Flat Feet is suspected as the cause of PseudoStenosis (or any other set of symptoms), it usually calls for professional evaluation and treatment. Often, orthotics or braces are all that are needed to control the biomechanical problems that are the source of the symptoms. Mechanical testing can help predict which treatment will be effective. With a mild-to-moderate or even a moderate-to-severe Flat Foot, my approach is to use a modified Low Dye strap, which is explained in detail in the appendix. The patient must keep this clean and dry for at least 3 days to ascertain improvement in function and symptoms.

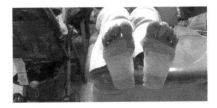

Picture 12.30. Modified Low Dye strap, with a 1/8-inch reverse Morton's extension.

If the Low Dye strap proves helpful, I ask the patient to keep it on for the several days between visits, for two reasons. Wearing it maintains the therapeutic improvement. Improving the spine function, and thus eliminating the pressure on the nerves for many days, gives the nerves time to heal. If the nerve inflammation resolves itself, the symptoms *may* not come back quickly! At the least, many people who find relief of nerve pressure over the course of many days enjoy relief that persists for the weeks that it takes for the permanent devices to arrive. Many patients, however, have recurrence without support, and they either suffer recurrence of symptoms or they return to be treated mechanically with an Unna boot or strapping while waiting for the permanent device.

There is another option, to provided over the counter non custom inserts, instead of strapping. This has some advantages. However, I feel that the strapping approach has the following major advantages:

> ## Introductory Thoughts on Orthotics
>
> *In the section on LLDx, I mentioned use of an **orthotic as well as a lift**. As will be clarified in this section, I find that a great many people with flexible Flat Feet experience great improvement with orthotics. The use of orthotics is also something of an art. Individuals may have tried orthotics before without improvement, or they may have been unable to tolerate the insert. Orthotics are often ineffective or uncomfortable when there is a cause of a flexible Flat Foot that has not been controlled. Two common causes of this situation are Equinus (usually caused by tight leg muscles) and Limb Length Discrepancy. Adding a lift to the shorter leg for a discrepancy, or adding lifts to both inserts in the case of Equinus, may solve the problem. After these problems are addressed, orthotics—maybe even your old orthotics—may then be comfortable and helpful. I hope you didn't throw them away!*
>
> *It also MUST be recognized that orthotics have many shapes and features. **Failure with a particular pair of orthotics does not mean that orthotics cannot work for you, only that the previous pair did not work.** This is especially true if they were provided by someone who did not have all the information and experience to solve your particular challenge. Show your provider this book. It may be food for thought for that provider and the right help for you!*

- The effect of strapping is just as good as a custom orthotic.

- Modifications to enhance the effect can be built into the strap.

- It facilitates compliance by allowing the patient to wear any shoes and still enjoy the benefit of the mechanical control.

- Most important, it induces compliance, by not being removable! Unless the person removes the strap, which is something they cannot hide, the strap is on full time.

- Since compliance is enhanced, success should occur within 1-3 days. If not successful, other treatment can be investigated, with the confidence that compliance was adequate.

Follow-up exam after strapping

A major reason to keep the strap on until the next visit is that it allows me to do my follow-up exam with confidence. People with Functional Hallux Limitus often have severe sensitivity along the bottom of a joint in the midfoot, the first metatarsal cuneiform joint. Successful elimination of this sensitivity suggests to me that the mechanical support we tested was adequate. If that area remains very sensitive, I consider the possibility that different mechanical control is needed.

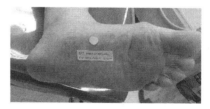

Picture 12.31. The circle shows the location of the bottom of the first metatarsal cuneiform joint (MCJt). This spot is often very tender when a person has symptoms associated with the mechanics of a flexible Flat Foot. If this area stays tender after strapping, I try more aggressive mechanical control.

The other specific areas that I routinely check in such cases are the areas of nerve hypersensitivity (as described in Chapter 6) that are found on physical examination. The second, third, and fourth intermetatarsal spaces, along with the tibial and femoral nerves, are often extremely sensitive to pressure in patients with either Spinal Stenosis or PseudoStenosis. This is a sign consistent with spinal nerve irritation from SS/PS. If nerve sensitivity improves with Mechanical Testing, this confirms that the biomechanical function of the foot affected the biomechanical function of the back that was causing the nerve sensitivity! In other words, *PseudoStenosis.*

If the nerve sensitivity does not improve, then it is more likely that the feet are not the primary problem causing symptoms, or that inadequate control (of either Flat Foot or LLDx) has been effected. If, however, the severe sensitivity disappears—usually in just a day or two—the patient and I both know that the strap has accomplished something great, that we have controlled the spinal nerve irritation causing PseudoStenosis symptoms. If sensitivity remains in either the nerves or the joints, we still have work to do!

After any treatment for either Spinal Stenosis or PseudoStenosis, for all of the clinical conditions that are mentioned in Section 3 of this book, I do a follow-up exam, checking both for areas of mechanically induced sensitivity and for those of nerve sensitivity.

Success with Strapping Suggests Likely Success with Orthotics

If strapping is helpful, orthotics are indicated. Occasionally, over-the-counter orthotics can be helpful. In most cases, with symptoms as significant as those addressed in this book I recommend custom-built orthotics fitted and provided by a podiatrist. This is not a place to skimp if you can at all afford it. It is much easier for me to suggest that a patient spend the money needed for orthotics when testing by strapping demonstrates the potential for improvement.

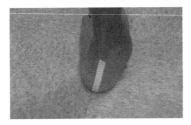

Picture 12.32. A Flat Foot with an everted heel. The tape shows the eversion of the heel with the foot bearing weight.

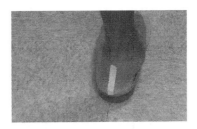

Picture 12.33. The same foot resting on a custom-built orthotic. Eversion of the foot is reduced even without the supportive structure of a shoe.

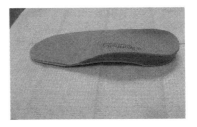

Picture 12.34. The orthotic used in this case to control symptoms coming from moderately severe Pes Planus.

I do not use orthotics routinely, but rather selectively. A *section on the decision as to whether or not to use orthotics is included in Chapter 19, "Understanding and Managing Arthritis through the Gift of Biomechanics."*

Unna Boots and Ankle Braces

If the Flat Foot is more severe or more rigid, I may test with an Unna boot, which is kind of like an ace bandage that stays moist after it is put on. This is an old treatment, long used to treat stasis ulcers on the inside of the ankle caused by vein problems. I have used Unna boots for years as a first line of treatment for certain conditions (such as Posterior Tibial Tendonitis) and to test to see if a brace will be helpful. I do this instead of sending the patient for physical therapy, believing that if we can realign the structures and remove the abnormal mechanical stress, the inflammation and pain will subside without medicine or therapy. The approach usually works quite well. To maximize the mechanical control, I may add a reverse Morton's extension or a Cluffy wedge to the Unna boot. I also add a heel lift if there is a Limb Length Discrepancy.

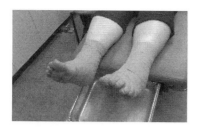

Picture 12.35. Unna boots applied, to test for likelihood of effectiveness of an ankle brace.

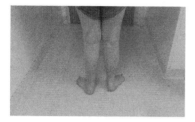

Picture 12.36. Severe Flat Feet associated with chronic back and leg pain, which improved with Unna boots.

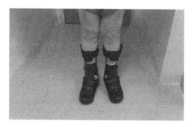

Picture 12.37. Immediate improved position with Arizona Hinged Braces. Chronic PseudoStenosis pain resolved with the use of these braces.

For clinicians applying straps or Unna boots, I share observations and techniques you *might* find helpful. These are found at the end of the book, in the appendix.

Treatment for the Flat Foot condition can have many benefits, not only in improved mechanics of the spine and the spinal nerve irritation that causes secondary foot or leg symptoms, but also in more direct improvement of a great many problems within the foot and leg. These will be addressed in Chapter 19, on arthritis.

StoryTime: Leslie is the young lady whose story introduces Chapter 1. She came to the office with a chief complaint of right heel pain, which had been bothering her for months. Further discussion revealed she also had jaw pain from TMJ, neck pain, back pain, leg pain, and foot pain, which had been present for many years. She could only walk one

to two blocks before severe pain set in, which often lasted for hours. By midafternoon, she was able to go upstairs only by crawling on her hands and knees.

Having had Lupus, a form of inflammatory arthritis, for over 30 years, all of her symptoms had been attributed to that disease. She'd been treated with physical therapy, steroids, and other medications, which had provided limited, short-term help.

Leslie walked better when pushing a grocery cart, which suggested the presence of Spinal Stenosis or PseudoStenosis. She also had a bilaterally symmetrical First Interspace Fine Sign, with severe sensitivity in the second, third, and fourth intermetatarsal spaces as well as along the posterior tibial and femoral and tibial nerves on both the right and left sides. Her symptoms involved jaw pain and headaches, and she had Hallux Extensus Interphalangeus and other signs of a pronation problem, but she had no evidence of an LLDx. I used a bilateral Low Dye strap to test for Flat Feet as a cause of PseudoStenosis, including modification with a Cluffy wedge and a reverse Morton's extension.

I saw her again three days later. **All the TMJ, neck pain, and back pain were gone, as was most of the leg and foot pain.** She was able to walk for blocks with none of the chronic pain, and was able to go up and down the stairs with no limitation. Almost all of the nerve sensitivity was gone. All this improvement occurred within three days!

Symptoms that had been diagnosed for years as having their source in Lupus had actually been caused by her biomechanical problems that led to PseudoStenosis. All the improvements were maintained with orthotics. Three of her interviews—on her first visit, on the visit a few days later, and then at another visit a few months later—can be seen on the website, WalkingWellAgain.com.

By the way, there are two completely separate points to learn from her story. One of the reasons her symptoms—all of which resolved so quickly—were so severe may have been her Lupus. It is known that inflammatory arthropathy, such as Lupus or Rheumatoid Arthritis, is more susceptible to symptoms from nerve compression, which is in part what had happened here. A valuable lesson.

Secondly, you may notice the fact that after the strapping, *almost* all the nerve sensitivity was gone. What was left was tenderness along the posterior tibial nerve on the right foot and along the third and fourth intermetatarsal spaces, in addition to the original heel pain that she came in with. I felt that she also had a Tarsal Tunnel Syndrome involving the Lateral Plantar Nerve, a condition described in Chapter 6. During her second visit, I casted her for orthotics and repeated the strap to maintain improvement. I also provided a topical anti-inflammatory cream for relief of the tarsal tunnel sensitivity. When that did not work, I gave her a cortisone injection into the area of the tarsal tunnel, which succeeded in relieving the foot pain. A year later, she had no recurrence.

I would not have been able to diagnose her tarsal tunnel condition accurately, with a specific pattern of nerve sensitivity, until we relieved the nerve sensitivity that was coming through the spine—in this case, from PseudoStenosis caused by flexible Flat Feet. Sometimes a few visits are needed to conduct a proper investigation and come to all the right conclusions!

CHAPTER 12F

Five Less Common Causes

Rigid and Nearly Rigid Flat Feet

Rigid Flat Feet are not as easily controlled as flexible Flat Feet may be. In my experience, orthotics usually do not work well with rigid Flat Feet, but an Ankle Foot Orthosis (AFO) such as the Arizona Brace described above might. It will not make the foot and ankle function normally, but it may improve function enough to improve back function and local arthritic symptoms. A description of local arthritic symptoms and concerns is included in Chapter 19.

By this stage, I hope you are aware of the spine-mediated symptoms, including back pain and Pseudo-Stenosis. If they improve with the Mechanical Testing of the Unna boot, an AFO might do the trick. If the symptoms do not improve with mechanical control, then this may be a situation in which PseudoStenosis needs to be managed with Positional Testing (Chapter 7) and Adjunct Measures (Chapter 8). Don't forget: if the Flat Foot is more severe on one side, consider Limb Length Discrepancy! For overall management of this condition, you will need an excellent physiatrist, podiatrist, orthopedist, physical therapist, or chiropractor, and quite possibly more than just one of them.

Recognizing and Treating Equinus

Equinus, as you may recall, is a limitation of adequate motion upward within the ankle joint. It is most often caused by tightness of the muscles in the back of the leg, involving the Achilles tendon complex. The limited motion within the ankle can also be caused by other soft tissue pathology or arthritic changes causing an actual bone block.

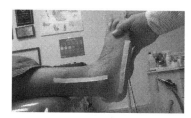

Picture 12.38. A repetition of picture 12.17, showing that the foot, when slightly inverted and pushed upwards, gets to 10 degrees short of the perpendicular.

The tight muscles can give rise to a variety of symptoms. There may be leg cramps at night. This is a common cause of "growing pains" in children, which, unless treated, often persist into adult life. Equinus can cause legs to tire with walking, mimicking claudication from poor circulation. If more severe, Equinus can cause an instability in which the person feels as if he is going to fall backward. It can create greater pressure on the front part of the foot, worsen pronation, and cause calluses or bunions. It is a common problem that makes orthotics or even braces too uncomfortable to wear.

There can also be a compensation that occurs in the knees, involving a backward curve in the knee called "Genu Recurvatum."

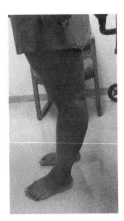

Picture 12.39. Genu Recurvatum.

When Genu Recurvatum occurs, the person's femur, or thigh bone, leans a bit forward proximally higher up. In order for the person to stand straight, he or she must increase the extension of the spine. This can cause narrowing of the spinal canal and lead to nerve sensitivity consistent with Spinal Stenosis.

In addition, Equinus is a force causing increased pronation (flattening) of the feet, causing an internal rotation of the leg structures, affecting the spine function. In other words, the presence of Equinus can worsen symptoms associated with Flat Feet, as reported in the previous sections of this chapter.

There are different ways to deal with the muscle tightness associated with Equinus. One is to accommodate the tightness by wearing shoes with significant lift in the heel or with a high heel, such as a cowboy boot. This eliminates the need for the backward curve of the knee and the secondary increased spinal extension.

It is also quite reasonable simply to add lifts to the bottom of orthotics, if Equinus makes them feel uncomfortable in the arch. Don't forget: you may need to add more lift on one side if there is a Limb Length Discrepancy!

If the person has severe Equinus and requires an ankle brace, the brace may cause pain in the back of the calf. This may be eliminated by putting felt padding on the top of the brace in the area of the heel.

Another way to treat the muscle tightness is to do stretching exercises, which sometimes work and sometimes do not, depending upon the origin and nature of the Equinus. **Greater details of my take on Equinus**

and stretching are expanded upon in Chapter 21, on nighttime symptoms.

An essential point to bear in mind: **if there are symptoms of SS/PS, with spinal nerve irritation and nerve sensitivity, stretching may worsen that sensitivity and set of symptoms.** While this can be addressed in many ways, I will share six.

One way is to alter the method of stretching. In normal stretching, there is some hyperextension of the spine, as seen in picture 12.40.

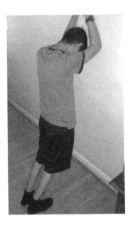

Picture 12.40. Standard stretching may hyperextend the spine and aggravate symptoms and sensitivity associated with SS/PS.

By standing farther away from the wall and placing the hands and elbows lower, one can stretch the tight leg muscles, flex the lower spine, and avoid hyperextending the spine. For some of my patients, this allows stretching without exacerbating SS/PS symptoms and sensitivity.

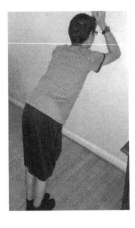

Picture 12.41. Stretching from farther away from the wall to allow pull on the Equinus without hyperextending the spine.

A second way to deal with the need to stretch in the presence of active SS/PS nerve irritation is to relieve the nerve sensitivity by doing Positional Testing first. Use the walker as directed, and perform the adjunct interventions as discussed in Chapters 7 and 8. Symptoms may disappear in a few days, but I recommend full-time use of the walker for at least a week before beginning the stretching exercises needed to resolve the Equinus. At times, physical therapy can help with stretching that an individual cannot manage alone. That is a reasonable option if you've had no luck on your own.

A third way of dealing with Equinus is to use a manipulation technique to increase flexibility within the ankle joint, which improves motion at the head of the fibula, in the area of the knee. This technique has been popularized in the United States by Dr. Howard Dananberg. I have personally used it only occasionally but have seen some individuals with improvement from using it.

A fourth way to treat Equinus is to use a standard night splint, which I have occasionally used with some success.

Options five and six are to reduce the Equinus medically or surgically. Botox injections have been reported to provide months of improvement in tight leg muscles. Surgical treatment can provide permanent correction, although the type of surgery of course depends upon the nature of the Equinus. Surgery is usually reserved for people who do not get relief with nonsurgical treatment, and it is often successful.

More details on Equinus are included in Chapter 21, on nighttime symptoms, since Equinus is such a common cause of nighttime leg cramps.

Altered Gait Caused by Stroke or Other Nerve Dysfunction

This is a complicated condition. There are so many different ways that a stroke or other neurologic injury can affect a person's gait, many of which can affect spine function and cause SS/PS symptoms. Treatment necessitates working with a good orthopedist, physiatrist, physical therapist, or podiatrist, or with a team.

Quick Resolution of Bilateral Equinus

In this book, there is frequent mention of the phenomenon of unilateral Equinus secondary to LLDx resolving completely with appropriate use of the proper-size lift. I've used this to follow treatment in hundreds of patients, and I find it essential for the management of LLDx.

There is a related pattern that I have seen less than 20 times but that has powerful implications.

*When there is significant bilateral Equinus worse on the short leg, with Pes Planus and significant symptoms, I (like many other podiatrists) strap as a test for the efficacy of mechanical control. In such a situation, I now add 1/8 inch for the heel of the longer leg, and 1/8 inch PLUS compensation for the measured LLDx for the shorter leg. **In such cases, I frequently see resolution of Equinus in both legs.***

I have explained that I believe that the asymmetric Equinus on the short leg is a subconscious attempt by the body to keep the spine level, and that removing the need (LLDx) results in resolution of the Equinus in 1–3 days. Similarly, I believe that the dysfunction of the Pes Planus (which may be felt consciously or subconsciously) may induce the body to try to reduce the pronation by supinating and plantar flexing the foot and ankle, inducing Equinus. By removing all the pronatory stress through the straps and the lifts, the need for the body to compensate is gone, and the Equinus may quickly resolve.

*In years past, I would have treated such a person quite differently. If stretching for the Equinus had not been effective, orthotics had not been helpful or tolerated, and physical therapy had not been helpful—and long-term symptoms were affecting the quality of life—surgery would have been the next option. This would have involved lengthening the Achilles tendon complex and correcting the Flat Foot deformity. And yet here in 2015, I find that the approach described above **sometimes** eliminates the bilateral Equinus in just a couple of days, allowing the individual to tolerate and benefit from orthotic or AFO control.*

I do not know how frequently this approach will work in such patients, but I felt it essential to present these details for orthopedic and podiatric surgeons to consider.

The first thing to consider is the origin of the lower-extremity symptoms. Are the actual symptoms caused by the stroke or another neurologic problem, or are they caused locally by the primary foot and leg dysfunction, or are they at least in part caused by SS/PS? The Grocery Cart Test is wonderful for clarifying this. If there is great improvement with a cart, there is most likely an SS/PS component to the limitations, and there may be great improvement with full-time Positional Testing and Adjunct Measures. This method can be diagnostic as well as therapeutic, because the spine inflammation from nerve compression usually resolves in a matter of days, demonstrating that the symptoms that improved clearly did not derive primarily from the stroke. **After all, if the symptoms and nerve sensitivity were from a stroke, using a walker for a few days would not change that!**

After a stroke, the affected extremity may have severe Equinus with a very tight Achilles tendon, which usually does not improve with stretching. In contrast to the above scenario, where the shorter leg has a tight tendon, this situation is functionally the opposite. It is often associated with contracture of the knee and restricted movement of the hip. The tight tendon actually causes the affected leg to function as the *longer* leg. Using a lift will not help the tightness go away. In such situations, I use enough lift ON BOTH SIDES to allow the patient to stand comfortably, and there is often an immediate improvement in terms of increased stability when standing. (Otherwise, patients often feel as if they are standing in a way that causes them to fall backward.) It is important to use the same amount of lift on the opposite foot, in order to not cause the body to function with an environmental Limb Length Discrepancy! Often patients must use a walker for stability, but they find that use of a walker combined with the amount of lift needed to compensate for the neurologically induced Equinus is very helpful.

There is an excellent article addressing changes that occurred in function of both lower extremities, after taping mimicked the Equinus associated with a stroke. It was published in *Gait and Posture* in 2004 by Michael Goodman and other authors, and is entitled "Secondary gait compensations in individuals without neuromuscular involvement following a unilaterally imposed Equinus constraint." Details of the article are included in the appendix.

Of course, even in a person who had a stroke or other neurologic injury, one should also check for Limb Length Discrepancy, because it is possible that the stroke affected a limb that was already shorter. I have seen this several times. I am NOT saying that the Limb Length Discrepancy is a result of the stroke, just that by percentages, *some* people who have strokes already have a Limb Length Discrepancy. In situations where there was Equinus caused by both LLDx and a stroke, there is a good chance at reducing the Equinus by treating for LLDx with enough lift, leaving only the Equinus component caused by the stroke. This often restores greater balance and reduces abnormal strain on the spine that can cause PseudoStenosis.

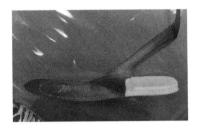

Picture 12.42. Lift added to brace for Drop Foot.

A lift may be incorporated into an ankle brace or orthotic, or the patient's shoes may need to be modified. Custom-made braces and off-the-shelf braces may both be used for people who have had a stroke. The decision as to which is appropriate should usually be made by a specialist.

I have seen several patients who developed a PseudoStenosis phenomenon because of the effect that this kind of problem had on the spine. **It was assumed that their nerve pain was from the stroke,** but either Positional Testing for SS/PS or Mechanical Testing for the local foot dysfunction (such as a brace or a lift) eliminated the pain. Therefore, even if a person has another possible cause of symptoms (such as Diabetic Neuropathy or a stroke), I believe it is essential that Spinal Stenosis and PseudoStenosis be considered and investigated.

StoryTime: Brandon W

Brandon W was a 34-year-old man who had a lifetime challenge of Cerebral Palsy. For interested clinicians, it was a mild case of Spastic Hemiplegic CP, including left arm contracture and Equinus, knee contracture, and mild steppage gait.

Colleagues, please do not get skeptical. Keep in mind that there are different patterns of Spastic Hemiplegic CP, and that this is only one single case. I do not know how widespread the ramifications are. However, also keep in mind that LLDx is common in CP.

Brandon had Equinus of –20 degrees of his left, affected leg, and my measurement suggested a ⅜-inch discrepancy. A CT Scanogram reported a 9-millimeter difference, exactly what my exam suggested. The visit after I strapped that amount to his left foot, examination showed that his Equinus was totally resolved: his ankle dorsiflexion was now 90 degrees, perpendicular. In addition, his mild knee contracture was completely resolved. He walked and stood better with just the lift. With a shoe with an 8-millimeter sole lift, these improvements were maintained.

The lesson? In this case, his Equinus resolved quickly, despite the presence of Spastic Hemiplegic CP. As with patients with Equinus related to strokes, I recommend evaluation and treatment for LLDx in patients with Spastic Hemiplegic CP. Such investigation should include the caveat of an appreciation that even partial improvement can be clinically helpful. Here I speculate. I wonder if LLDx plays a role in the Equinus pathology and gait challenges of many people with Spastic Hemiplegic CP.

A video interview from Brandon's second visit is available on WalkingWellAgain.com.

Neurologic impairment is usually not a condition that patients can treat themselves. I strongly recommend that you follow up with a physiatrist, or with a podiatrist with special interest in these conditions, to investigate further.

Altered Gait Caused by a Painful Condition

Painful conditions of the foot, the ankle, or any other part of the lower extremity may cause a person to walk differently. **Any walking pattern that causes you to walk differently in order to avoid pain may be called "guarding."** Sports doctors generally advise athletes to recover to the point where they no longer need to alter

Cerebral Palsy

Another type of neurologic dysfunction that causes some gait abnormalities similar to those caused by a stroke is Spastic Hemiplegic Cerebral Palsy (CP), which is a condition causing damage to the motor centers of the developing brain. It occurs either during pregnancy or delivery or during the first three years after birth. The resultant problems are usually not progressive.

In Spastic Hemiplegic CP, one side of the body is affected, the hemiplegic side. In 2010, an article* was published noting that the hemiplegic side was shorter than the other by more than 15 millimeters in 25% of teenagers studied. They suggested that the Limb Length Discrepancy should be addressed clinically. I laud the article and insight.

Please note the criterion they note for a problematic LLDx. It is 15 millimeters, the same 3/5 of an inch listed in the article on LLDx in army recruits mentioned at the beginning of this chapter. There is a consideration among authorities that an LLDx that large must be present for there to be problems. I repeat for the umpteenth time: I find that there are often symptoms and physical findings associated with even a 2-millimeter difference.

Without speculating on frequency, as my experience is too limited with this group, I will present that I have had a few patients with documented Spastic Hemiplegic CP in which a clinically valuable amount of the Equinus resolved after compensation for LLDx, allowing for more normal gait, or after use of a brace allowed more normal gait. LLDx should be investigated in all patients with this form of CP.

* Riad J., Finnbogason T., Broström E. 2010. "Leg length discrepancy in spastic hemiplegic cerebral palsy: A magnetic resonance imaging study." J Pediatr Orthop. 30 (8): 846–50.

* J Pediatr Orthop. 2010 Dec;30(8):846-50. Leg length discrepancy in spastic hemiplegic cerebral palsy: a magnetic resonance imaging study. Riad J[1], Finnbogason T, Broström E.

their gait to avoid pain, since any abnormal gait pattern would make them more susceptible to new injury. The same holds true for patients with a painful foot or leg who walk in a compromised manner to avoid pain. This altered gait may cause strain in other joints and altered function in the back.

This condition leads to a complicated situation that has a few possibilities.

1. The lower-extremity pain is caused directly by local pathology.

2. The pain in the lower extremities is partially caused by Spinal Stenosis, which is exacerbating the local problems.

3. The pain in the lower extremities is partially caused by PseudoStenosis, in which the altered gait induced by painful foot or ankle condition causes spinal dysfunction, which in turn causes nerve sensitivity that exacerbates the pain from the local problems.

4. Both Spinal Stenosis and PseudoStenosis are present, in addition to local pathology.

So, how do you tell if there is a PseudoStenosis or Spinal Stenosis component? By now, if you have read through the book, you may know the answers.

A positive First Interspace Fine Sign is suggestive of SS/PS. There is no reason for those nerves to be so sensitive because of localized foot or ankle pain. Just keep in mind the other possibilities presented earlier, in Chapter 6 in the section entitled "Basic Podiatry: Other Common Nerve Sensitivity Patterns."

A positive Positional History and/or a rapid response to Positional Testing strongly suggest either SS or PS. Significant relief of foot or leg pain in the presence of a painful foot condition suggests that SS/PS plays a part in the symptoms. There would be no reason for a walker or the Professor Position to relieve the pain of, for example, foot arthritis.

But wait. For long-term management of this condition, we need to distinguish between SS and PS. How to check? When it comes to suspecting Limb Length Discrepancy or Flat Feet, it is possible to do Mechanical Testing and see if that eliminates pain. Similarly, you can identify the cause of pain that *may* be causing the PseudoStenosis, treat it, and just wait a day or two. If the treatment is successful, it may reduce or even eliminate all SS/PS symptoms.

Several times, I've had patients come in with severe foot pain from porokeratosis, a form of callus that can be very deep and painful, and a classic Spinal Stenosis presentation that was actually PseudoStenosis.

StoryTime: Reena was a 33-year-old woman who came in complaining of severe foot pain with deep calluses called "porokeratosis." In addition, her back hurt, her legs hurt with standing, the nerves in her feet and legs were sensitive, and the calluses were very painful. How could I determine if her severe pain was from the calluses alone, if there was a primary problem with her spine that was causing the back and leg pain, or if the way she walked was causing the back problem—a PseudoStenosis presentation?

In her case, it was easy. I aggressively trimmed and padded the deep calluses. A few days later, as expected, the pain from the calluses disappeared. In addition, her back pain was gone, the leg pain that had caused such difficulty when standing or walking was gone, and the severe nerve sensitivity was gone.

In my mind, the sequence confirms that the problem had been PseudoStenosis. Had Reena undergone spine surgery, the operation would not only have been unnecessary—it would quite likely have failed.

There was recurrence of all symptoms when the calluses came back, so Reena will need either periodic care or surgery to treat the calluses.

Similarly, I have had patients with Sinus Tarsi Syndrome that caused PseudoStenosis, including back and leg pain and nerve hypersensitivity. This condition involves pain in a joint just below the ankle, although it often feels as if it is *in* the ankle. Sinus Tarsi Syndrome often develops because of an ankle injury, although it may not show up for months afterward. It is a not-uncommon cause of persistent pain after ankle injury or surgery. Twisting the ankle (suffering a mild sprain) can cause a flare-up of severe pain, sometimes weeks or months after the initial injury.. The joint below the ankle is often severely sensitive.

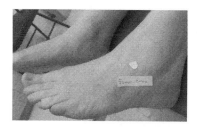

Picture 12.43. Circle identifies the sinus tarsi.

Sinus Tarsi Syndrome can cause ankle pain and aching in the front of the lower leg, but not pain in the back or thigh or even calf—at least not directly. However, if an altered walking pattern causes PseudoStenosis, all those other body parts can hurt. Again, I have had people for whom all these areas were severely painful for a long time, and who experienced relief from all their symptoms soon after injection of the sinus tarsi, without recurrence. Sinus Tarsi Syndrome often has long-term relief with injections, and may also be successfully treated with use of either an orthotic or an ankle brace.

StoryTime: Elsie was a 70-year-old woman who presented with back and leg pain that had developed gradually over a period of about 9 months, beginning in the wake of a mild ankle sprain. The pain prevented her from walking more than the length of a block. She also experienced some discomfort in the left ankle.

Examination showed a Limb Length Discrepancy, asymmetric Equinus, and severe nerve sensitivity. Suspecting that the Limb Length Discrepancy was the cause of her symptoms, I provided a lift. The results were not as good as I'd hoped. The lift provided only mild help, allowing her to walk two blocks before she had to stop and sit down because of back, leg, and ankle pain.

It was time for a reevaluation. The Equinus was gone, but the nerve sensitivity persisted. This time, however, I recognized severe sensitivity in the sinus tarsi, which I injected with cortisone. A few minutes later, all the "ankle" pain was gone. Even better, the following week Elsie reported resolution of all the ankle pain, as well as the pain in her leg and back. My exam showed that all nerve sensitivity had disappeared as well. Just three days after the injection, she went out to a shopping mall for hours! In her case, spinal and secondary leg symptoms had been caused by Sinus Tarsi Syndrome and the resultant altered gait. Months later, she had no recurrence.

StoryTime: Augustine presented with pain that had been ongoing for several years in her spine, right leg, and right foot. She had fractured her right ankle 15 years earlier, which required surgery. She'd taken anti-inflammatory medicine for years and had had several epidural injections in the spine. The injections provided only short-term help for a few days or no help at all. My exam showed a Limb Length Discrepancy, with the right leg shorter by about ⅜ of an inch. There was an asymmetric Equinus, and nerve sensitivity in both legs. I found tenderness in the sinus tarsi and the ankle joint, especially along the screws that had been used to repair the ankle.

Hoping the pain had just been caused by the Limb Length Discrepancy, I provided a lift for her shoe. Although Augustine at once stood with greater balance, the lift did not help mitigate her back or leg pain. Considering the ankle and sinus tarsi arthritis, I applied an Unna boot. Home run! She was immediately able to stand and walk without foot or leg pain, and much of her back pain disappeared as well.

Several days later, she returned to report that all foot, leg, and back pain was gone. I casted her for a brace, which arrived a few weeks later. Once she was without the Unna boot, all the pain returned. She did fine with the brace, although it irritated the screws in her ankle from the surgical repair, so I sent her back to the surgeon to have that taken care of.

Augustine's case is one in which ankle arthritis and sinus tarsi pain altered her gait enough to bring on PseudoStenosis symptoms. With a hinged brace that eliminated ankle pain and dysfunction, her gait also improved, and all the symptoms were controlled.

Two videos of Augustine's visits are available on WalkingWellAgain.com.

These are just some of the painful conditions that I have seen many times cause PseudoStenosis, with resolution of all signs and symptoms of the back and lower extremities just by the treatment of one problem in the foot. There are many others. It is not necessary to list them. **It is only necessary to be aware that a painful foot or leg problem should always be addressed when investigating for Spinal Stenosis or PseudoStenosis.**

Lower-Extremity Arthritis as a Cause of PseudoStenosis

Arthritis is a wily character. It disguises itself easily and can hide its origins behind a plethora of painful symptoms.

There are many distinct ways in which arthritis can blend with Spinal Stenosis or PseudoStenosis.

- Any altered gait caused by the arthritis can cause the spine to function improperly, thus giving rise to spinal arthritic pain or nerve irritation. In the absence of actual Spinal Stenosis, this would certainly be a manifestation of PseudoStenosis.

- Altered gait may aggravate true Spinal Stenosis.

- The definitive hip or knee arthritis may cause local pain but no aggravation of back function or spinal nerve activation.

- The lower-extremity arthritis symptoms, including the hip or knee, are actually secondary to Limb Length Discrepancy or Flat Foot problems. Tending to the underlying problems may completely or at least significantly resolve the arthritis issue.

Arthritis is a very complicated condition. How to categorize and evaluate arthritic symptoms is addressed in great detail in Chapters 18 and 19.

When a patient with any severe lower-extremity symptom experiences even a temporary improvement—through injections or other treatment options—the upshot may be that the patient begins to walk more normally. This in itself can reduce or eliminate the secondary spine dysfunction. **I believe strongly that any painful condition in the foot, ankle, knee, thigh, or hip should be investigated and hopefully addressed before the person decides on spine surgery—to eliminate the possibility of a PseudoStenosis contribution to the overall pathology.**

PseudoStenosis: Final Thoughts

Chapter Summary . . . Until Now

Allow me to summarize these last two chapters and then present four supplemental and yet essential concepts. I've thrown a lot of material at you, and I want to make sure my conclusions thus far are very clear.

"PseudoStenosis" is a term I have coined that refers to a condition in which lower-extremity dysfunction causes the spine to malfunction in a way that may mimic **Spinal Stenosis**. As such, PseudoStenosis may be responsible for a wide variety of symptoms, either mimicking or exacerbating all the conditions listed in Section 3 of this book. The symptoms may be viewed as overlapping, or at times may be misdiagnosed when there are multiple conditions present. These include arthritis, Peripheral Neuropathy, arterial circulation problems, venous circulation problems, Fibromyalgia, Restless Leg Syndrome, and others.

Often, treating the lower-extremity dysfunction (which, in the case of a suspected Limb Length Discrepancy, may be done by the patient himself) can provide rapid and dramatic relief of symptoms and physical signs that would otherwise be considered to be coming from Spinal Stenosis. Other possible causes should be investigated in all patients with Spinal Stenosis symptoms.

In the majority of cases, treatment for possible PseudoStenosis is something that I do in my office before starting treatment for actual Spinal Stenosis. Mechanical Testing with lifts, straps, or Unna boots may provide rapid relief. If it does, this suggests a long-term treatment plan. Using lifts for Limb Length Discrepancy, or

lifts to modify old orthotics, may provide effective Mechanical Testing. Otherwise, you may need professional help for Mechanical Testing or treatment for suspected PseudoStenosis.

It is reasonable to start Positional Testing with the walker and all Adjunct Measures to get relief of symptoms, if you have to wait for treatment of PseudoStenosis. Of course, I believe that Positional Testing should almost always be the initial treatment for actual Spinal Stenosis.

PseudoStenosis combined with actual Spinal Stenosis is a very dangerous combination. Because the symptoms are mediated through the spine, spinal treatment such as physical therapy and epidural injections can provide good temporary help, suggesting that the spine is the actual primary problem. When the causes of PseudoStenosis are not considered before spine surgery, the persistence of the actual root of the problem may cause the surgery to fail or the symptoms to recur, no matter how well the surgery is performed. Therefore, biomechanical evaluation and treatment should generally be implemented before spine surgery is attempted. This treatment may improve the likelihood of long-term success in patients who need surgery, and may obviate the need for surgery in many others.

I share this view with you as a strong conviction. However, please remember that I am just presenting my opinion, and that it is not at all standard treatment in managing spinal pathology. Do not be shocked if it has not been included in your treatment plan until now. After all, that's the whole purpose of this book!

There are two more ideas and two great stories that I'd like to share to wind up this long chapter.

The ideas, for both clinicians and the lay public, are on the need to consider this new diagnosis and on the value of Mechanical Testing as a way to negate the need for a leap of faith.

(The material originally included for clinicians at the end of this chapter—details of strapping and Unna boots and my full Examination Form—has been moved to the appendix.)

StoryTime: Hold the Blame

This story is different from all the others in the book. It's a bit funny, and the lesson is indirect.

A young woman of 18 was brought in by her mother for a toenail problem. She had High-Arched Feet, fairly rigid. Although she had no pain, we discussed the fact that her foot type did not absorb shock well, but rather transmitted the shock higher up the leg. I told her that shoes with good shock absorption or with silicone lifts could be useful for preventing long-term back, hip, or knee problems. I also mentioned casually that this foot type could also cause a loud footstep that could be misinterpreted as an ANGRY way of walking.

The teen turned to her mother. Turning both hands into fists, she raised them high in the air and shook them, yelling, "SEEEEEEEEE!" On her face was an emotional release, as she finally found support that she was not walking loudly on purpose, as she'd apparently been accused of doing for many years.

I immediately put on my "counseling hat" and assured the mother that the daughter's foot type caused the loud footstep, and assured the daughter that there was no way for her mother to have known this. This was not a time for blame, but for moving forward.

Why is this story relevant to *Walking Well Again*? A great many people with PseudoStenosis have had severe symptoms present for years. Many have had many medical evaluations, along with tests, such as MRI, circulation tests, tests for neuropathy, blood work for possible arthritis, and so on, without ever finding a cause. Many have had extensive treatment that did not solve the problem. Some may have been accused of exaggerating their symptoms or of just being lazy. For years.

Now you can consider a new condition as the possible cause of so many symptoms. I assure you that PseudoStenosis can cause almost all of the symptoms described throughout this book. You, too, may have been accused of exaggerating or creating symptoms. On the other hand, the physicians have been in the mother's situation, as there was no way for them to have known this before, since this approach is not yet established in medical literature. This is not a time for blame, but rather for moving forward. If you suspect that PseudoStenosis MIGHT be a problem, have it checked out!

Mechanical Testing

This next section, for both clinicians and patients, is about **Mechanical Testing** with strapping and Unna boots for symptoms caused by pronation. **Mechanical Testing is a way to eliminate the need for a "leap of faith."**

Imagine. You, the patient, have an appointment with a podiatrist. Perhaps you've come about the kind of serious, long-term problems that are addressed in this book, or maybe you've come in for one of the significant problems that are more standard for podiatry, such as an ingrown nail, heel pain, a bunion, etc. In either case, the doctor asks some questions, conducts an examination, and tells you that he or she can probably improve your long-term and disabling symptoms, which on the surface seem unrelated, but which are likely caused by your foot function. GREAT! But there's a catch. Treatment will cost several hundred dollars for orthotics, or even more for ankle braces. Here is where a leap of faith comes into play.

You might understandably ask yourself some questions. Is your doctor being honest, or is he just trying to sell you something? Why didn't your other doctors suggest this over the years? Does your insurance pay for orthotics, and if not, why not? Is the kind of success that the doctor is talking about actually possible? If treatment helps, how much will it help? Can mechanical control with orthotics or ankle braces actually improve long-term symptoms that have been present for years? What if you had orthotics before and they did not help? Will they work for you this time?

All valid questions.

As a treating clinician, when I evaluate a patient and decide that there is a good chance that orthotics or braces will resolve his symptoms, I have a dilemma as well. **After all, I am not sure**. I just *think* that the symptoms will improve with this kind of care. Orthotics cost hundreds of dollars, braces are closer to a thousand dollars, and both take weeks or longer to arrive. How can I ask someone to spend so much money and wait weeks for an answer, when I am not confident of the results?

Mechanical Testing instead of a Leap of Faith

This is where Mechanical Testing with straps or Unna boots is such a blessing. If the testing works, there is improvement within just 1–3 days, at which point both patient and doctor can be confident of the likelihood of long-term improvement with orthotics or braces, which provide the same mechanical control that the test does. I can then cast and order devices with confidence.

I will often replace the strap or Unna boot, sometimes even keeping symptoms controlled in this way until the orthotics or braces arrive. Occasionally this is not needed, as even a few days of good mechanical control can provide a reduction of inflammation that persists for days or weeks after the support is removed.

The important point is that within a few days, both patient and clinician will have an excellent idea as to whether or not the biomechanical intervention tried can work, and they can use that knowledge to direct long-term treatment.

What about the "leap of faith"? I use this set of techniques to help not only foot and leg arthritis symptoms, but also PseudoStenosis symptoms that can mimic or exacerbate neurogenic claudication, arthritis, neuropathy, poor circulation, and all of the other conditions mentioned in this book. Believing that this is possible constitutes a leap of faith. **Mechanical Testing allows us to know if that leap is justified! It answers all the clinical questions mentioned above.**

For both patients and clinicians I will share a great story, including a lesson learned from one of my many mistakes.

StoryTime: This anecdote refers to both arthritic pain and PseudoStenosis. Patsy P came in for treatment of an ingrown nail, but discussion revealed that she had had chronic pain with her feet and legs for many years, which made it hard for her to walk, stand, and, especially, climb steps. She also had had chronic back pain since she was a teenager, as well as headaches and progressively severe neck pain. Finding only limited and temporary help from medications, injections, and therapy, she was resigned to taking strong narcotics three times a day. By the way, she reported walking much better pushing a grocery cart.

Physical examination showed, among many other things, severe flexible Flat Feet bilaterally, Hallux Extensus Interphalangeus, and severe sensitivity along the plantar aspect of the first metatarsal cuneiform joint. She also had a severe First Interspace Fine Sign on both feet and nerve hypersensitivity in her legs, with no signs suggesting Limb Length Discrepancy. I was not sure if we should first treat for Spinal Stenosis or for PseudoStenosis, but chose the latter and strapped her up, including a reverse Morton's extension.

The next week, Patsy happily reported to my staff that almost all of her foot and leg pain was gone, so they prepared her room for me to cast her for orthotics. Since it was a busy day, I walked in and casted her, and prescribed an aggressively controlling orthotic. AS SHE WAS LEAVING, I remembered to ask about her other symptoms, the back, neck, and headache pain. When I heard that those symptoms were no better, I sent her back to the treatment room, and we applied Unna boots to both feet and ankles. Several days later, she reported a home run. Her feet and legs stayed fine, and the back and headache problems she had had for over 40 years disappeared. Only moderate neck pain remained. I felt she needed more control than orthotics could give, so I left the Unna boots on and sought approval from her insurance company for the more expensive Arizona Hinged Braces. Approval came in a week later.

Whoops. The day she came in for casting for the braces, the orthotics arrived. My staff had sent out the casts for orthotics, because I had never told them not to. Since they were there, I provided the patient with the orthotics, with curiosity.

She used the orthotics for several weeks until the Arizona Braces arrived. She had maintained the same improvement in foot and leg pain as was obtained by the strapping, but had not maintained the improvement of long-term back and headache symptoms. They were back to the level of the previous 40-plus years.

I provided the Arizona Braces. A happy ending. The braces did the trick and eliminated the back and headache symptoms. Six months later, all symptoms were still resolved. She often used the orthotics for more limited activity and used the braces if she was going to be more active. No more narcotic use, unless she was having bad pain with her neck, a much less common occurrence. Patsy P's interview is on WalkingWellAgain.com.

There are three lessons to be learned from this story. First of all, at least in this case, the improvement obtained with orthotics followed that of the straps, and the improvement with the gauntlet braces followed that of the Unna boots. Second, the symptoms of both arthritis and PseudoStenosis, even if present for decades, may improve within days of rebalancing the faulty biomechanics. Chapter 19 is aptly named "Understanding and Managing Arthritis through the Gift of Biomechanics."

The third lesson is stressed in Chapter 19 but is fitting to stress here as well. **In order to optimally treat the problems that can be associated with Flat Feet, you have to recognize what those problems might be.** Please, do not misunderstand me. I am NOT saying that all patients with chronic headaches, knee pain, local back pain, and neurogenic symptoms consistent with Spinal Stenosis symptoms have their problems caused by Flat Feet. I am saying that some do, and that if that may be the case, it should be investigated using the rapid, safe, and inexpensive techniques of Mechanical Testing.

* * * * *

For patients, their families, and other laypeople, I hope these chapters on PseudoStenosis have provided you with the needed information to consider the many lower-extremity problems that can affect SS/PS symptoms, and to seek the help you need in dealing with symptoms that are addressed in the next section of this book.

Clinicians, I hope that this has also been helpful for you. At this point I want to reiterate that most of the biomechanical observations of this book are not original on my part. In the Appendix, I present a list of published articles that support some of the findings of this chapter and those of Chapter 19. These two chapters are strongly interrelated; for those seriously considering the insights of this chapter, I recommend studying that chapter as well.

CHAPTER 13

An Overview of Supportive Devices

With Positional Testing, use of the proper type of walker, properly set and properly used, often results in very significant improvement within just a day or two. That improvement can be seen in patients' overall ability to stand and walk, their decreased level of pain, and their changed sleep patterns. Using a walker is a safe, inexpensive, and rapid way to improve your quality of life.

> ## For Clinicians:
> ## About Walkers in Medical Offices
>
> *I believe that having walkers in the office is essential for any clinician actively treating symptoms of the spine or lower extremities addressed in this book. Testing for improvement with Positional Testing and identifying the optimal height for any individual patient are essential steps in pain investigation and management. It is necessary to have the various types needed, including walkers that can accommodate both short and tall people, to properly prescribe the optimal walker height, as well as to demonstrate quickly to the patient the potential for rapid improvement. To treat the conditions listed in this book, you must have the necessary tools, including walkers.*

That's why I strongly encourage patients to allow themselves to be open to using a walker despite possible concerns about how they look. For most people, use of a walker is only temporary or at least only temporarily full time. A major part of the battle is the willingness to use the walker, so I am glad you are here.

By the way, the emphasis I put on using a walker is the exact reason why I rarely provide them in my office. I don't want to be accused of "selling walkers" since I push so hard for their use.

Are You Strong Enough for a Walker?

Before addressing the question of what type of walker would be best for you, first decide if you have the strength and balance necessary to use a walker. If you have been able to walk for a few minutes without a walker, or even with one, it is likely that you will be able to use a walker successfully during the Positional Testing protocol.

If, however, you have been unable to walk for even a few minutes with or without support, then before you begin Positional Testing you should have an evaluation and the help of a good physical therapist. In this situation, you may need help gaining balance, strength, and confidence to begin. Failure to obtain that help could result in falls and injuries. **I therefore repeat: if you have not been able to stand or walk for even a short time, then get professional help before beginning.**

> *If you need to see a physical therapist or other professional to help you begin to walk, that does NOT necessarily mean that you should not use the flexion position for Spinal Stenosis. Your therapist may not concur. At the time of this writing, therapists usually disagree with me. In fact, all too often a therapist will change the walker to the standard height as suggested in the standard literature, after which I change it back. Eventually, the patient will make the final decision based upon what proves most helpful. That's fine with me. If you do need a therapist to help you begin walking again, please show the therapist this book. You, the patient, may know almost immediately which position feels the best. So by all means include the therapist when making your decision—but at least give my recommendations a try.*

Maybe Two or More Walkers

Sometimes a patient will initially need more than one walker. You might need a second walker for a second floor or basement. You might walk best with a rollator walker but be incapable of moving it down the steps to get out of the house or of putting it into a car. In such cases, you might need a standard folding walker with wheels and skis when navigating alone, since it is so much lighter.

I stress again, for good reason, that the handle height of the walker is crucial in Positional Testing. Let's review the common types of walkers and explore the advantages and disadvantages of each of them in specific situations.

The Four-Wheeled Rollator Walker

The walker that I recommend most often is the four-wheeled rollator walker. This walker has several advantages.

First, most models are quite easy to push for most people. Second, this type of walker has a seat that you can sit on. People who previously were unable to walk

the hoped-for distance may have found themselves "trapped"—that is, in so much pain that they were unable to continue walking, and not in good enough shape to sit on the ground and get up again. Without a chair to sit on, they were in an untenable situation.

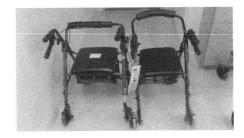

Picture 13.1. Four-wheeled rollator walkers, junior size.

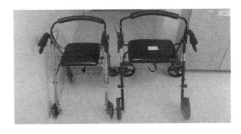

Picture 13.2. Four-wheeled rollator walkers, standard and bariatric sizes.

Having a seat on the walker removes the fear of being "trapped" and keeps a person from becoming what I once described as a "Spinal Stenosis Cripple." This phrase is not meant in a negative way. It simply recognizes the fact that the inconsistent walking limitation characteristic of that disease process prevents some people from walking even short distances if there is no place to sit along the way. The walker seat removes that limitation. This is a major advantage.

This is not, however, the main advantage of using a walker with a seat for successful Positional Testing. **The main advantage is that the seat can be used as a tray to transport objects.** I want the patient initially to strive to use the walker one hundred percent of the time. If there is a need to carry packages or laundry, or even move food from the kitchen to the dining room, the walker seat can be used as a tray so that the walker may be used full time. **This is the greatest advantage of the drop-down seat: the ability to use the walker full time.** After all, full time means full time!

Apart from the various brands that are manufactured, there are also multiple types of this four-wheeled rollator walker, geared to different body weights and heights. As explained in Chapter 7 on Positional Testing, **the most crucial aspect of using a walker is the handle height**. Thus, even though some patients are too heavy to qualify for using a standard or junior (pediatric) walker, it is vital that the handle height be considered the most important factor.

This is true even if a person is too wide to sit on the walker or is heavier than the walker is certified for. For example, if someone weighs 270 pounds but is only 5'2", that person needs the junior walker for Positional Testing, even if that walker is only approved for someone weighing 220 pounds or less. The weight limit is only for sitting, and I would sacrifice the patient's ability to sit in order to ensure the right height, keeping the seat for use as a tray. This is especially important since the severe walking limitation that the individual has lived with for years may be dramatically improved in just a few days, rendering the ability to sit on the walker seat much less important.

> *My goal is to help a patient achieve the proper spinal position and to control the SS/PS symptoms. I have, however, had a few patients who felt the positional benefits were limited and preferred to have a wide walker that allowed them to sit when necessary, rather than a low walker that induced a flexion position. If there is a question as to which walker to get, I usually lend the patient a walker that induces flexion first, to allow them to experience the benefits of my choice of flexion position.*

Many manufacturers have at least three models of four-wheeled rollator walkers. There may be a standard walker, whose handle height is usually between about 32 and 37 inches. This is usually fine for people above 5'6". Remember that these numbers are only approximate.

The next walker is the junior (pediatric) walker. Here, the handle height may go as low as 28 or 29 inches and raise up to about 34 inches. This is an appropriate walker for people from about 5' to about 5'9".

The bariatric walker is designed for people above approximately 275 pounds. Different versions come in different heights.

As with all the other walker types, there are some disadvantages to the four-wheeled rollator walker when compared to the other walkers listed below. These disadvantages will become clear in our discussion of the other walkers.

The Three-Wheeled Rollator Walker

I originally recommended this walker for most of my patients, though I now do so less frequently. Even so, it has a few major advantages over the four-wheeled walker. The main disadvantage is obvious. This walker does not have a drop-down seat to sit on or to use as a tray. A few versions do, however, have a small tray available for carrying small items like food, but the carry-on area is definitely much smaller than on a four-wheeled rollator.

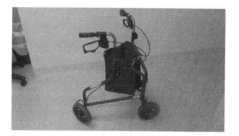

Picture 13.3. A three-wheeled rollator walker.

What are the advantages of the three-wheeled walker? First, it is slimmer and therefore easier to fit through narrow areas. It is intrinsically narrower than the four-wheeled version, and by adjusting a part in the front it can be made even more so.

Second, some versions are lighter than the four-wheeled walkers. Some patients have difficulty lifting a walker in and out of a car, and those few pounds can make a big difference.

Finally, because of the way it folds, this walker is actually easier to fit in a backseat or trunk of a car. For all these reasons, I still at times recommend the three-wheeled walker. As always, achieving the correct height is the most essential point of all.

The Standard Folding Walker

The last kind of walker that I'll address here is the standard folding walker. Most versions of this standard walker do not have a drop-down seat to enable the user to transport items and to walk without fear of being stuck with no place to sit. However, this walker is significantly lighter and easier to stow in a car than either a three- or four-wheeled walker. Some seniors are still independent enough to drive themselves around but not strong enough to lift a rollator walker. They may not be quite strong enough to lift a rollator walker up a few steps if they go for a walk alone outside the house. For these people, having a lighter standard walker is valuable.

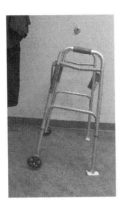

Picture 13.4. Standard folding walker with wheels in the front and sliders in the back.

Standard folding walkers come in different versions. For most people, the easiest one to use has wheels in the front and skis in the back (see picture 13.4). This walker is almost as easy to push on most flat surfaces as a wheeled walker, but it is not as good for uneven or rough surfaces. I most often use this as a primary walker for individuals under approximately 5', as this walker comes in a pediatric version that has a minimum height of 26 inches, in contrast to the rollator walkers I now use, which have a minimum height of 28.5 inches.

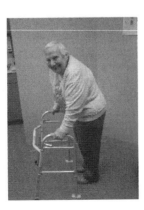

Picture 13.5. At 4'8", this person is still able to achieve a comfortable flexion position with a pediatric walker at 26 inches.

At times, there is value in setting this standard walker to a slightly lower height in the back section. Patients often have a tendency to stand inside the walker and not flex the spine. By setting the back section slightly lower, the handle is angled and the patient is forced to stand farther back and lean into the walker, thereby flexing the spine.

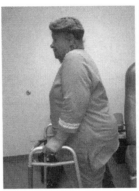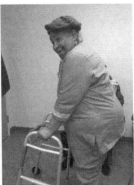

Picture 13.6. These pictures demonstrate how altering the configuration of the walker by lowering the back section may induce the individual to stand behind the walker and lean forward.

For individuals with balance difficulties, a walker without wheels may be necessary. This type of walker has the disadvantage of requiring the patient to lift the walker with each step and turn. However, even if this kind of walker is needed for stability, having it set to the proper height to induce slight lumbosacral flexion is also of real value. Once again, if there is ANY question as to the person's ability to use a walker without falling, a good physical therapist would be the best choice for aiding in the process of increasing the person's walking ability.

Other Walker Types and Walker Attachments

Another valuable type of walker is a platform walker, which has arm supports that help a person that does not have full use of one or both arms because of orthopedic or neurological problems. Imagine someone who has a weak or contracted arm as a result of a stroke and is unable to use a regular walker. This walker has a platform to lean the arm on and help stability. I have ordered this type of walker or handle only a few times, but for such a person it makes the difference between being able and not being able to use a walker properly.

There are many other types of walkers you can find online or at a durable medical equipment dealer. I mention the ones that I use, but if you need another type, just be sure to get guidance by an expert.

There are many attachments for walkers, such as cup holders, seats, trays, and arm rests. Anything that makes the walker easier to use is worth investigating.

Use of a Cane

Finally, there is the cane. Canes are very valuable walking aids. They do not, however, usually add great walking-distance ability or reduce SS/PS pain for most individuals with Spinal Stenosis. That particular observation is corroborated by a 2010 article* that reported that the cane does not improve walking-distance ability in patients with Spinal Stenosis. A cane is not as good a tool as a walker, but nonetheless it may be helpful for patients with SS/PS. Why?

As I have said, after full-time Positional Testing, individuals may reduce or totally eliminate the use of the walker, depending upon their improvement or the attainment of their goals. Again, I recommend using the walker for long walks initially after the Positional Testing phase, especially as you try to increase your walking distance. **However, for those suffering from ANY balance problems—not uncommon in older adults—a cane has an important role to play in improving balance and reducing the risk of falls.**

If you have not yet done so, *please* read the section at the end of Chapter 10, "Should You Use a Walker or Cane Long Term?"

*Comer et al. 2010. "The effectiveness of walking stick use for neurogenic claudication: Results from a randomized trial and the effects on walking tolerance and posture." Archives Phys. Med. Rehabil. Vol. 91. January 2010.

Ordering a Walker Through my Website

Compared to many other products, walkers are not a high profit item. Therefore, at least in my area, pharmacies may not carry the variety needed to serve the needs of the entire population.

On my website, WalkingWellAgain.com, I will have links to the specific walkers that I recommend for use.

If you can purchase the right walker locally, that is usually preferable. It may be covered by your insurance, and you can try the walker out. If you cannot get what you need (a low handle height, for example), or if the cost is much higher at your local pharmacy than online, then acquiring the walker through my web site may be of value.

You may check out our current recommendations at WalkingWellAgain.com, at the store section.

Radiology

Much of a physician's work involves playing medical detective. The doctor must study the patient's symptoms like a sleuth unearthing clues. With the help of some of the techniques I outline in the previous chapters, I can often unmask the culprit that has been causing my patient so much pain and discomfort. On occasion, especially for symptoms that persist despite best efforts, the doctor must resort to using various other tools to

Patients and Family: A Brief Summary Is All You May Need

This chapter explains a few important points in some detail. Often, that amount of detail is not needed for individuals seeking pain relief. **In this box, I briefly present the main points, and leave it up to you to decide if you want to read further or instead move on to the relevant clinical conditions presented in the next chapters (Section 3).**

1. *Spinal imaging is usually only needed if conservative care fails, if the diagnosis is unclear, or in case of urgency or trauma.*

2. *If an MRI does not show expected pathology, a second opinion by another radiologist might be valuable.*

3. *Some Spinal Stenosis–related pathology is not always demonstrated by an MRI.*

4. *There is significant potential value in flexion/extension X-rays.*

5. *All patients with Spinal Stenosis pathology should be investigated for PseudoStenosis.*

6. *If details of a suspected Limb Length Discrepancy are not clear, imaging such as a CT Scanogram or teleoroentgenogram can be helpful. There may be, however, a margin of error of a few millimeters.*

7. *Just as Spinal Stenosis and PseudoStenosis can mimic or worsen so many conditions, there are also other medical conditions that can cause similar symptoms. Three I present are Cervical Myelopathy, CIDP, and NPH, which are not rare and which are usually treatable. Further evaluation by a medical specialist such as a neurologist or physiatrist may be helpful in cases where the diagnosis is not clear or where the symptoms are not resolved.*

assist in the investigation. A detective has a magnifying glass and a forensic lab. My fellow medical practitioners and I have imaging scans.

Radiology is a wonderful tool to aid in the diagnosis and management of Spinal Stenosis and related conditions. Like most tools, however, it has limitations. In fact, I only order an MRI or CT scan occasionally—for fewer than one out of every ten patients with the conditions addressed in this book.

Let's talk about the great benefits of spinal imaging, its significant limitations, and what to consider if your test results come back negative. We will also seek clarity as to why spinal imaging is usually unnecessary in the first place.

Types of Spinal Imaging

There are two different types of imaging of the spine. (I do not include standard X-rays, as they are not detailed enough to clarify most presentations of Spinal Stenosis. Flexion/extension X-rays do have some value and will be discussed later.)

MRI (**m**agnetic **r**esonance **i**maging) is a test that, without any radiation, can provide a clear picture of the structures of the spine. It shows the bones, as well as the ligaments, discs, joints, and nerves, in good detail. It is the gold standard of spinal imaging.

What are the limitations of an MRI?

For one thing, MRI cannot be used in the presence of certain metal implants, which would distort the image. Some types of metal can be dislodged by the magnetic fields, indicating a need for caution with certain types of implants, including delicate clips from surgery. Occasionally, an MRI has to be ordered with contrast dye, such as when there is suspicion of scarring around the nerves after spinal surgery. The use of contrast dye occasionally has side effects or complications and is limited in patients with kidney disease. Dye should not be used in patients taking Metformin (Glucophage) for diabetes or related conditions without their temporarily stopping that medication. Otherwise, an MRI should have no effect on the body.

The MRI's sister test, the **CT** (**c**omputerized **t**omography, or CAT) scan, also provides great detail, although it is not quite as good for soft tissue as the MRI. A main advantage of a CT scan is that it can be used in the presence of metal implants such as screws or plates from previous surgery, although there could be some distortion. It does, however, expose the patient to radiation, which can be associated with a very slight increase in cancer risk, and therefore should be ordered with a degree of caution. To make a CT scan as accurate as an MRI may require the use of contrast dye, which comes along with the same precautions listed above.

Finally, X-rays of the back may be helpful. Certain changes seen on standard X-ray views would suggest Spinal Stenosis or related conditions, but they would do so without the depth of MRI or CT scans. One non-standard view that can be helpful is called a "flexion/extension view"; it is discussed below.

When to Order Spinal Imaging

Overall, I do not order spinal imaging very often. If the patient gets good relief with conservative care (Positional Testing for Spinal Stenosis or Mechanical Testing for PseudoStenosis), I refrain from ordering imaging. There is rarely reason to order expensive tests unless treatment is to be guided by them. If I can obtain elimination of symptoms with conservative care, why make a patient or insurer spend the money?

I felt validated when, in 2011, the American College of Physicians came out with a position paper stating the same policy. It said that spinal imaging was not necessary unless it was needed to direct invasive treatment because conservative care proved ineffective, or if there was doubt about the working diagnosis. Therefore, for most people, an MRI or CT scan is unnecessary, particularly since, according to a 2009 report in *SPINE* (Kalichman, L., et al. 2009. "Spinal stenosis prevalence and association with symptoms: The Framingham Study." *SPINE* 9 (7): 545–50.), 47.2% of all patients over sixty years old have at least some Spinal Stenosis.

If Spinal Stenosis symptoms persist despite good conservative care, or if they quickly recur after a temporary improvement, spinal imaging may then be ordered. **Remember, however, that even if you have symptoms of Lumbar Spinal Stenosis and the MRI or CT scan demonstrates Spinal Stenosis, you still have not confirmed that Spinal Stenosis is the cause of the symptoms. You have not ruled out PseudoStenosis.** This is essential to bear in mind, because temporary improvement with Spinal Stenosis treatment does not rule out

PseudoStenosis. Even if you improve with injections in the back, you still might have PseudoStenosis. Surgery could then fail. If you are not clear about the importance of this caveat, please review Chapters 11 and 12.

It is also possible that symptoms could be caused by another unrelated condition, even in the presence of Spinal Stenosis. The symptoms could arise from neuropathy, myopathy, poor circulation, arthritis, Cervical Stenosis, or another condition, even if the spinal imaging shows Spinal Stenosis. Expert clinical judgment is essential, especially if Positional Testing was not helpful.

Four Common Reasons Spinal Imaging May Be Negative

Now for the flip side of the picture. What if an MRI is ordered and comes back negative, when Spinal Stenosis is strongly suspected by an expert? This, in my opinion, could be the result of one of four common possibilities presented below.

1. MRI Interpretation Is Not Quite Standard

The report does not reflect the pathology. In other words, the radiologist did not identify the full pathology visible. In one of my two 2003 articles on Spinal Stenosis, I advised caution, noting that "competence at reading CT and MRI images is not uniform. In strongly suggestive cases, it is recommended that an expert read the images or review tests read as negative."

Similarly, a more recent report (2008), published in the journal *SPINE* from the investigators at the large Spinal Stenosis Outcome Research Trial (SPORT), concluded that inter-reader reliability may have only "moderate to substantial reliability," depending upon the spinal pathology being investigated. This is a diplomatic way of saying the same thing.

Getting a second opinion from a musculoskeletal radiologist who specializes in spinal imaging or from a neuroradiologist might be a good idea. I have had many patients for whom a second opinion verified the presence of a suspected pathology. If there is doubt, a second opinion can be of great value.

2. The MRI Does Not Show the True Problem

While symptoms are coming from lumbar spine pathology, the MRI report is negative because there is no abnormality visible on the MRI. Are you confused? You're not alone. This is an unclear situation. I will share with you some of the concerns presented in the literature.

Two published observations may shed light in this situation. They address Spondylolisthesis, a condition where one vertebra shifts onto another because of instability. In such a circumstance, because of the mobility of the vertebrae, the shift is only seen in certain positions. Here are two tools that may help clarify this confusion. The first tool, which is known as "axial loading," may be utilized by performing the MRI while the person is in a vertical position, simulating the standing position, which is often most symptomatic. It may also be done by using an apparatus to exert pressure on the collarbone, which in turn puts pressure on the spine and simulates standing. Articles published in *SPINE* have reported that many people who have symptoms of LSS but unimpressive MRI findings reveal much greater pathology with axial loading. Again, the most common problem brought to light with this method is Spondylolisthesis, instability causing one vertebra to shift onto another. Be aware, however, that axial loading during spinal imaging is not universally available.

The second tool calls for the radiologist to be aware of an indicator known as the "Distended Facet Sign," a swelling of the facet joint between two vertebrae. This sign is described as being a sign consistent with the presence of the Spondylolisthesis shift, even if the shift itself is not seen. Either of these insights can sometimes be used to help unmask pathology that is truly present but not seen in a standard MRI.

A concern about positioning during spinal imaging

In order to maximize patient comfort during MRI or CT imaging of the spine, the technician may place a pillow or other bolster under the patient's thighs or knees. This is precisely the maneuver that can relieve stenosis-induced symptoms. Making a patient more comfortable is an intended act of kindness . . . but I am concerned that avoiding the very position that causes the discomfort may mask important findings. It may be better to provide the patient with pain medication if necessary, to allow him to tolerate the discomfort of lying flat.

> ### *Flexion/extension X-rays*
>
> *The MRI offers a wealth of detail and has much value. It is, however, a static test, one that shows the spine in a single position. As mentioned above, the position that the individual is placed in may have an effect on the results.*
>
> *There is an additional investigation that can be helpful. Flexion/extension X-ray views can be taken of the spine from the side (lateral) position, with the individual leaning forward and with the individual leaning backward. Though this test does not provide nearly the amount of detail that can be obtained by the MRI, it is nevertheless useful because it may show if there is an instability between the vertebrae that is not always shown clearly on the MRI. It is another part of the puzzle. It is of particular value in checking for spondylolisthesis if axial loaded MRI is not available.*

3. The Constant Imperative: It might be PseudoStenosis

A third possible reason for there being SS symptoms and negative spinal imaging is that there is no significant Spinal Stenosis, and the symptoms are actually caused by PseudoStenosis. I find this to be a very common phenomenon. The symptoms are exactly the same as those of Spinal Stenosis and are mediated through the spine (caused by pressure in the nerves of the back). The actual cause, however, is that the feet and/or legs are not working properly, causing spine dysfunction. The approach I advocate mandates that for most patients this be thoroughly checked before spinal imaging. However, if this is not done, and spinal imaging is done and is negative, *the next crucial step is a careful scan of the feet and legs*!

By "scan," I do not mean an MRI or even an X-ray, but rather a thorough examination by an expert in podiatry, physiatry, orthopedics, physical therapy, or chiropractic medicine, who has a special interest in biomechanics and who can properly examine the feet and legs and the way the patient stands and walks. I reiterate what I have already shared in this book: It is *routine* that people who come into my office with signs

and symptoms of Spinal Stenosis have excellent improvement with management of the pathology causing PseudoStenosis. It is thus possible that the MRI is negative and the symptoms stem from PseudoStenosis. **It is also quite possible that the MRI is positive and shows spine pathology, but the symptoms *still* stem from PseudoStenosis.** Even when there is severe pathology present, PseudoStenosis can be at the root of some symptoms.

Radiologists who may have skipped to this chapter: I am referring to PseudoStenosis as described in Chapters 11&12. Please see the end of Chapter 11 for an explanation.

PseudoStenosis Continued: About Radiology and Limb Length Discrepancy

A perfect method of evaluating all details of Limb Length Discrepancy does not appear to be available at this time. Nevertheless, when combined with a detailed physical examination, radiologic evaluation can be extremely helpful. I personally order radiologic evaluation when there is need for additional information, but I keep in mind a realistic margin of error of 2 or 3 millimeters or more. Reasons I order tests include, but are not limited to, the following:

- Lack of expected improvement with a lift and other treatment
- Lack of mechanical changes in the feet, leading to suspicion of a functional LLDx
- Inconsistency of the apparent discrepancy, being different on one day as compared to another, suggesting the presence of a functional LLDx, as well as or instead of a structural LLDx
- Need for evaluation for a major discrepancy, one of over 9 millimeters, ⅜ of an inch
- Disagreement between medical professionals
- Desire to seek corroboration of diagnosed pathology for the encouragement of the patient

Tests I use included CT Scanograms (non-weight bearing views) and Teleoroentgenograms (weight bearing Long Leg Studies) [Picture14.1] and weight bearing x rays of the pelvis and lumbar spine both with and without lifts, to compare height of the femoral head, iliac crest and see the effect upon spinal position.

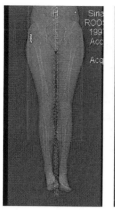
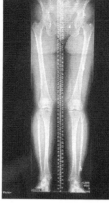

Picture 14.1. CT Scanogram (non weight bearing) and Teleo-roentgenogram (weight bearing).

Radiology testing, Limb Length Discrepancy (M21.70)

Patient _____ Date _____

_____ CT scanogram

_____ Teleoroentgenogram _____lifts, see below

_____ AP & Lat x-ray, pelvis & lower lumbar spine

_____ Please report on asymmetry of the femoral
head & iliac crest, & position of the lumbar spine.

	1. ___MM ___ ft	2. ___MM ___ ft
AP Views	3. ___MM ___ ft	4. ___MM ___ ft
	5. ___MM ___ ft	6. ___MM ___ ft

Other _____

Please contact our office
with any questions.   _____

Signature

Picture 14.2. Radiology request for LLDx.

Under different circumstances, different tests have specific value. If there is a flexion deformity of the knee (sagittal plane deformity), a test may be ordered to include a lateral view. I usually order tests after initial treatment for LLDx, as sagittal plane abnormalities of the knee sometimes improve with treatment. If there is a frontal plane deformity, the weight-bearing teleoroentgenogram could provide optimal clinical information. If there is pathology in the foot causing different limb height, or scoliosis or a hip rotation problem causing a functional Limb Length Discrepancy, this will not be identified by a CT Scanogram. Under that circumstance, a full-standing lower-extremity series, including the pelvis, for LLDx and scoliosis, could provide optimal information. If deformity, injury, or surgery of the foot is suspected to contribute to the LLDx, bilateral weight-bearing lateral X-rays of the foot and ankle

could be taken, measured, and contrasted in addition to the CT Scanogram.

If radiologic evaluation or indirect measurement by the treating clinician has established likely amount of LLDx, a second weight-bearing view would allow evaluating the effect of a lift on pelvic position, thus supporting selection of the lift height chosen. If scoliosis is present and flexible, immediate improvement in that condition might be noted as well.

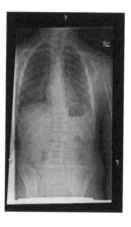

Picture 14.3. AP spine X-ray showing scoliosis in a 15-year-old boy.

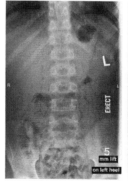
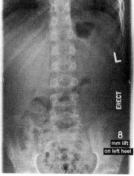

Picture 14.4. These X-rays, of the same person shown in Picture 14.3, show the change that occurred in the scoliosis with 5- and 8-millimeter lifts. Clinical examination (indirect measurement) suggested that 8 millimeters was optimal. A CT Scanogram also suggested an 8-millimeter difference.

As in the case above, when in doubt, I often order both CT scanogram and x-rays of the lower lumbar spine and pelvis with multiple lifts of different heights.

A second factor to be emphasized is the expected imperfect accuracy of the test selected. In some journal articles addressing this issue, accuracy is often lauded as successful when the differences between interpretations

The Pelvic Bones and Position Affect the Support of the Spine

At times there is confusion because of disagreement between clinical examination and radiologic findings. *The leg with common signs of being shorter clinically, including a less pronated foot and tighter Achilles tendon, and corresponding to the lower iliac crest, may be reported to be longer on both ct scanogram and weight bearing x rays of the lumbar spine and pelvis. I have had patients in which I obtained good clinical relief by using a lift on the shorter appearing leg, only to be told that it was longer leg on radiologic exam. In some cases, the radiologist had noted that the head of the femur was higher in those longer legs, but upon requested review noted that the iliac crest was lower, corresponding to my clinical findings.* **Therefore, specifically requesting that the position (symmetry) of the iliac crests be included in the report could be helpful.**

The reason for this dichotomy may be unclear, and could include a deformed pelvic bone (including an anomaly of the ilium), a sunken, subluxed, or arthritic acetabulum, an atypical 5th Lumbar or sacral plateau causing a functional scoliosis, or post surgical changes. It might also be caused by a pelvic rotation, which might respond to therapy, manipulation, or other clinical treatment. **Pathology of this nature could lead to a structural or functional discrepancy of the support of the spine, even if the limb (head of the femur to floor) itself is not involved.**

Radiologic review along with consultation with an excellent physiatrist, chiropractor, physical therapist, or orthopedist surgeon may be helpful in this type of case, although there still may not be clarity even with expert help.

Regarding the important decision of how to treat, I feel that increased caution should be exercised in treating children and younger adults with atypical presentation. In contrast, when dealing with older symptomatic individuals, expert clinical examination and strong clinical benefits may supersede unclear radiologic findings in determining treatment.

of radiologic tests are less than 3 millimeters. My own observation is consistent with that range, in that there is often a difference of 2 or 3 millimeters or more when the tests are interpreted by different radiologists.

I will present that the criteria for success in interpretation may be different in different circumstances, and they may differ from my own. For pediatric orthopedists addressing severe LLDx deformity of up to several centimeters, getting to within a single centimeter difference successfully allows the patient to have independent and active ambulation, a medical miracle that must be lauded. Orthopedists repairing severely deformed and arthritic hips and knees could measure and take into account the discrepancy, and should certainly justifiably note success when the patient has a functioning joint and independent and active ambulation.

I laud the skill and dedication of those professionals, but my clinical practice focuses on different goals and symptoms. Even if the deformity is not obvious and is not a surgical condition, I feel strongly that even a 2 or 3 millimeter difference can affect all the conditions

listed in Section 3 of this book. I have had hundreds of people improve with just a 2 or 3 millimeter correction, so the difference that is still common with current technology of radiologic evaluation can have great clinical implications.

Therefore, I feel strongly that the radiologic findings are a valuable guide and are part of the puzzle, but they should not have the final say in determining the presence of a small but significant LLDx, nor should they determine the exact amount of lift needed to provide optimal relief for an individual.

4. Totally Unrelated Etiology; A (Very) Few Examples

A fourth possible explanation for SS/PS symptoms in the absence of positive spinal imaging is that a condition completely separate from Lumbar Spinal Stenosis or PseudoStenosis is responsible for the symptoms. While many conditions have overlapping symptoms, I will present only a few. For this type of evaluation, you need a truly good neurologist or physiatrist. Beyond the conditions dealt with in individual chapters in Section 3 of this book (i.e., neuropathy, arterial circulation, swollen legs, Restless Leg Syndrome, and arthritis), here are a few more to consider, each of which I have identified at least a few times over the years. This is not a comprehensive list. In fact, I am sure it is just a beginning. However, each of these conditions can often be successfully treated.

1. **Cervical Stenosis/Cervical Myelopathy** is a condition in which the narrowing occurs not in the lower spine, but in the neck area. The resulting symptoms can resemble those of Spinal Stenosis, including difficulty walking because of leg weakness, loss of balance, and numbness in the feet and legs. I had one such patient who saw fairly good but only temporary improvement with Positional Testing, and who had a negative spine MRI but severe Cervical Stenosis. One of the hallmarks of Cervical Stenosis is the presence of pain in the neck or pain radiating into the arms or legs, which may be exacerbated by flexion of the neck. This phenomenon is called "Lhermitte's Sign." There may be weakness in the hands as well, including difficulty fastening buttons and a tendency to drop things. There may be hyper-reflexia—increased deep-tendon reflexes. If this is the case, treatment of the neck should be managed by an expert such as a physiatrist, an orthopedic surgeon specializing in neurosurgery, or a neurosurgeon.

2. Difficulty walking because of weakness in the legs can be an indicator of a brain problem called **"NPH, Normal Pressure Hydrocephalus."** Suspicion of this condition is based on a triad of symptoms, although all three are not always present. They are the following: walking difficulty, incontinence (inability to control urine flow), and dementia. The amazing thing about this condition is that it is a reversible form of dementia. One can test for NPH by imaging the brain and, if suspected, drain cerebrospinal fluid by a spinal tap. Drainage may lead to temporary improvement in all three areas, including the dementia. If that is the case, placing a shunt from the brain to the abdomen to reduce pressure in the brain can provide long-term relief.

3. There is a form of neuropathy called **"CIDP, Chronic Inflammatory Demyelinating Peripheral Neuropathy."** The presentation may include weakness and wasting of the muscles in the thighs, difficulty standing and walking, as well as other symptoms. This condition is reported to occur eleven times more frequently in diabetic patients than it does in the general population, and it can often be resolved with intravenous medication; it is thus a frequently reversible form of neuropathy.

The Need for Additional Medical Investigation

The managing physician in this medical whodunit must assiduously follow the clues. If a patient suspected of stenosis has no improvement with Positional Testing and has spinal imaging that comes back essentially normal, and thorough investigation reveals no significant lower-extremity problems affecting the spine, it is time to focus on the other possibilities. There are many conditions that can cause the symptoms in the lower extremities. As this book makes clear, I find that Spinal Stenosis and PseudoStenosis are the most common, but if workup and treatment are not helpful, the patient should be seen by an appropriate practitioner for additional investigation.

The Bottom Line:

Applying SS/PS Knowledge to Common Medical Challenges

CHAPTER 15

Peripheral Neuropathy and (Maybe) SS/PS: An Essential Investigation

Peripheral Neuropathy (PN) is a diagnosis commonly given that is often either incorrect or only partially correct. This chapter provides a very basic introduction to Peripheral Neuropathy and will help you determine whether Spinal Stenosis or PseudoStenosis (SS/PS) plays a significant role in your neuropathy symptoms—a situation that arises far more often than you might think.

This understanding is vital, because if SS/PS *does* play a significant role in causing your symptoms, it is very likely that the protocols described in this book will provide a rapid reduction of those symptoms.

Chapter 25 briefly presents treatments for symptoms of Peripheral Neuropathy that I find are often quite helpful. This chapter, however, deals only with the overlap and misdiagnosis of neuropathy and SS/PS.

> ### For clinicians: My right to opine
> *The challenge of diagnosing the cause of neuropathy and other lower-extremity symptoms, and of helping the patients who suffer from them, is what led me to focus my efforts on this clinical problem. You may wonder how I feel qualified to present so definitively my findings in this field. At the end of this chapter, you will find a list of my articles on this challenge that have been published in peer-reviewed journals between 1997 and 2013. Each listing includes a summary of my findings.*

The Overlap of Symptoms

The term "neuropathy" refers to a condition in which there is dysfunction of the actual nerves. Peripheral Neuropathy, by definition, involves nerve tissue excluding the brain or spinal cord, primarily in the lower or upper extremities.

Common symptoms include the following:

- Numbness (loss of sensation)
- Burning sensation or pain
- Shooting pain
- Deep ache and discomfort
- Loss of balance
- Difficulty walking
- Worsening of symptoms at night
- A cold and stiff feeling
- A pins-and-needles sensation, also called "paresthesia"

What makes diagnosing Peripheral Neuropathy a challenge in day-to-day practice is the fact that **most of the above-mentioned symptoms can also be caused by Spinal Stenosis and PseudoStenosis**.

Many Causes of Peripheral Neuropathy

The advice in this chapter, on how to identify and manage the possible SS/PS component, applies to all of the causes. This book does not guide identification of the cause of true neuropathy, just the SS/PS component!

Here is a partial list:

Diabetes (the most common cause)	Rheumatoid Arthritis
Kidney or liver problems	Other inflammatory arthritis
Hypothyroidism	Chemotherapy, anti-cancer drugs, or other medications
Vitamin deficiencies	
Alcoholism	Infections such as HIV/AIDS, Lyme disease, diphtheria, or leprosy
Heavy metal poisoning	

Neuropathy may also be labeled "idiopathic," which means that the cause is unknown. This allows an official diagnosis when in fact there is no real clarity as to the cause. All too often, in my experience, the neuropathy symptoms are actually caused by SS/PS—as you shall soon see.

For details of physical differentiation, please see Chapter 6.

Details of physical presentation of neuropathy and patterns of symptoms are primarily addressed in Chapter 6, on physical examination. I do not want you to get bogged down with those concepts, as they are not essential for the path of the patient. For the clinician and the very curious, those interested in greater detail, please review Chapter 6.

There are so many potential causes of Peripheral Neuropathy! I do not want to give the impression that I am trying to oversimplify the diagnosis and management of neuropathy. Not infrequently, despite a fair amount of experience and success, I need to refer a patient to a neurologist to have an in-depth evaluation as to the cause of the existing Peripheral Neuropathy. There are whole chapters of medical textbooks, and even entire textbooks, that focus on neuropathy. **If there is a lack of clarity about what is causing neuropathy symptoms, an evaluation by a good neurologist can be very helpful.** I am not an expert in neuropathy, only in the insights and techniques shared here in this book.

Picking Up the Gauntlet: The Challenge of Differentiation

In that this book revolves around the accurate diagnosis and management of Spinal Stenosis and PseudoStenosis and their role in affecting other conditions, this section on Peripheral Neuropathy is one of the most important chapters of all. For many patients diagnosed with neuropathy, their Spinal Stenosis or PseudoStenosis either strongly contributes to the symptoms or, frequently, is entirely responsible for them.

Patients may wonder why there is such difficulty in getting a clear diagnosis. They may ask, "Can't there be clarity just from a type of nerve test to tell if the symptoms are from neuropathy?" The answer is a definitive *no*.

Nerve-conduction tests only check for large-fiber neuropathy. Small-fiber neuropathy can be identified with a newer test, the Intra-epidermal Nerve Fiber Biopsy. However, even if this test is positive, it does not mean that there is no Spinal Stenosis or PseudoStenosis contributing to the symptoms!

An MRI of the spine may identify Spinal Stenosis, but that does not mean that Spinal Stenosis is causing the neuropathy symptoms. In addition, PseudoStenosis can be present and is often the main problem, whether or not there is also true Spinal Stenosis or true Peripheral Neuropathy present. This important diagnostic challenge can often be quickly resolved with the information of this book.

Common Patterns of the Cause of Peripheral Neuropathy Symptoms

1. Peripheral Neuropathy, with no other contributing factor.

2. Peripheral Neuropathy, with Spinal Stenosis contributing to the overall symptoms

3. Peripheral Neuropathy, with PseudoStenosis contributing to the overall symptoms

4. Peripheral Neuropathy, with both Spinal Stenosis and PseudoStenosis contributing to the overall symptoms

5. Either Spinal Stenosis or PseudoStenosis causing all of the symptoms, with no actual PN present

6. Other foot or leg pathology, including local nerve entrapment affecting neuropathic symptoms, with or without Peripheral Neuropathy, Lumbar Spinal Stenosis, or PseudoStenosis present

7. Other pathology, such as Cervical (neck) Stenosis, with or without neuropathy

8. A Peripheral Neuropathy other than that diagnosed—for example, CIDP in a patient diagnosed with Diabetic Neuropathy

Prevalence of Misdiagnosis

The misdiagnosis of Peripheral Neuropathy is a very widespread problem. A report on my in-office study published in *Diabetic Medicine* in 2004 identified this. I reported that **over 60% of the people who presented with a diagnosis of Diabetic Neuropathy and moderate-to-moderately-severe neuropathy symptoms had Spinal Stenosis contributing to the symptoms.** I did not recognize PseudoStenosis at the time, but would now include that category as well.

I have seen this pattern in my office practice over the past fourteen years.

This diagnostic problem is not simply in cases involving Diabetic Neuropathy. SS/PS is often the cause

of symptoms in patients diagnosed with other causes of Peripheral Neuropathy as well, including chemotherapy-induced neuropathy, AIDS-induced neuropathy, idiopathic neuropathy, and others. I have had many patients with these conditions who saw significant improvement of their symptoms within 1–3 days of treating the SS/PS component.

Using the Insights of This Book to Investigate Lower-Extremity Symptoms

As I mentioned in the beginning of this chapter, everything that has been written in previous chapters of *Walking Well Again* has been in preparation for this next step—of identifying and managing lower-extremity symptoms caused by SS/PS. While Positional Testing and Positional Therapy are great for lower-back symptoms of Spinal Stenosis, as a podiatrist, my greatest interest, and that which compels me, is the ability to identify and successfully treat lower-extremity symptoms coming from Spinal Stenosis and PseudoStenosis.

Six Tools of Investigation

The keys to strongly suspecting and actually diagnosing that a person has SS/PS contributing to his neuropathy symptoms can usually be QUICKLY pinned down by methods that I describe in previous chapters:

1. Positional History as the initial step, to identify the likely SS/PS component (Chapter 5)

2. Positional Testing after a positive Positional History, to potentially provide relief of symptoms in 1–3 days (Chapter 7)

The above two protocols will likely clarify whether either Spinal Stenosis or PseudoStenosis contributes to, or even entirely causes, the neuropathic symptoms. For a complete evaluation, you will need the following:

3. The LuSSSExt scale (Chapter 3), to facilitate the understanding and tracking of symptoms

 (The section on foot symptoms is most relevant to those investigating Peripheral Neuropathy symptoms.)

4. The physical examination (Chapter 6), to provide details that support the diagnosis of likely SS/PS, and also to permit the following of improvement with treatment

(In differentiating neuropathy from SS/PS, the First Interspace Fine Sign and the Loss of Protective Sensation scale are most valuable, although all eight clues have value.)

5. Investigation of the role PseudoStenosis may play in causing neuropathy symptoms (Chapter 12)

6. The Adjunct Measures (Chapter 8), for optimal Positional Testing and Positional Therapy

Using these six tools can help both clinicians and patients identify and treat SS/PS symptoms that mimic neuropathy. Use them aggressively! **For clinicians, there is a copy of my full Intake and Examination Form in the appendix of this book.** I have spoken to several podiatrists and physicians from around the country who have had great success with material learned from my articles and lectures, and I assure you that this book provides much more detailed and thorough guidance.

I only order an MRI or CT scan of the lumbosacral spine if Positional Testing and Therapy for Spinal Stenosis, and Mechanical Testing and Therapy for PseudoStenosis, do not provide long-term success. Spinal imaging should be ordered only if invasive therapy is being considered, or if there is a strong doubt as to the proper diagnosis. If the person has excellent improvement with conservative management and the symptoms do not return, then there is no need for invasive treatment or expensive testing.

Very often, patients have both Peripheral Neuropathy *and* Spinal Stenosis. In such patients, there may be residual numbness, paresthesia (pins-and-needles sensation), or even burning pain that persists even after overall successful treatment of SS/PS. This may reflect the actual Diabetic Neuropathy or other Peripheral Neuropathy present. For these patients, there may be a very good or excellent, but not complete, relief of symptoms. Though the disabling symptoms—including an inability to walk well, stand well, or sleep well—may be completely gone, some annoying symptoms linger. In these cases, there are some interesting treatment approaches with which I've had a great deal of success when dealing with true Diabetic Neuropathy. They are described in Chapter 25. In addition, if the SS/PS symptoms are improved, I believe the patient would then be more likely to have good improvement with the medications currently approved for neuropathic pain, such as Cymbalta or Lyrica.

Diabetic Neuropathy: A Natural Misdiagnosis

Well over a thousand patients in my practice, previously diagnosed with Diabetic Neuropathy, have been dramatically helped by addressing the underlying Spinal Stenosis or PseudoStenosis cause of symptoms. The presence of SS/PS is the most common cause of misdiagnosis of neuropathy that I see in my practice, and it is quite understandable. Little of the scientific literature specifically addresses this diagnostic challenge. Since my own articles have not yet made it into the mainstream literature, one cannot blame doctors for not knowing about them. **It is important not to point the finger of blame on this misdiagnosis.**

Whenever a patient has neuropathy symptoms and a diagnosis of diabetes, it is natural to assume that the two are related, since diabetes is the most commonly reported cause for neuropathy. Also, in that the path of Diabetic Neuropathy is reported as being quite variable, unusual patterns could still be caused by it. Diabetic Neuropathy is hard to evaluate using testing techniques; some recently developed new tests are still being investigated.

According to almost all the literature, Diabetic Neuropathy cannot be reversed or modified. Instead, emphasis is placed on good diabetes control and on medications to mask the painful symptoms. In other words, common protocol is to make the diagnosis, encourage good management of diabetes through medications, diet, and exercise, and prescribe a pill to mask the symptoms. If this is how you have been managed, in my opinion you are not receiving optimal treatment, though it is the present-day standard of care.

In contrast, I aggressively investigate for Spinal Stenosis and PseudoStenosis, and then deal with the remaining symptoms by trying the treatments described in Chapter 25. With all of these approaches, some two-thirds of my patients who presented with a diagnosis of Diabetic Neuropathy have seen very good or even excellent improvement. Here are a few of their stories:

StoryTime: Susie T was a woman in her 60s who came in for a diabetic foot evaluation. Her diabetes, which she'd had for 38 years, was being treated with insulin under the supervision of an excellent endocrinologist, and her blood sugars had been well controlled for many years. During the

Positional History, she reported neuropathy symptoms in her feet, involving burning and discomfort that occurred at night in bed. Her legs became tired with either standing or walking for more than 5 minutes. There was moderate back pain, also relieved by sitting.

I conducted a physical examination. Despite her many years of diabetes, she had good, healthy exam results in so many ways, without a loss of sensitivity to either light touch or vibration. She had nerve hypersensitivity in both feet and legs and a positive First Interspace Fine Sign.

Because she had a mild Limb Length Discrepancy, I initially provided her with a lift and directed her to use the Adjunct Measures—with limited success. Susie reported a mild improvement in nighttime symptoms and an ability to increase her walking distance to over a block. Nice, but not that nice. I added full-time Positional Testing with a walker. HOME RUN! All the nighttime pain, burning, and tingling attributed to neuropathy were gone. Her back pain vanished. She gradually increased her walking over a period of a few weeks, and was eventually able to walk up to one mile, rest for a few minutes, and then repeat. She transitioned to Positional Therapy, reduced her walker use to only long walks, with no recurrence of back, leg, or foot pain, either by day or by night.

In Susie's case, all her symptoms were due to SS/PS, not neuropathy. Perhaps a nerve biopsy might have shown some neuropathic changes, but I had a clear clinical answer and—just as important—success in treatment.

Two of Susie's interviews are available at Walking WellAgain.com.

StoryTime: Grace D, 80, came to see me with a primary complaint of neuropathic pain that had become progressively worse over the past 5 years. The worst progression had taken place in the previous 2 years, after she had a knee replacement on each leg. As a diabetic, she saw a world-class specialist in Diabetic Neuropathy. Nerve testing and biopsies confirmed the presence of Diabetic Neuropathy, but her symptoms did not improve with standard medications.

Grace had fallen twice in the preceding year, and she frequently shifted from side to side when standing. She could walk one or at most two blocks before her feet hurt so much that she had to stop, but she walked better pushing a grocery cart. Physical findings helped me quickly conclude that she had SS/PS, in addition to possible neuropathy. She had a severe First Interspace Fine Sign; a severe but atypical loss of sensation, with a score of "9 A (12222)" on both feet; and a VPT of "90" on the right and "35" on the left. She had severe Flat Feet as well as a Limb Length Discrepancy.

Before treating Grace for possible Spinal Stenosis, we implemented Mechanical Testing for Pseudo-Stenosis by strapping both feet and providing a lift for the shorter leg. She returned to the office 4 days later and reported elimination of foot pain, leg pain, and difficulty standing and walking. Her nighttime symptoms were gone, too. Unsure about whether she would need orthotics or a brace for the Flat Feet, or just good shoes and a lift for the shorter leg, I had her use only the lift. At the next visit, there was no return of the symptoms; she was doing fine with just the lift (although symptoms did return a couple of months later, which required repeat strapping). Her LOPS score had reduced to "3 (11100)" bilaterally. The VPT was "20" bilaterally.

While the patient certainly had some Diabetic Neuropathy, her long-term severe symptoms were due to PseudoStenosis caused by her Flat Feet and Limb Length Discrepancy.

Videos from Grace's first, second, and third office visits can be viewed at WalkingWellAgain.com.

StoryTime: Barbara S was a woman in her 60s who presented with severe neuropathic pain that had been present for a few years. She'd had a left knee replacement 4 years earlier, and now had pain in her right thigh as well as in her back. Going up and down stairs was difficult for her. She'd been diagnosed with Diabetic Neuropathy, but oral medication was not effective. Her burning pain was severe—a "10" out of 10. She could only walk a maximum of half a block but did better when pushing a grocery cart. Pain in her feet made it very hard for her to sleep. Barbara had been depressed and, for pretty good reasons, was very inactive.

The exam showed a positive First Interspace Fine Sign, worse on her longer right leg, and Equinus of her shorter left leg. I provided a lift that improved her balance immediately, prescribed a walker set at 29 inches, and advised her of the Adjunct Measures. I was hopeful.

At her next visit, Barbara was moderately better. She could walk two blocks before the burning pain set in. The right thigh pain had resolved, and the back pain was better. There was also significant improvement in her sleep patterns. Her balance was better, and she had a much easier time going up and down stairs. My exam showed that the Equinus was gone and the nerve sensitivity was equal on both sides. HOWEVER, she had not yet obtained a walker. By her next visit, she had a walker and was doing well, both physically and emotionally. All the burning had stopped, and her sleep was not affected by pain at all. She could walk over a mile with the walker without difficulty.

A year later, Barbara needed the walker only for walking long distances of over several blocks, and was able to walk miles without difficulty when she used it. Happily, she lives an active, pain-free life again.

The lesson? Her Limb Length Discrepancy after the knee replacement obviously had a lot to do with the PseudoStenosis and the actual Spinal Stenosis that had caused the neuropathic symptoms. Of course, I don't know if that discrepancy was present before the replacement, or if it was just present afterwards Perhaps she was simply not strong enough after the surgery to continue compensating for the discrepancy that had been present long term.

I have no criticism for the knee replacement surgery; her replaced knee was doing great. However, there was need to address the resultant Limb Length Discrepancy with a ¼-inch lift. And yet, numerous medical sources opine that a discrepancy of "only" ¼ of an inch is not that important. I disagree.

Unfortunately, I did not video Barbara's first visit. There are, however, three interviews from her following visits on WalkingWellAgain.com.

After Positional Testing or Mechanical Testing, any residual symptoms can then be reevaluated. At that point, the wisdom of using the LuSSSExt scale beforehand becomes apparent, because repeating the LuSSSExt scale helps the patient understand which symptoms have been resolved by managing the SS/PS and which symptoms remain.

Sometimes the residual symptoms are from Peripheral Neuropathy, and further neuropathy evaluation is indicated. At times, however, the symptoms are the result of Tarsal Tunnel Syndrome, a Morton's Neuroma, or a biomechanical problem of the foot or leg. *For these conditions, evaluation by either a good podiatrist or a foot and ankle orthopedic surgeon can be very helpful. If symptoms persist, I strongly recommend that the patient undergo further evaluation.*

What about Loss of Sensation from SS/PS?

I'd like to share something which is of particular interest to patients with Peripheral Neuropathy and loss of sensation. The burning, tingling, electrical shooting sensation, and overall pain from SS/PS frequently improve dramatically within 1–3 days of treatment. Numbness, the actual loss of sensation, sometimes improves very quickly, but not always. Sometimes it does not resolve or reach maximal improvement until at least 10 days after Positional Testing or Mechanical Testing. Therefore, for patients who have persistent loss of sensation, I recommend being strict with all Positional or Mechanical Testing techniques used, with reevaluation after at least 10 days, before concluding that the abnormal sensation is from the Peripheral Neuropathy. Monitoring the reduction of light touch sensitivity and vibration sensitivity can be done as described in Chapter 6.

Why Return to a Doctor Who Did Not Help You Before?

Before positional management, the SS/PS symptoms may have been so strong, and areas of sensitivity so widespread, that any evaluation that did not consider SS/PS may have been ineffective. Once the majority of symptoms and areas of sensitivity are better, however, an evaluation can become very helpful.

It is therefore reasonable to go back to a good doctor, even if he or she did not help you before.

The concepts of PseudoStenosis, the effect of both Spinal Stenosis and PseudoStenosis on neuropathic symptoms, and the benefits of positional or mechanical management for those symptoms are not (yet) well-known concepts. Once the SS/PS symptoms are quieted down, the doctor can begin to look for the other common causes that he or she is certainly familiar with.

Perhaps you will explain to that doctor how much you benefited from the approaches presented in this book, so that he or she can consider them for other patients. Keep in mind, however, that most doctors do not like to be told how to do their job by nonprofessionals. Occasionally I will have patients share something of medical value with me, but often their offerings do not have value for my practice. Please understand that, and be diplomatic when you approach your doctor.

Chemotherapy; Idiopathic and AIDS-Related Neuropathy; and SS/PS

I have had patients who unquestionably had neuropathy caused by chemotherapy received for cancerous conditions. Their symptoms began after chemotherapy, and Peripheral Neuropathy is a known possible complication of the medication. And yet, SS/PS may play an important role here, too. How is that possible?

SS/PS can have a **hyperalgesic** effect on any problem in the lower extremities. "Hyperalgesic" means that there is an increased sensitivity to discomfort. For example, someone with SS/PS may complain of increased discomfort when his or her toenails are cut. In a similar vein, a person with genuine chemotherapy-induced neuropathy may have mild neuropathy symptoms in the hands but more severe symptoms in the feet, because of the effect that SS/PS has on the feet. After a couple of days of using a walker, the symptoms in the feet may be just as mild as those in the hands. I have seen over fifteen such cases when dealing with chemotherapy-induced neuropathy.

By definition, idiopathic neuropathy is neuropathy with no known cause. Extensive blood tests must be done to exclude uncommon as well as common causes

of neuropathy. Nerve tests are usually conducted as well. These tests are not pleasant, but they do sometimes provide essential clinical guidance. However, in idiopathic neuropathy they do not, by definition, provide the answer. Nerve tests may indicate nerve changes of unknown origin. More frequently, they may show no change at all, with nothing to support the diagnosis of neuropathy other than the patient's set of symptoms. While the newer test that I described earlier in this book, the Intra-epidermal Nerve Fiber Biopsy, may or may not show changes, it does not as yet provide a specific diagnosis.

Please do not misconstrue the following paragraph as suggesting that idiopathic neuropathy does not exist. I have seen many people with true Peripheral Neuropathy (which sometimes responded to treatment, as explained in Chapter 25) that had no identified cause despite evaluation by excellent neurologists. The condition unquestionably exists.

That being said, I have seen dozens of patients diagnosed with idiopathic neuropathy for whom SS/PS was the true cause of symptoms. Remember, the symptoms of these two conditions overlap greatly. **Without focusing on the positional phenomenon of SS/PS, it would be impossible to perceive the difference clearly.** These patients usually saw significant improvement within a few days of positional or mechanical management, which eliminated symptoms that had been present and, in some cases, disabling—for years.

StoryTime: Martin was an 80-year-old man who was diagnosed with idiopathic neuropathy after undergoing heart surgery. The operation lasted several hours, and he woke up with neuropathy, which he said doctors attributed to one of the many drugs used during his surgery. He continued to have pain for years, pain which was exacerbated by walking, standing, and lying in bed. All blood tests came back negative, as did all nerve studies. He had minimal back discomfort, so no one considered the possible presence of SS.

My evaluation of Martin revealed a positive Positional History, distal nerve sensitivity patterns consistent with SS/PS, and no loss of sensation, despite the diagnosis of Peripheral Neuropathy made many years earlier. Within 3 days of Positional Testing with a walker, plus the Adjunct Measures, both his symptoms and nerve sensitivity disappeared. He had no recurrence at all after the full 10-day Positional Testing phase. His mild back symptoms were also relieved. Years later, he still had no recurrence of his symptoms.

I have seen several similar cases, in which a person developed neuropathy symptoms after a long surgery, symptoms which then improved after Positional Testing. I consider it likely that staying in one position on the operating table for many hours caused compression and inflammation of the spinal nerves. All such patients had been labeled as having idiopathic neuropathy.

Here is another story about a misdiagnosed case of idiopathic neuropathy, a complicated one.

StoryTime: Merle T was a woman in her 60s who presented with severe neuropathy symptoms in both feet, going back 5 years. She had a feeling of marbles in the bottom of her feet. The sensation was present even when she sat down but was much worse when standing or walking, which prevented her from standing or walking for more than a few minutes. The symptom also troubled her in bed at night.

She'd had a fracture of her right ankle 30 years earlier, which had been treated with 6 months of cast immobilization, and that ankle had become more stiff and painful over the same 5-year period in which she experienced neuropathy symptoms. She reported poor balance, with many near falls, but no actual spills. An MRI had identified Spinal Stenosis, but epidural injections proved ineffective. She walked only moderately better with a grocery cart.

Other symptoms included an asymmetric LOPS— "4 A (11110)" on the left foot and "7 A+ (21211)" on the right—and an asymmetric Equinus—0 degrees on the left and –30 degrees on the right. She had a ¼-inch addition to her right orthotic, but the physical exam suggested a discrepancy of about ¾ of an inch. I found a positive First Interspace Fine Sign on both feet, though it was a little worse on the left. However, her right posterior tibial nerve was the most sensitive of all her nerves. This was not a simple presentation.

I strapped a ⅝-inch lift to Merle's right foot, which helped her to feel more stable. Next, I ordered a walker for the Spinal Stenosis component of her pain. A week later, she reported only mild improvement. She said she'd been feeling moderately better for a couple of days, but then her strap became wet and the felt had compressed. She had not yet received the walker. I provided firm ⅝-inch lifts for several of her shoes, which she used and found helpful. She was even better once she got the walker. Much of the "marbles" feeling was gone, and she was able to walk a few blocks before her feet began to hurt. She was sleeping much better, too.

One area still hurt a lot. She had right ankle stiffness, right heel pain, and soreness along the outside of her right foot. My exam showed that none of the nerves in her feet and legs were hypersensitive, except for the posterior tibial nerve and the third and fourth interspaces on the right foot. Considering Tarsal Tunnel Syndrome, involving a nerve entrapment of the Lateral Plantar Nerve, I injected her twice. The ankle stiffness, heel and foot pain, and nerve sensitivity resolved. Within weeks, she was walking up to three miles nonstop with the walker, and taking walks of a few blocks without it. Success!

Life is full of curveballs. Merle subsequently suffered a stroke. Fortunately, it was a minor one. It slowed her down, and she began experiencing moderate foot pain again, with that feeling of walking on marbles. It turned out she had been using shoes without lifts, and no walker! Resuming use of the walker and lifts provided immediate relief. She was soon walking comfortably again. A few months later, I had to repeat the injection for Tarsal Tunnel Syndrome.

Here are the lessons. Lift height, like walker height, is essential. Both of those interventions made a big difference for this patient. But Merle did not regain her prior status until the Tarsal Tunnel Syndrome was addressed with injections. The ankle stiffness and pain, which became noticeable at the same time as her neuropathy, was probably the straw that broke the camel's back, causing the altered gait that made this severe PseudoStenosis/Spinal Stenosis–combination flare up. Until that problem was addressed, she still could only walk a few blocks. Afterwards, she could walk for miles!

There is an unwritten rule in radiology: if you find one fracture, you still need to look for the second. The same is true with PseudoStenosis. There may be a Limb Length Discrepancy or Flat Feet, but there also may be another problem that needs to be addressed as well before recovery can be complete. In Merle's case, both Spinal Stenosis and two causes of PseudoStenosis had to be addressed before her long-term "idiopathic neuropathy" symptoms were resolved.

Merle's interview is available on WalkingWell Again.com.

StoryTime: Michael was a 48-year-old man who presented with painful corns on both feet. Further discussion revealed that he had had burning and tingling and cramping in his feet and legs . . . for about 16 years. He was told repeatedly that the neuropathy symptoms were caused by HIV/AIDS and by the medications used to control this disease process. He took Neurontin, but that provided only minimal help. He had a maximum walking distance of one block, which left him in pain for several minutes after he sat down.

Fortunately for Michael, his corns hurt. My examination of Michael suggested a slightly shorter left leg. Standing, his left hip bone was lower. His left Achilles tendon was tighter, and the nerve sensitivity was far greater in his longer right leg, all signs consistent with PseudoStenosis caused by Limb Length Discrepancy. I provided him with a ⅛-inch lift for his left shoe. When he stood, he immediately felt better. I gave him several lifts to use in all his left shoes. He returned after a few days and reported that his symptoms had resolved in just 1 day. A few weeks later, he was still fine, and thrilled to have relief after so many years of pain and limitation.

By the way, Michael did have some neuropathy. He persisted in having an LOPS score of "2 (11000)," being unable to feel the 5.07 monofilament in his toes or in the balls of his feet. This is certainly consistent with small-fiber neuropathy, which could have been caused by either the disease process or by

the medications. It was just not the ONLY problem, and certainly not his main one. In his case, PseudoStenosis caused by a Limb Length Discrepancy, superimposed upon a mild neuropathy, was the cause of his symptoms.

I interviewed Michael at his second visit but decided not to use the recording for privacy's sake. At his third visit a few months later, he strongly suggested I use the video for education purposes, as he was committed to HIV counseling. I repeated an interview, and expect to post both interviews at WalkingWellAgain.com.

SUMMARY

Peripheral Neuropathy, Spinal Stenosis, and Pseudo-Stenosis share many identical symptoms. These symptoms can have a severely limiting effect on a person's quality of life and activity level. In patients with either a suggestive Positional History or suggestive physical findings, either Spinal Stenosis or PseudoStenosis is most likely present and contributing to the symptoms.

I must state this as clearly as possible. For patients with significant neuropathy symptoms, part of the initial evaluation should include an investigation for SS/PS. This includes taking a good Positional History and a good clinical examination, including the LOPS pattern, nerve sensitivity patterns, and a search for possible causes of PseudoStenosis. If there is any cause for suspicion, employ Positional Testing or Mechanical Testing.

With Spinal Stenosis, PseudoStenosis, or both, Positional Testing can provide rapid and dramatic relief from painful symptoms, even if they have been present for many years. Burning and shooting sensations, nighttime pain, and inability to walk all may improve quickly. Actual numbness or loss of sensation may take longer to reach maximal improvement.

For PseudoStenosis, one may see equally dramatic improvement of neuropathy symptoms with Mechanical Testing, such as the use of a proper lift for a shorter leg, strapping or an Unna boot for Flat Feet, or correction of any other condition causing an altered gait pattern that affects spine function.

Patients with PseudoStenosis, as well as those with more severe Spinal Stenosis, may have a recurrence of symptoms after discontinuing walker use. If this oc-curs, a physical exam should be conducted by a good podiatrist, physiatrist, orthopedist, physical therapist, or chiropractor, preferably one familiar with the con-cepts of this book, who can search for possible causes of PseudoStenosis. If improvement is poor or incomplete, please review the ideas in Chapter 12.

Some actual neuropathy symptoms may be helped through the measures described in Chapter 25. I only turn to those measures, or other standard medications commonly used for neuropathy symptoms, after I have ruled out SS/PS.

> *If the recommendations of this book do not pro-vide help, the patient should see a neurologist or physiatrist with interest in Peripheral Neuropathy. He or she may be able to provide optimal medical management or be able to determine if there is a type of treatable neuropathy or related condition that can be identified. A brief introduction to three of those treatable conditions (CIDP, NPH, and Cervi-cal Stenosis) is presented at the end of Chapter 14.*

For Clinicians: My Right to Opine

As promised, here is a list of my peer-reviewed articles addressing neuropathic symptoms.

1. **Spinal stenosis: A common cause of podiatric symptoms.** *1997.* Journal of the American Podiatric Medi-cal Association. *This article stresses the prevalence of Spinal Stenosis in causing or exacerbating any foot and leg symptoms, including neuropathy.*

2. **Neurogenic positional pedal neuritis: Common pedal manifestations of spinal stenosis.** *2003.* Journal of the American Podiatric Medical Association. *This article provides details on the symptoms of Spinal Ste-nosis as they present in the foot, and includes an introduction to physical findings and on what I would later label "Positional History" and "Positional Testing." It reports the many similarities of pedal presentation of neuropathy to Spinal Stenosis.*

3. **Value of a grocery cart and walker in identification and management of lumbar spinal stenosis in diabetic patients presenting with peripheral neuropathy or claudication.** *2003.* Diabetes Care. *This letter presents an introduction to what I will later label "Positional History" and "Positional Testing" in dif-ferentiating both neuropathic and arterial symptoms from those of Spinal Stenosis in diabetic patients.*

4. **Diabetic neuropathy or spinal stenosis: Prevalence of overlap and misdiagnosis.** *2004.* Diabetic Medi-cine. *This letter presents details of an in-office study in which over 60% of patients with moderate-to-moderately-severe Diabetic Neuropathy had Spinal Stenosis contributing to or entirely responsible for their neuropathic symptoms.*

5. **Nocturnal neuropathic symptoms in diabetic patients may be caused by spinal stenosis.** *2005.* Dia-betic Medicine. *This article identifies the pattern of Spinal Stenosis frequently causing nocturnal symptoms mistaken for neuropathy, and it reports insights on differentiation and management.*

6. **Lumbar spinal stenosis: Can positional management alleviate pain?** *2008.* Journal of Family Practice. *This article provides then-current details of both Positional History and Testing, as well as results of a retro-spective review of fifty-three patients treated in my office with documented Spinal Stenosis and symptoms, many of which were neuropathic. Coauthored with Dr. Charles Hennekens, author of Epidemiology in Medi-cine and (then) the fifth-most quoted medical author in the world over the prior five years.*

7. **The professor position and the single stance flexion test may clarify the effect of lumbar spinal ste-nosis or pseudostenosis on lower-extremity symptoms.** *2013.* Journal of the American Podiatric Medical Association. *This article explains two immediate forms of Positional Testing, and also presents the concepts and introductory details of PseudoStenosis, including its ability to mimic or exacerbate all lower-extremity symptoms of Spinal Stenosis, including neuropathy.*

I would love to hear some of the great stories that result from people using this material to investigate neuropathy symptoms. Those willing to share their stories may write to me via my website, WalkingWellAgain. com. Good luck!

For the clinician and the very curious

The Alternate Diagnosis: Neurogenic Positional Pedal Neuritis (NPPN)

Neurogenic-Induced Claudication (NIC) is the term commonly used to describe symptoms of Spinal Stenosis as they present in the leg. NIC is frequently mistaken for vascular claudication from Peripheral Arterial Disease (PAD). Differences in these two conditions are detailed in Chapter 16.

Neurogenic Positional Pedal Neuritis (NPPN) is a term I coined to describe the symptoms in the feet caused by Spinal Stenosis. It is most frequently mistaken for Peripheral Neuropathy, but may also be mistaken for poor circulation, muscle or local nerve pathology, or arthritis. To clarify this term, understand that it is "neurogenic" because symptoms are caused by compression of nerve, "positional" because the spine position often controls the pressure on the nerve and is thus the key to diagnosis and treatment, "pedal" because the symptoms present in the feet, and "neuritis" because symptoms most often present as nerve-type pain such as neuropathy.

I want to share a mistake, or perhaps more kindly to myself, an evolution. I began to consider the potential for a separate diagnosis of PseudoStenosis approximately in 2008, six years after the article entitled "Neurogenic Positional Pedal Neuritis" was published in the Journal of the American Podiatric Medical Association. If I knew then what I know now, I would have said that NPPN could be caused by either Spinal Stenosis or PseudoStenosis, in that they both may present identically.

In my office, a diagnosis I use is frequently one of the following:

1. NPPN caused by Spinal Stenosis
2. NPPN caused by PseudoStenosis
3. NPPN caused by both SS and PS

For this chapter, the first step is to recognize when symptoms consistent with Peripheral Neuropathy are actually NPPN, and the next step is to identify the true cause of NPPN in order to optimize treatment. Both conditions can be helped by Positional Testing, but for long-term success, the patients who have PseudoStenosis should have that condition treated as well.

Peripheral Arterial Disease and (Maybe) SS/PS

As I pointed out in the previous chapter, a mistaken or only partially correct diagnosis can be a source of much unnecessary pain and discomfort. Here is another common diagnosis to add to the list: **claudication from Peripheral Arterial Disease (PAD).**

Many people suffer from symptoms of claudication—the aching, tired feeling in the legs that is brought on by walking. All too often, such patients believe—and perhaps have been told by a physician—that their problems are caused by poor circulation, and that no help, other than surgery, is available.

I believe that, on the contrary, many of these people can easily be helped. For many of them, either Spinal Stenosis or PseudoStenosis contributes to their symptoms. In this chapter, I will provide an overview of possible patterns involving such individuals; I will explain how to identify those that may be helped; and I will shed light on what can be done for them.

Background Information

The following background information will help a layperson understand the basics of the disease process. If you are just interested in the quickest past to direction on how to evaluate your situation, you may jump to the section after picture 16.3, "Four Common Patterns to Address."

Poor circulation usually refers to what is called "Peripheral Arterial Disease (PAD)," which is usually caused by arteriosclerosis, or "hardening of the arteries." This occurs because a fatty substance called plaque accumulates on the inside of the walls of the arteries. The arteries become stiffer and narrower. Less blood flows through the arteries, and the arteries are not able to expand well because of the stiffness. When an area of your body needs more blood, such as when your leg muscles work harder while walking, blood flow is not adequate to bring the extra nutrients and necessary oxygen to supply the muscles, and it becomes easier for your muscles to tire. Eventually, if circulation becomes severely constricted, there may not be enough blood to handle even limited activity, or to allow for the proper healing of injuries. This is a more severe medical challenge, which should be managed by a vascular surgeon.

Arterial Testing

How can circulation be measured? An old and established method is a test called an "ABI," or "Ankle-Brachial Index." In this test, the blood pressure is taken at both arms and ankles; the ABI result is the ankle pressure divided by the brachial (arm) pressure. For example, if the blood pressure at the ankle is 120 and the blood pressure in the arm is also 120, the ABI would be 120/120, or 1.0, which is normal. In contrast, if the brachial pressure measures 120 but the ankle pressure is only 80, the index would be 0.66, which is abnormal. A classic guide to normal and abnormal measurements follows.

- is completely normal.
- to 1.2 is the classic normal range.
- 0.9 to 1.0 is the low normal range.
- 0.8 to 0.9 represents a mild reduction in circulation.
- 0.5 to 0.8 shows moderate PAD.
- Below 0.5 indicates severe PAD.
- Above 1.2 (some say 1.3 or even 1.4) suggests calcification of blood vessels and possible cardiovascular disease.

This test is not as dependable in presenting a clear picture of available circulation in diabetic patients with calcification of blood vessels as other tests available. One other test is the TBI, or Toe-Brachial Index, in which the pressures and waveforms of the toes are used instead, as the blood vessels of the toes are not usually affected by calcification.

In an ABI, a noninvasive vascular examination, cuffs that measure the blood flowing in the limbs may be placed on the toes, ankles, legs, and thighs. See picture 16.1.

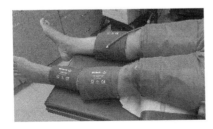

Picture 16.1. Some cuffs in place.

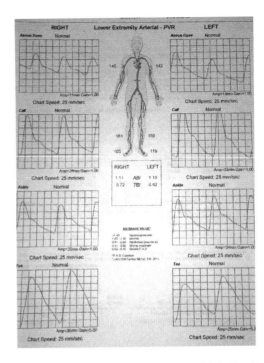

Picture 16.2. In the test of this report, multiple levels have good pressure and waveforms, indicating good arterial flow.

A thorough vascular test evaluates the pressures and waveforms in the vessels in the thighs and legs, in addition to the ankles and toes. In the example shown in picture 16.3, the circulation was more reduced in the thigh than in the calf or ankle, and this was only identified by checking multiple levels.

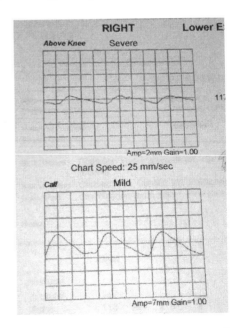

Picture 16.3. In this report, there is a reduced blood flow in the blood vessels in the right thigh, which required surgery.

Four Common Patterns to Address

For the purpose of dealing specifically with walking challenges, here is a basic classification of four types of patients with circulation problems:

1. The first patient has only mild-to-moderate circulation reduction and is still able to walk well without claudication.

2. The second patient has only mild-to-moderate circulation reduction but also has significant symptoms that cause difficulty with walking.

3. The third patient has moderate-to-severe circulation reduction and significant activity limitation.

4. The fourth patient has, in a less common pattern, moderate-to-severe circulation reduction but is able to be at least moderately active without claudication or pain.

I know this is too simple, but it provides a framework to use. Here is a look at the groups listed above, one by one.

Mild PAD without Walking Limitations

If you are a person who falls into the first group, with only a mild reduction in circulation and no walking limitations, you might not be looking to this book for help. Wonderful! However, the fact that you are reading this section suggests that you have a concern. I have two recommendations for you. ***First, stay active.*** Walking can maintain or even improve your circulation. The usual advice for circulation problems has always been to walk as far as you can to the point of experiencing uncomfortable symptoms, rest, and then repeat. I would NOT recommend this for someone with Spinal Stenosis—but for someone with mild or even moderate PAD *only*, it is sound advice. Being active can include walking, cycling, swimming, or playing tennis, golf, or any other sport of your choice. Use it or lose it. Stay active!

Second, recognize that mild circulation problems can become more severe, so they should be taken seriously. I am not suggesting surgery for mild problems, but rather aggressive preventative treatment. Such treatment involves managing your "risk factors" (the behaviors and medical conditions that can lead to arteriosclerosis, the blockage of blood vessels). These factors include smoking, diabetes, high blood pressure, and hyperlipidemia.

> *Regarding smoking, it is clear that even two cigarettes a day can have an adverse effect on circulation and may delay healing after surgery. For most smokers, there is no way other than to stop "cold turkey." If you want to protect your circulation, not only the circulation in your legs, but also in your brain, lungs, heart, and other organs, the decision to stop smoking is one of the most important decisions you will ever make. If you want to stop but have difficulty, there is help available. Ask your doctor, or check for smoking cessation programs through your local hospital.*

Other PAD risk factors—diabetes, high blood pressure, and hyperlipidemia—can usually be improved through a combination of exercise, food control, and medication. Consult with your primary care provider for help. With each of these issues, an ounce of prevention is worth much more than a pound of cure.

Finally, it is important to know that even a mild circulation deficit can be associated with heart disease. A thorough cardiac evaluation may be in order, so be sure to discuss this with your primary care provider.

Mild PAD with Significant Walking Limitations

The second group of individuals has only mild circulation reduction but significant limitation of activity. In a way, this pattern is very common, yet in another way, it is very uncommon. What do I mean by that?

It is my observation that patients with only a mild circulation deficit—with an ABI of 0.8 or higher—should not experience significant claudication symptoms. If they do, I feel that there is another factor causing the symptoms, most commonly either Spinal Stenosis and/or PseudoStenosis (SS/PS). The symptoms would thus be "neurogenic," caused by nerve involvement.

There are two ways to evaluate whether the problem is coming purely from limited circulation or if SS/PS is playing a big role. The first way is to pay close attention to the details of your symptoms. If when you walk and your legs get tired, you can get relief by standing straight, then poor circulation is most likely causing the problem. **If when you walk and your legs**

get tired, you get relief only by sitting down, leaning against something, or taking the Professor Position (see Chapter 6), then SS/PS almost certainly plays a major role in your symptoms.

> Many people report that they can stand and rest to obtain relief of leg discomfort. When pressed, however, they admit that they have to stand **and** lean against something. That pattern suggests SS/PS.

There are other distinguishing signs as well, based on your symptoms. People with poor circulation often experience much more difficulty walking up a hill than down one, while those with SS/PS may actually walk better uphill and have more difficulty going downhill, because of the effect on the position of the lower spine. Patients with SS/PS may ride a stationary bicycle without producing claudication symptoms in the legs. If the problem is arterial, the same symptoms occur when riding a bike as when walking. A chart that points out these differences is presented here. It is modified from my 1997 and 2003 articles on Spinal Stenosis that appeared in the *Journal of the American Podiatric Medical Association*.

Those paying attention throughout this book may notice that this chart focuses on many of the questions asked in the Positional History, as presented in Chapter 5.

The Grocery Cart Test

A second way to clarify whether symptoms stem from poor circulation or from SS/PS is your reaction to Positional Testing, as described in Chapter 7. To test this, you do not need to use a walker, although that may turn out to be the necessary temporary treatment. Identifying whether the symptoms are related to a circulation issue or to SS/PS may be made crystal clear with the Grocery Cart Test.

This is a test in which you examine your walking capability with and without wheeled support—in this case, a grocery cart. People who suffer from poor circulation do not walk better when pushing a grocery cart. In fact, sometimes the strain of pushing a cart continuously makes it harder to walk, and they actually cover *shorter* distances.

People with either Spinal Stenosis or PseudoStenosis usually walk much better when pushing a grocery cart—as long as they are above about 5'2". People below that approximate height walk better only if they hold the cart far in front of them or rest their arms on the bar of the grocery cart, as this puts them in a position where they are leaning forward and opening the spine. The details of the Grocery Cart Test are presented at the very end of Chapter 7.

To be effective, the Grocery Cart Test must take place with **uninterrupted walking**. Why is that? People

Comparison of Vascular Induced and Neurogenic Induced Claudication and Related Syntoms

Evaluation	Vascular	Neurogenic
Claudication Distance	Consistent	Often inconsistent
Pain Relief	Standing and resting	Must sit, lie down, or lean on something, to flex the spine
Walking up Slope	Pain	Often causes less pain
Walking down Slope	Pain	Often causes more pain
Riding Bicycle	Pain	Often causes no pain
Walking with a Wheeled Walker	Pain if walking continuously	Often no pain if leaning forward
Walking on a Treadmill	Pain	Often no pain if leaning forward
Walking with a Grocery Cart	Pain if walking continuously	Often no pain if leaning forward
At the Checkout Counter	Pain free	Often painful
Circulation Evaluation	Shows significant deficit	May or may not show deficit
Back Pian	Irrelevant	Frequent, but not always
Night Pain	Severe cases only	Frequently a problem

who have poor circulation often mistakenly think that the grocery cart helps them walk better. Shopping involves short walks and stops to browse or to pick up selected items. If the normal claudication distance—the distance someone needs to walk in order to start having leg symptoms—is half a block, about 250 feet, and that person stops every 100 feet in the grocery store, the symptoms will never have a chance to arise. Anyone might then mistakenly think that the grocery cart helped them, while it was actually the frequent stops involved in shopping that did the trick. If you stop to talk or shop, the test is invalidated. You must test your ability to walk without interruption to ascertain whether the cart truly makes a difference. If there is any question, redo the test.

If the cause of symptoms does turn out to be either Spinal Stenosis or PseudoStenosis, you might be amazed at the results of the Grocery Cart Test. I have had patients who for years could not walk half a block. However, when pushing a grocery cart they were able to walk through an entire store once, twice, or even three times on the first try. Changing the spine position helped bring about an almost magical improvement in their walking, suggesting that the problem derived primarily from SS/PS rather than from PAD. **The Grocery Cart Test, when coupled with a thorough physical examination for PseudoStenosis, can help prevent the need for tens of thousands, or even hundreds of thousands, of unnecessary MRIs to see if Spinal Stenosis is contributing to symptoms.**

The Checkout Counter Sign

Another aspect of grocery shopping led to an insight that I have used in my discussions with patients for years, but which I define for the first time while writing this book. I call it the **"Checkout Counter Sign."** People with poor circulation feel fine at the checkout counter because there is no increased demand on their legs. Their circulation is not challenged, and they are able to stand comfortably. In contrast, people with Spinal Stenosis and/or PseudoStenosis will often walk throughout the entire grocery store symptom-free with the aid of a shopping cart. When they get to the checkout counter and are no longer leaning on the cart but rather standing straight, this position may quickly bring about a recurrence of their symptoms. Those symptoms are relieved when they lean on the cart, a pattern patients often acknowledge when carefully questioned.

Through the information provided in this section, you should be able to find much greater clarity as to whether your symptoms are a result of poor circulation or of Spinal Stenosis or PseudoStenosis.

The Next Steps

If you suspect that you might have PseudoStenosis (Chapters 11 and 12), first check for Limb Length Discrepancy, as it is by far the most common cause. Otherwise, see a good podiatrist to check out the other possible causes and treatments for PseudoStenosis. Strapping or using an Unna boot for Flat Feet, or providing other treatments for other causes, can eliminate the symptoms in just a couple of days.

Even if you have PseudoStenosis, you may also choose to undergo Positional Testing with a walker. You might get great temporary or even long-term relief. The only downside of this approach is that you may not have all the findings in physical exam, as they may be improved by Positional Testing. Improvement will prevent you from undergoing Mechanical Testing to determine the success of mechanical management in relieving symptoms. However, if your symptoms are resolved long term, that exam is not so important. If your symptoms return, the exam for PseudoStenosis and Mechanical Testing will again be valid.

If you choose to use Positional Testing, read the instructions in Chapters 7 and 8. Follow the instructions regarding use of the walker and the other methods of reducing spinal nerve pressure that I have recommended. Many people see dramatic improvement in ALL related symptoms in just 1–3 days.

Not only should you be able to improve your walking with a walker, but there is also **a very good chance that temporary use of the walker can provide long-term relief** (Chapter 10). I have had a great many patients with a mild circulation deficit who, I determined, had SS/PS as the primary cause of their symptoms, and who returned to an absolutely normal walking capacity after Positional Testing with a walker. The ability to walk blocks or miles, often without a walker, is common after successfully treating Spinal Stenosis.

StoryTime: Felice M was a 68-year-old woman who came in for a toenail problem but had plenty more to discuss. For many years, she'd been suffering from severe back, foot, and leg pain that made it very hard for her to stand or walk for more than a few minutes. She was on narcotics—three or four times a day—and had been told that her pain was from Diabetic Neuropathy and circulation problems. She walked much better when pushing a grocery cart. She had pain in her feet and legs every night in bed, which made it difficult for her to sleep.

Examination showed good pulses and skin temperature, and the overall appearance of her feet and legs was normal. However, she had severe sensitivity in all of the nerves in her legs bilaterally, with the exception of the first intermetatarsal space. In other words, she had a bilateral First Interspace Fine Sign. This was strongly suggestive of Spinal Stenosis.

I had Felice get a walker and use all the Adjunct Measures. I instructed her about modifying her sleep position and what to do about stairs, standing, the shower, and the kitchen. When I saw her one month later, all of her back, foot, and leg pain was gone. She was able to walk up to a half an hour at the mall without difficulty, and her entire mood and way of life had undergone a radical change.

Incidentally, the walker was a little bit too high, so she had arm and shoulder pain when she walked a lot. I adjusted the walker so that it was comfortable for her, and she did very well afterward.

The lesson? For years, Felice had been told by doctors that her walking limitation was from a circulation problem. It was, however, a clear case of Spinal Stenosis. To be honest, stories like this motivated me to begin writing about Spinal Stenosis.

Two videos, one of Felice's first visit and one of her second visit, can be viewed at our web set, WalkingWellAgain.com.

I do not mean to sound like a broken record, but I must stress the following: **even if you temporarily experience complete relief with the grocery cart or walker, you may still have PseudoStenosis.** Follow the instructions in Chapter 12, on PseudoStenosis, to evaluate yourself. You may either treat yourself—for example, with a heel lift for a Limb Length Discrepancy—or be treated by a professional, such as a podiatrist, physical therapist, physiatrist, or orthopedic surgeon.

Moderate-to-Severe PAD with Claudication

What of the third group of people, those with a moderate-to-severe circulation deficit and a real walking limitation? What can be done for them?

I must present two ideas right up front. **First, if you have such a severe circulation deficit that you have ulcers or infections that do not heal, or if you have even mildly cool, pale, or dusky feet, then you must be seen and managed by a vascular specialist.** It is quite possible that surgery can be performed that will improve your circulation. While twenty years ago such surgery usually involved an open bypass, newer procedures are now able to improve circulation in a much less invasive manner, with less risk and less time needed for recovery. If there are physical signs of a severe circulation deficit, see a vascular specialist who is up to date on these great new, innovative techniques.

Signs that you, the patient, can observe that are consistent with poor circulation:

1. *Loss of hair on the toes*
2. *Loss of hair on the feet and up into the legs*
3. *Paleness of the skin of the toes and feet*
4. *Blue color in the toes or feet*
5. *Weak or absent pulses*
6. *Thinning out (atrophy) of the muscles in the legs*
7. *Shiny skin on the toes, feet, or legs*
8. *Painful ulcers that do not bleed and that are slow to heal*
9. *Dusky discoloration of the toes*

The more of these signs that are present, the greater the likelihood that there is a real and significant circulation problem. It is essential that someone with these signs get a professional vascular evaluation.

However, even for those people with a moderate-to-severe circulation deficit along with pain in the legs aggravated by activity, it is quite possible that SS/PS may also play an important role in the symptoms. Having a problem with your circulation does not rule out another concurrent contributing cause of symptoms.

I have had many patients whose circulation test identified poor circulation, who had significant difficulty walking short distances—and who saw valuable improvement in their overall symptoms and ability to walk with Positional Testing for Spinal Stenosis or Mechanical Testing for PseudoStenosis.

The Grocery Cart Test, the Adjunct Measures to Positional Testing, and my newly named "Checkout Counter Sign" (which at the time of this writing is all of thirty minutes old), should guide you as to whether SS/PS likely plays a role in your overall symptoms. **The previous section concerning evaluation of people who have only a mild reduction in circulation but still experience symptoms, applies just as well to a patient with a moderate-to-severe circulation deficit.** Anyone who has difficulty walking because of poor circulation should, in my opinion, take the Grocery Cart Test and thus investigate whether SS/PS contributes to the overall symptoms.

If, for example, Spinal Stenosis prevents you from walking a quarter of a block, and your circulation deficit prevents you from walking a full block, then simply managing the Spinal Stenosis could improve your walking distance fourfold! Also, when Spinal Stenosis is present, one has to sit or lean to obtain relief, so removing the symptoms caused by the Spinal Stenosis could considerably improve the patient's ability to be active. **Therefore, I recommend that people with a moderate-to-severe circulation deficit follow all of the suggestions presented in the previous section.**

I want to stress that enjoying such a benefit is not a solo treatment. In all circumstances, whether or not the patient improves with Positional Testing for Spinal Stenosis, it is vital that a primary care doctor or cardiologist aggressively manage the patient's risk factors for poor circulation.

How SS/PS May Affect Vascular Surgery

There is, however, an important caveat in evaluating the need for vascular surgery. The vascular specialist may decide on surgical intervention not only on the basis of test results and risks of not healing, but also on the basis of the person's symptoms. Someone with reduced circulation and with leg symptoms so severe that

they prevent walking could reasonably be considered a candidate for surgery.

Managing Spinal Stenosis or PseudoStenosis can dramatically reduce your symptoms, and symptoms could be a factor in the decision on whether or not to have surgery.

StoryTime: Dr. William P, aged 67, came in for treatment of a painful fungus nail. Discussion revealed that he had back and right-leg pain and had been walking poorly since suffering a stroke 15 years earlier. He had no nighttime symptoms, but his back hurt a lot when he got out of bed. He could only walk half a block and had poor balance—all attributed to the stroke. Because of concern for his circulation, he'd had a stent placed in his right leg, but that procedure did not improve his symptoms.

My initial examination identified flexible Flat Feet, a unilateral Equinus, and an asymmetric First Interspace Fine Sign. Indirect measurement suggested a ½-inch Limb Length Discrepancy. Suspecting a PseudoStenosis component, I strapped both his feet and included a ⅜-inch lift within the strap for the shorter leg.

Soon afterward, William was hospitalized for complications from a medication, and I did not see him for months. At our next meeting, he related that he'd had good improvement of symptoms for the few days after his first visit, followed by a rapid recurrence after the straps were removed. This time, I provided him with some ⅜-inch lifts for his shoes. A few days later his back and leg pain was gone, and he was able to walk for blocks without pain. It had also become much easier for him to get out of bed in the morning. At his next visit, all his symptoms were still gone, as were all signs of PseudoStenosis.

The lessons? First of all, I am confident that William's doctor would not have performed surgery for the circulation if there had been no blockage. In William's case, however, it seems that the pain was due not to his circulation, but to the Limb Length Discrepancy and to PseudoStenosis.

I have stressed that PseudoStenosis should routinely be considered before Spinal Stenosis surgery is implemented. Similarly, SS/PS should be routinely considered before arterial vascular surgery, if the deficit is not severe. Symptoms may play a big role in deciding whether surgery is needed. If symptoms are relieved another way and the person can be active, surgery may not be needed. It is important that this decision be guided by a doctor.

The second lesson is a big one. William did not have an orthopedic injury or surgery that would have caused this Limb Length Discrepancy to develop. He'd most likely had it all his life. It was just that in years past, he'd been strong enough and healthy enough to compensate for it by altering his own body mechanics to avoid the onset of SS/PS symptoms. After the stroke, he was no longer able to do that. His back and leg pain, along with his difficulty standing and walking, developed after the stroke—and were blamed on the stroke.

The way I see it, however, the real problem was William's shorter leg and his inability to compensate for it as he'd been able to do in the past. The stroke did not *cause* the problem. The stroke deprived him of the strength to compensate for it. The lift brought him back (almost) to the way he'd been before. He was then able to stand and walk without the back and leg pain that arose after his stroke.

Dr. William P's interview is available on our web set, WalkingWellAgain.com.

StoryTime: Shirley, 72, was a diabetic woman who presented with years of symptoms, including an inability to walk comfortably for more than a quarter of a block. She had back pain as well as severe right leg pain. My exam showed a Limb Length Discrepancy, so I provided her with a lift. She reported good improvement of the right leg pain at her next visit. Her back, however, was only mildly better, so I treated her with Positional Testing, including the use of a walker. She returned with a total resolution of back pain and leg pain, but could only walk one block before her thigh became very tired.

I then did an ABI to test Shirley's circulation. All of her blood vessels showed a decent flow—except for the major vessel to . . . her right thigh! Shirley was accordingly referred to a vascular surgeon.

As spring turned into summer, she started wearing shoes without a lift for her shorter leg. Immediately, the severe right leg pain returned. She was quite relieved to come back to the office and get new lifts for her summer shoes!

The lesson? Be persistent, and consider that there may be multiple conditions. In this case there was PseudoStenosis, Spinal Stenosis, and PAD, all in one patient. It is necessary to reevaluate the patient after each intervention, and to be willing to start from scratch. Ask questions, and reevaluate the physical signs as if each visit is the first. A patient, step-by-step approach is something that both the clinician and the patient must be willing to embrace.

By the way, Shirley did have resolution of her right thigh claudication symptoms when she had a stent placed in the appropriate vessel. Modern techniques of vascular surgery are such a blessing—as long as they are used for the right person, of course!

Shirley's interview is available on our web set, WalkingWellAgain.com.

Moderate-to-Severe PAD without Claudication

The fourth and final group of patients have documented moderate-to-severe circulation deficit but no symptoms. This situation is a double-edged sword.

On the one hand, a lack of symptoms allows a person to walk at least to some degree and to remain active. This is obviously great for independence and activity level, and it helps in managing medical conditions such as diabetes. In this respect, a lack of symptoms that limit activity is indeed a blessing.

On the other hand, those who have a moderate-to-severe circulation deficit but no claudication symptoms in the legs may have such significant neuropathy that they simply do not feel the aching or cramping that their muscles would otherwise be transmitting to the brain. **This is a form of silent claudication,** with a circulation deficit in which the muscles have been depleted to the point where there should be symptoms, but these symptoms are not being felt due to a lack of normal nerve function.

Cardiologists identify a similar condition called **"silent heart disease,"** in which a person has a circulation deficit that should bring on the heart symptom known as "angina." However, because of an autonomic neuropathy, the person doesn't feel any symptoms and therefore is not aware that any heart disease is present. This person is at high risk for a cardiac incident, but lacks the warning symptoms.

StoryTime: Today I saw a patient in my office for follow-up who is, thank G-d, doing well. A few years ago, I tested his circulation, despite his lack of claudication symptoms and despite the fact that he could stand and walk without complaint. His X-rays showed calcification of his blood vessels. His circulation test, the ABI, produced poor results. My clinical exam suggested both small-fiber and large-fiber Diabetic Neuropathy. I voiced an opinion that he might be at high risk for a heart attack, because any heart disease could be just as silent as

---

For the clinician and the very curious

Stationary Neurogenic-Induced Claudication

Long after this chapter was written, I considered that an additional classification of claudication symptoms, called "Stationary Neurogenic-Induced Claudication (SNIC)," might have value. This is the presence of the aching, tired feeling of the legs that mimics vascular claudication, but is present when a person is standing in one place, such as at the checkout counter, and not when walking.

This is meant to contrast with and to facilitate differentiation from two other conditions: Intermittent Claudication (IC), which presents with leg aches from walking that are relieved by standing and resting, and Neurogenic-Induced Claudication (NIC), which classically presents with similar symptoms from walking but which requires sitting or leaning forward to achieve relief. While SNIC may certainly be caused by standard Spinal Stenosis or any form of PseudoStenosis, it appears to be a common finding in patients with a Limb Length Discrepancy, who often report that it is harder to stand in one place than to walk. This finding may not be pathognomonic, but it is a strong clue and a finding worth soliciting. This new classification, SNIC, may make this pattern easier to solicit and record.

---

his leg circulation disease. The patient was not happy about the idea of consulting a cardiologist, but once I got his internist on board he agreed to have an aggressive cardiac evaluation. Within two weeks he underwent heart surgery—a quadruple bypass. He was informed that he'd already had at least two silent heart attacks and could have died at any time.

A few weeks ago, he came in because of neuropathic pain that interfered with his sleep. The pain was actually coming from his spine, caused by a mild Limb Length Discrepancy. He began using a lift and within a few days was sleeping peacefully again. He came in today and thanked me, and also reminded me of the story that had happened a few years back—not that I had forgotten. Seeing this patient reminded me of just how much I love my job!

If you have any questions regarding the severity of a circulation deficit, you should undergo circulation testing, with an ABI, for example. If there are major changes in your ability to be active or in the appearance or sensation of your feet, you should have expert evaluation.

Any person who has significant peripheral circulation problems or erectile dysfunction, even in the absence of cardiac symptoms, should be evaluated by a cardiologist to see how he or she can best be managed. This might even involve surgical treatment. While it might seem overly aggressive to consider surgical treatment when there are no symptoms, a good cardiologist can establish whether the person is at high risk for a heart attack, and can decide whether or not aggressive treatment is necessary.

SUMMARY

Poor circulation is a serious condition, as well as a risk factor for heart disease, and should be taken seriously. However, I believe it is quite common for the symptoms of poor circulation to be affected by the presence of Spinal Stenosis or PseudoStenosis. Investigating and treating SS/PS may dramatically improve a patient's symptoms and his or her ability to be active. All it takes is the understanding that the symptoms may stem, at least in part, from SS/PS, followed by evaluation and appropriate treatment.

It is my hope that this chapter has led the reader, either patient or clinician, to look at the claudication symptoms and the relationship between PAD and SS/PS in a new way. If you have success, I would love to hear from you! Please contact me via my website, WalkingWellAgain.com.

CHAPTER 17

Painful Peripheral Edema

Peripheral Edema, or swelling of the legs, is a common condition. And, as with neuropathy and poor arterial circulation, the discomfort attributed to this condition may commonly be caused by Spinal Stenosis or PseudoStenosis.

> Before we talk about the pain in the legs associated with edema and how relief of those symptoms can often be achieved in a matter of a few days, I must emphasize what this chapter is **not** about. **It is not about diagnosing the cause of your swelling.** For that you must see a physician with expertise—either an internist, a cardiologist, or a vascular specialist. If the swelling comes from an arthritic condition, you may need a podiatrist, orthopedist, or physiatrist. Some causes of swelling are only an annoyance, while others may be an indication of a serious medical problem or risk. Get a personal evaluation by the appropriate specialist!

Basic Information on Edema

This section provides basic information about the causes and types of Peripheral Edema. If you are not interested in this background information and are just interested in the quickest path to direction on how to evaluate your situation, you may skip to the section "Painful Edema."

Peripheral Edema has many possible causes. It frequently stems from dysfunction of the veins in the legs (varicose veins or thrombophlebitis) and may be affected by poor arterial circulation or the by lymphatic system, any of which could affect one or both legs. It may result from fluid retention arising from problems in the internal organs, such as the kidneys, lungs, liver, or heart. The swelling may be affected by how much salt you have in your diet or what medication you take.

It may also be caused by biomechanical problems such as arthritis, tendonitis, or bursitis, but those causes would usually result in more of a local or limited area of swelling, as compared to diffuse swelling of both legs, or occasionally one leg. An injury, a local vascular problem, or even a mass in the pelvis are more likely to cause diffuse swelling in just one leg.

The more common presentation of edema is **pitting edema**, in which the swelling is not firm. It often reduces after sleeping. When this condition is present, a finger pressed firmly into the skin will cause a depression (pit) to form, which persists after the pressure is removed. Less common is **non-pitting edema**. Here, pressing on the skin and the underlying tissue does not result in a depression, which means that the swelling is much firmer. This is often associated with Lymphedema, chronic or severe venous insufficiency, or Myxedema associated with Hyperthyroidism.

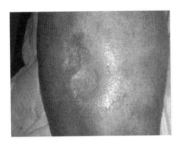

Picture 17.1. Pitting edema shows a depression (pit) where pressure is placed.

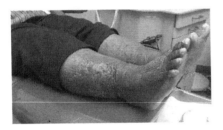

Picture 17.2. Non-pitting Lymphedema is firm, and does not create a pit where pressure is placed.

Painful Edema

I'd like to focus on the symptoms that may be present with edema. **While the medical literature reports that Peripheral Edema may be accompanied by significant aching and heaviness, I believe it is unusual that these symptoms are caused solely by the edema.** Most people with edema have no symptoms at all, or only mild ones. This is usually the case when the cause

of the swelling is medical (fluid retention because of a heart, liver, kidney, or lung problem), venous insufficiency, or even Lymphedema.

Among patients with diffuse edema, a subset experiences fairly severe discomfort with edema in the legs. It is difficult for them to stand, to walk long or sometimes even short distances, and sometimes even to sleep comfortably.

> ### When the edema and its cause <u>might</u> be the source of pain
>
> I am not saying that edema itself is **never** the cause of symptoms, just that in my experience it generally is not. The edema (or the condition causing it) may be the actual cause of the discomfort if there is an inflammatory condition such as Rheumatoid Arthritis, a mechanical condition such as degenerative arthritis or tendonitis, a blood clot, or severe edema. However, even in those conditions, SS/PS should be considered

Discomfort May Prevent Edema Treatment

Many of these people have another problem. **They have an overall sensitivity in the legs that makes it too hard for them to tolerate compression therapy,** whether from support stockings, wraps like a "CircAid," or intermittent compression pumps, which pump fluid from the legs. For these patients, symptoms can be disabling, and they may not be able to tolerate the conservative treatment available. They may have been told that surgery for their veins is the only possible resolution. The swelling in their legs may progress from a more mild pitting edema to a more severe non-pitting edema, because they are not able to tolerate compression therapy comfortably. Over the course of years, the soft tissue in their legs may become firm, a change known as "dermatofibrosclerosis." People with this condition often have real discomfort in their legs when standing or walking. The appearance of their legs may be identical to that of legs with Lymphedema, shown in picture 17.2.

HOWEVER . . .

SS/PS: Commonly the Real Cause of Pain

I mentioned earlier that the swelling is not, in my opinion, the usual cause of the leg discomfort. The cause of the discomfort is usually Spinal Stenosis, PseudoStenosis, or both.

Six Tools of Investigation

The keys to strongly suspecting and actually diagnosing that a person has SS/PS contributing to his neuropathy symptoms can usually be QUICKLY pinned down by methods that I describe in previous chapters:

1. Positional History as the initial step, to identify the likely SS/PS component (Chapter 5)

2. Positional Testing after a positive Positional History, to potentially provide relief of symptoms in 1–3 days (Chapter 7)

The above two protocols will likely clarify whether either Spinal Stenosis or PseudoStenosis contributes to the lower-extremity symptoms. For a complete evaluation, you will need the following:

3. The LuSSSExt Scale (Chapter 3), to facilitate the understanding and tracking of symptoms

4. The physical examination (Chapter 6), to provide details that support the diagnosis of likely SS/PS, and also to permit the following of improvement with treatment

    (As is presented later in this chapter, the First Interspace Fine Sign is of particular value in evaluating patients with painful edema.)

5. Investigation of the role PseudoStenosis may play in causing extremity symptoms (Chapter 12)

6. The Adjunct Measures (Chapter 8), for optimal Positional Testing and Positional Therapy

The clinical presentation brought on by Spinal Stenosis and PseudoStenosis may include an aching and tired feeling, and sometimes neuritic symptoms such as tingling or burning brought on by walking and even standing. Does this sound familiar? These may be symptoms that have been diagnosed as coming from edema.

I need to share two points as we approach this diagnostic challenge. First, although I do not believe it to be true, it seems like common sense to view swelling of the legs as the cause of discomfort experienced with standing and walking. It is obvious, almost a "no-brainer." And yet I disagree.

Second, the information shared here has not, to the best of my knowledge, been published in any journal. The reason I share this information is that there is no cause to blame your doctor or any other professional for not knowing this. It is not in the literature!

Potential Improvement with Proper Treatment

By using the six tools above, you can go through the process of considering, examining for, and then testing for SS/PS. If you are working with a foot specialist, any condition causing PseudoStenosis can be investigated and treated. If you are on your own, you may treat for Limb Length Discrepancy or simply use Positional Testing, which of course could work for either Spinal Stenosis or PseudoStenosis.

If either Positional Testing or Mechanical Testing proves effective, you will be able to walk better, stand better, and even sleep better—within just 1–3 days.

Here are two amazing additional things to think about.

First, while it is common for people who do Positional Testing full time to experience relief from their symptoms in just 1–3 days, **10 days of Positional Testing will often provide relief that lasts for weeks, months, or years**. Therefore, after you stop using a walker, you may still have the same edema—but enjoy a total elimination of your symptoms! I have seen many patients who had been diagnosed with pain coming from edema who have held true to this pattern. To me, it seems to prove that the edema was not causing the symptoms in the first place!

Second, along with the elimination of painful symptoms, there may also be an elimination of sensitivity. Many people with this combination of conditions (edema and either Spinal Stenosis or PseudoStenosis) find that pressure really bothers their legs, thus preventing them from using any kind of compression therapy. This sensitivity to pressure can be expected to disappear once the other symptoms are gone, which, as I've noted, can happen in just a few days. When that happens, you may then be able to make use of compression therapy—support stockings, wraps, or intermittent compression pumps—that you could not tolerate before. This, in turn, can often reduce the actual swelling of the legs.

StoryTime: Martha B was an 82-year-old woman who presented with severe difficulty standing and walking for more than three minutes at a time. This difficulty had persisted for many years and was attributed to severe Lymphedema. Though she did not have back pain, she had nerve sensitivity in her thighs, legs, and feet, and she had a classic and symmetric First Interspace Fine Sign. She had severe edema and had been unable to tolerate any compression, even support stockings, because of leg sensitivity.

Suspecting Spinal Stenosis as the cause of her symptoms, I prescribed a walker to treat her with Positional Testing, plus the Adjunct Measures. Within a few days, she was walking and standing better than she had in years. The nerve sensitivity was completely eliminated. She began an exercise program by walking in her apartment building, and was soon able to walk back and forth from one end of the hallway to the other, passing thirty apartments without difficulty. By her 3-month follow-up, she could walk the corridors with just a cane, but used the walker whenever she left the building. She tolerated compression with an Unna boot and was able to tolerate a compression pump when she needed it for treatment of edema and ulcers. Years later, she is still pain free and walking well.

Two of Martha's interviews are available on WalkingWellAgain.com.

Positional Testing May Be the ONLY Good Choice

The value of Positional Testing as an initial treatment of choice must be emphasized. Many people with chronic edema have risk factors such as heart disease or phlebitis, and are on anticoagulants such as heparin, Plavix, Pradaxa, Xarelto, or even aspirin. Such medication can increase the risk for complication from an epidural injection by causing bleeding into the spinal area. In order to have an epidural, a patient must stop taking medication for a period of time sufficient to reduce that risk of complication. This in turn puts the patient at greater risk for the cardiac issues or phlebitis or embolism to plague him or her again. The patient may be temporarily placed on a low-molecular-weight heparin such as Lovenox, in order to keep lower risks. Positional Testing carries none of those risks.

Physical therapy is a commonly used form of intervention for Spinal Stenosis. However, many patients are not conditioned enough to go through such therapy for Spinal Stenosis. Physical therapy usually takes weeks to work, if it works at all.

In such patients, there is a tremendous increased benefit of Positional Testing as a treatment for Spinal Stenosis. None of the risks of injections apply. There's no need to go off anticoagulants. There are none of the struggles of physical therapy, nor is there the need to wait weeks to see hoped-for improvement. **Positional Testing, in my mind, is almost always the best first treatment for true Spinal Stenosis. In situations like these, it is clearly the fastest and safest intervention possible.**

Exploiting Nerve Sensitivity

(For a more detailed explanation of information related to this idea, please read Chapter 6, on the physical exam for SS/PS.)

Frequently, people with painful legs associated with edema suffer from a great deal of sensitivity to pressure or any unpleasant stimuli. Because the tension caused by the swelling goes around the entire leg, there can be sensitivity around the entire leg. All areas of the leg may be quite tender.

This is in contrast to people with leg pain from Spinal Stenosis who do not have diffuse edema. Using the nerve sensitivity pattern reported in Chapter 6, one sees that Spinal Stenosis patients often have severe sensitivity along the nerves, such as the tibial nerve, which is on the inner side of the calf, or the femoral nerve, which is on the inner side of the thigh. These areas could be painful because of nerves, but could also be painful because they are next to veins, and when veins have clots or are inflamed, they can also be quite tender.

In fact, if there is great sensitivity along a vein, as well as swelling, it suggests that there may be a thrombophlebitis (blood clot) in one of the deep veins. This is a serious condition, and if suspected, should be investigated by a radiologic test, such as a doppler ultrasound exam.

That sensitivity along the course of both the vein and the nerve could certainly also be present in someone with both SS/PS and diffuse edema. **There are two strong clues, however, that may help clarify the picture.**

First, in someone with Spinal Stenosis and/or PseudoStenosis there is usually sensitivity not only in the calf or thigh, but also in interspaces 2, 3, and 4 of the involved foot. This is the "First Interspace Fine Sign" described in Chapter 6. There are no major veins here as there are in the legs, so one would not expect great sensitivity in this area from vein pain.

(Caution! This does not mean that someone with this pattern cannot also have a blood clot—just that SS/PS is likely present as well.)

Second, if Positional Testing for Spinal Stenosis or PseudoStenosis, or Mechanical Testing for PseudoStenosis, proves to be effective, **the sensitivity of all the nerves listed above almost always disappears in just 1–3 days along with the symptoms.**

Sensitivity can disappear, though the edema remains. This scenario strongly suggests that something other than the edema is at the root of the pain. I believe, and feel supported by the quick response in dozens of such patients, that the true cause of the sensitivity is SS/PS.

Keep in mind that if the symptoms of Spinal Stenosis return quickly after you stop Positional Testing and transition to Positional Therapy, it could very possibly mean that PseudoStenosis is a contributing cause. This should be checked.

Two Immediate Positional Tests

Two tests are available to immediately investigate the effect of SS/PS on diffuse leg pain otherwise attributed to edema. These tests are effective for individuals who have discomfort within a few minutes of standing. They are the **Professor Position** and the **Single Stance Flexion Test**, the details of which were published in the *Journal of the American Podiatric Medical Association*, March 2013 issue, and **which are described in this book in Chapter 6, which I suggest you review**. Because these two tests are so good for evaluating this exact kind of symptom, I will explain here their logic as well as a few of their details.

If a person has leg pain when standing or walking and obtains relief of symptoms by leaning on a grocery cart or walker, I agree that *it is logical* to conclude that the relief comes from the reduction of one's weight on the lower body. This is a claim that I have heard many times from therapists and doctors. **However, I present that this logical conclusion is not correct.** These two tests support my theory and, I hope, will convince you to investigate this for yourself.

By leaning forward and opening the spine, one achieves a relief of symptoms similar to that obtained by leaning pushing a grocery cart or walker. **Both of these tests show that it is the position of the spine that reduces the leg pain, not the reduction of weight bearing**. Pain is not caused by the weight (pressure bearing on the leg or legs) or by the standing position of being vertical that increases the gravity, affecting the swelling of the legs. Neither of those two factors is altered by leaning forward. If these maneuvers help, it strongly suggests that Positional Testing could be of great benefit. Use these tests for an opportunity to have an immediate insight as to whether Positional Testing may help you!

Pain May Be Gone, but Swelling May Persist

Back to the actual edema in the legs. Unfortunately, patients with the fibrotic firm swelling of the legs may not respond as well to compression therapy as do those patients with less advanced edema. However, though the swelling may linger, the discomfort may completely vanish—allowing you to resume Walking Well Again!

StoryTime: We usually think of painful swelling as a condition that affects only older people. Not true.

Tara T was a 27-year-old woman who presented with pain in the ball of her left foot. She also had fairly severe and firm edema and pain in her left leg, along with difficulty standing or walking, that had begun 15 years earlier when she'd fallen and injured herself. Tara had suffered many leg infections and had spent time in renowned hospitals. The established diagnosis was Lymphedema that was causing both her swelling and pain.

My exam showed a Limb Length Discrepancy and Flat Feet. There was an asymmetric Equinus in the shorter right leg and a painful callus in the ball of the foot of the longer left leg—a common presentation. I found nerve hypersensitivity in both of her feet and legs. I trimmed the callus, padded it, added a lift for her shorter leg, and strapped both feet.

A hole in one! At her next visit, she reported that all of her leg pain was gone. She was able to stand and walk without difficulty for the first time in more than a decade.

Here is a practical management insight. Since I was uncertain whether the patient needed just a lift or also orthotics, I provided lifts and had her return a week later. She still felt somewhat better, though not nearly as good as she'd felt with the strapping. We therefore had orthotics made for her Flat Feet and included a lift for the Limb Length Discrepancy. After that, she did great.

The lesson? The obvious cause of symptoms is not necessarily the true cause. Straightforward biomechanical care, such as the kind that can be provided by any good podiatrist, was all that was needed. The cause of the swelling was not found—but we did discover that it was not the swelling that had caused her severe symptoms, and we then relieved those symptoms.

Tara's interview is available on WalkingWellAgain. com.

StoryTime: Dee was a woman I treated for many years for tender, curved thick nails. She also had chronic severe swelling of her legs. I mention this story because of the unusual diagnosis, Lipedema. This condition usually involves excess fat being deposited from the waist down into the legs, but not past the ankle. It does not cause swelling in the feet, as would usually be found in Lymphedema. Lipedema often runs in families and is reported to often be painful.

In Dee's case, her legs were painful. She had difficulty walking and standing because of an aching, tired feeling in her thighs, legs, and feet, until she underwent Positional Testing with a walker. Within days, her chronic discomfort was gone. The swelling was unchanged. She used the walker for a couple of weeks and then stopped.

Years later, improvement is maintained. Lipedema in Dee's legs is present, but symptoms are gone.

Obviously, her symptoms were from SS/PS, not Lipedema.

Above I mentioned that Lipedema is frequently reported to be painful. I therefore question how many patients with painful swollen legs from this and other conditions would have great relief of pain and improved ability to stand and walk by treating SS/PS. I think that when the research on this is eventually done, there will be a lot of grateful patients and surprised clinicians.

Tibial Tendonitis and Swelling

Sometimes people have mildly diffuse swelling around the entire ankle or lower leg but primarily along the inside of the ankle (see picture 17.3). This presentation is often mistaken for Peripheral Edema or even arthritis, but it is actually a form of tendonitis, involving the posterior tibial tendon.

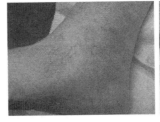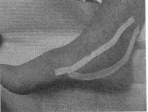

Picture 17.3. In that the swelling is hard to see in this picture, I have used tape to outline where swelling and tenderness are usually the greatest.

I want to make two essential points about Posterior Tibial Tendonitis. First, it is often associated with a Flat Foot deformity. If you have read this far, you know that it is often found in the longer leg of an individual with a structural Limb Length Discrepancy. Therefore, successful treatment often requires adding an appropriate lift for the opposite side. You read that correctly. If the tendon is painful in the left ankle, putting a lift in the right shoe is often very helpful!

Second, I offer a word of caution regarding treatment. I usually treat this condition with a Low Dye strap (as a test for orthotics) or an Unna boot (as a test for an ankle brace). However, as mentioned above, if there is symptomatic Spinal Stenosis or PseudoStenosis, the nerves and overall soft tissue of the leg may be so sensitive that the Unna boot is not tolerated, being too painful. In such situations I address the SS/PS, and only after resolution of the overall sensitivity and nerve sensitivity do I apply an Unna boot to address the swelling and sensitivity of the tendon. Otherwise, there is a painful ankle and an unhappy patient!

A Word on Vein Surgery

I do not mean to suggest that surgical treatment of vein pathology is never indicated. Sometimes it is necessary for certain individuals, especially if there are venous stasis ulcers or there is severe edema that does not respond to conservative care. Some may also choose to have surgery done for cosmetic reasons, because of the appearance of unsightly varicose veins. Surgical treatments available include venous stripping, ligation (tying off individual perforating veins), sclerotherapy (injecting to seal off smaller veins), and other methods. Minimally invasive surgical treatment by vascular surgeons is much more refined than in years past, which may lead to quicker recovery. This is a field in which great advances have been made in surgical treatment.

Surgical treatment may improve symptoms that are in part caused by SS/PS. Those who read earlier chapters understand that SS/PS can cause exacerbation or worsening of symptoms from other conditions, ranging from ingrown toenails to Peripheral Neuropathy or, as we will soon address, arthritis. The same is true with painful edema. There may be mild edema symptoms that SS/PS is making much worse. Getting rid of the obvious problem, such as an ingrown nail or venous edema, may also provide good relief of symptoms, as there is then no painful condition for SS/PS to exacerbate. Thus, even if SS/PS contributes to one's symptoms, there may be reasonable cause to correct the other problem. It might be successful! However, if Positional Testing for Spinal Stenosis or Mechanical Testing for PseudoStenosis relieves all or even most symptoms, then that may change the equation in deciding whether surgery is indeed necessary. If there is a question, it can be discussed with your primary care provider.

Keep in mind that if spine-mediated symptoms or sensitivity improve, you may then be able to tolerate the support stockings, compression pump, or Unna boot that had been difficult to tolerate in the past.

Nighttime Edema and Pain

Regarding nighttime symptoms and sleep positions, pain associated with edema is a situation in which the **efforts to make things better can actually make things worse**. The overall approach to nighttime symptoms is explained in greater detail in Chapter 20, but I will give you a few details here.

As you now understand, body position greatly affects symptoms caused by both Spinal Stenosis and PseudoStenosis. That is why, in my 2003 (*JAPMA*) article, I labeled the foot symptoms "Neurogenic **Positional** Pedal Neuritis."

Individuals with significant edema with or without nighttime symptoms are often advised to elevate their legs to help reduce the edema. Gravity will help pull the swelling down. I am not going to disagree with this universal advice. And yet . . .

Pillows put under the feet or calves can induce a stretch on the nerves in the back of the legs going up to the spine that can exacerbate nerve sensitivity. The position may help reduce the swelling, but it can also make SS/PS symptoms much worse! I instead tell my patients that if they sleep on their back, they should put a pillow or two under the knees and thighs (see picture 17.4). They can also put a pillow under the feet or legs to direct gravity, but for symptoms, that may not be important. What is important is to open up the spine, which the pillow under the knees and thighs does, without putting stretch on the nerve. In contrast, a pillow under the feet or calves may induce that stretch if the knee is not flexed. Helping one problem, the swelling, can therefore aggravate another problem, the spinal nerve irritation. Now that you are aware of that, you can address this problem. For greater detail, see Chapter 20, on nighttime symptoms.

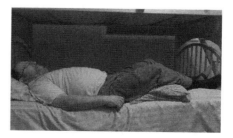

Picture 17.4. A pillow under the knees may open the spine of a patient with either Spinal Stenosis or PseudoStenosis and may relieve symptoms.

SUMMARY

1. This chapter is for people who suffer from chronic edema. If there is a new or acute problem, it is essential to seek medical care to discover the cause.

2. In my experience, in the great majority of patients with painful swollen legs, the pain derives primarily from Spinal Stenosis, PseudoStenosis, or a combination of both.

3. These patients may have too much leg sensitivity to tolerate compression treatment, such as support stockings, leg wraps, or intermittent compression units.

4. Nerves along the leg and in the foot may be hypersensitive and may improve rapidly with positional or mechanical treatment, which would then allow for compression therapy.

5. Improvement in symptoms when walking with wheeled support (grocery cart, baby carriage, walker, or even treadmill) suggests that Positional Testing can be of great benefit.

6. All people who only temporarily improve with Positional Testing should also be evaluated for PseudoStenosis.

7. The Professor Position and the Single Stance Flexion Test can both quickly demonstrate that the position of the spine, and not only weight-bearing and gravity, contributes to the symptoms.

8. Many people with either Spinal Stenosis or PseudoStenosis experience long-term improvement of their discomfort and walking ability with positional management. Some use the walker long term, while many can reduce or even stop walker use completely.

9. It is best to review the details of the other chapters in this book if you now suspect that SS/PS may be contributing to the symptoms. As an amateur medical detective, it's vital that you look at *all* the clues. Remember, educating yourself is the first step on the road to recovery!

10. There are circumstances where surgery for veins is indeed indicated, but there may be great value in using the information of this chapter fully before surgery is scheduled.

11. The same sleep position that can improve edema may make spinal nerve sensitivity and symptoms worse. Optimize your sleep position to address both problems.

Good luck! I look forward to hearing success stories from both patients and clinicians. You may contact me through my website, WalkingWellAgain.com.

CHAPTER 18

Arthritis: Clarifying a Common Conundrum

Arthritis. Such a powerful word, and so much a part of the everyday life of so many people, that it seems to stand alone. It is certainly a word and a reality that deserves a chapter all its own. Unfortunately, for many it is a word and a diagnosis that causes them to change the way they live.

But I will share a secret with you. The symptoms of lower-extremity and spinal arthritis, although real, can often easily be helped—without medication, injections, or surgery.

Considering Where the Pain MIGHT Be Coming from

The key is to clarify the pattern of your symptoms and to discover the following:

1. What pain comes directly from arthritis—in other words, from local joint changes—with or without soft-tissue inflammation

2. What pain derives from or is affected by spinal nerve involvement caused by either Spinal Stenosis (SS) or PseudoStenosis (PS)

3. What mechanical problem (Deforming Force) caused and might still be affecting the arthritis

4. What mechanical problem could be preventing the arthritis from improving

5. What pain stems from a systemic disease process, such as Lyme disease, Crohn's disease, Fibromyalgia, Polymyalgia Rheumatica, Chronic Fatigue Syndrome, or any of the myriad other conditions that can affect arthritis development and symptoms

Both SS and PS may have a powerful impact on arthritis symptoms—and both may be easy to treat. Without an understanding of the material in these two essential chapters, recognizing the root cause of the symptoms so that appropriate treatment can be administered is often an impossible challenge, a conundrum. It is my belief that following the paths presented in Chapters 18 & 19 can provide clarity and rapid pain relief for many of those who suffer from symptoms of arthritis.

Symptoms that can be affected by the patterns listed above are quite wide ranging. They can include any of the following:

- Arthritis and tendonitis of the foot and ankle, with or without significant deformity

- Knee arthritis or tendonitis

- Hip arthritis or back arthritis

- Neck or jaw pain, shoulder pain, pain radiating down the arms, and even headaches related to foot and leg dysfunction (These patterns are less frequent but not uncommon.)

- A pattern of diffuse aching that can be diagnosed as Fibromyalgia or any other medical condition associated with arthritis symptoms

Keep all these symptoms in mind as you proceed with your evaluation, and pay close attention to the changes that occur with treatment, which are often directly related to biomechanics, as is presented in Chapter 19.

Degenerative arthritis does not occur in a vacuum. Except in the case of some sort of damaging injury (which may be an acute, one-time injury or a chronic stress such as that caused by physical labor), most "wear-and-tear" arthritis develops because of imperfect biomechanics. This concept is explained in Chapter 12, on PseudoStenosis, as it may affect the spine. This chapter and Chapter 19 present that the same poor mechanics that can cause PseudoStenosis in the spine may also cause lower-extremity degenerative arthritis involving the foot, ankle, knee, and hip.

A portion of the information needed to understand the salient points in this chapter has already been presented in the chapters on PseudoStenosis. **For clarity's sake, Chapters 11 and 12 need to be read along with this chapter and Chapter 19.** Some information presented elsewhere in this book is either repeated or expanded upon here as well, to address the essentials from an arthritis standpoint.

When your doctor tells you that you have arthritis, the diagnosis may not be wrong; it may be merely incomplete. This is because there are so many possible factors to consider. The vital point to remember is that there are often better ways to address painful symptoms than with pills, therapy, injections, or surgery.

Two Stories to Get You Going

StoryTime: This is an old one, dating back to 1991. I was just beginning to appreciate the effect of Spinal Stenosis on patients at a very basic level. A patient was referred to me for surgical correction of a very painful hammertoe with a corn. He'd been sent to me by his endocrinologist, who was managing his diabetes. This patient had severe sensitivity with the corn, much more than most people experience. Even back then, I was committed to non-surgical treatment whenever possible. I trimmed the corn and asked him to return for a follow-up visit in a month, or sooner if necessary.

After only a few days of relief, he came back for surgical scheduling. I was surprised that it hurt so much and that the pain had returned so quickly. With further discussion, I began to suspect that the symptoms he had, which had been attributed to Diabetic Neuropathy, were actually caused by Spinal Stenosis. After some serious back-and-forth with his endocrinologist, we obtained an MRI that showed Spinal Stenosis, and the patient received an epidural injection. In just a couple of days, all the neuropathy symptoms were gone, and so was the pain coming from the corn! That pain never returned at the same level as before. From that point on, the pain was no more than mild and responded to periodic trimming, like that of a normal corn.

There is much to learn from this episode. Spinal Stenosis can not only cause back pain and mimic other foot and leg conditions, but can also make an existing condition in the feet or legs much more painful. In other words, Spinal Stenosis can be the villain that both causes pain and exacerbates it. This patient had a corn that hurt because of the Spinal Stenosis. **Similarly, many people with actual arthritis of the feet, ankles, knees, and even hips experience much more painful symptoms due to Spinal Stenosis or PseudoStenosis.**

Before we get to the "meat" of the chapter, here is another quick story—a much more recent one.

StoryTime: Charlotte F came into my office complaining of severely sensitive ingrown toenails. Discussion revealed that she had not been able to walk even one minute without some pain in almost 7 years, and could only walk for a few minutes before she was forced to sit down. She'd been diagnosed with Rheumatoid Arthritis and was being managed by a very good rheumatologist with the most modern medicines. Her symptoms included stabbing back pain, severe knee pain with some changes often seen with Rheumatoid Arthritis, and chronic leg and foot pain that worsened with brief standing or walking.

My evaluation suggested the presence of Spinal Stenosis and PseudoStenosis (caused by a short leg) in addition to the Rheumatoid Arthritis. A lift in her shoe helped her stand in a more balanced way, but she still had significant pain. When I had her walk with a walker, she felt immediate improvement in her back, leg, and knee. She was thrilled! It was a Friday afternoon and I did not have the heart to make her wait until Monday to get a walker, so I lent her one of mine.

Charlotte had an appointment to return on Monday. I was quite anxious—and hopeful. I was not disappointed. She reported that on Saturday (the day after I'd lent her the walker) she went to the park with her grandchildren for the first time since she'd moved to the neighborhood 3 years before. On Sunday, she went to the mall for three solid hours. Three hours! She told me that she made sure to sit down every forty-five minutes, as she did not want to overdo things. All the sensitivity along the nerves was gone. She was still in some pain from the arthritis in her knees, but her overall symptoms were, for the first time in almost 7 years, quite manageable.

If you're looking for encouragement in your own situation, there's a treat in store for you. Charlotte's interviews are on my website, WalkingWellAgain.com. You can see her at her first visit, and then again a few days later. These rank high among my favorites.

Six Crucial Points to Consider

1. **Many people are labeled as having arthritic pain when the primary pain is actually mediated through the spine, through either Spinal Stenosis or PseudoStenosis.**

2. **Frequently, the genuine arthritis that is present in the lower extremities affects the mechanics of the spine, which causes nerve compression similar to that found in cases of Spinal Stenosis. In other words—PseudoStenosis.**

3. **Many patients with genuine local arthritis suffer much harsher symptoms because of the presence of Spinal Stenosis or PseudoStenosis.** Spinal nerve sensitivity can cause any lower-extremity pathology—from nerve pain to circulation pain to arthritis pain—to be experienced with greater intensity. In such circumstances, treating the Spinal Stenosis (either with Positional Testing or by direct spine treatment such as epidural injections) or tackling the source of the PseudoStenosis (with Mechanical Testing) can quickly reduce or even eliminate pain believed to be caused by arthritis.

StoryTime: Yvette B was a woman in her 30s who presented with a chief complaint of fairly severe bunion pain in the right foot, of about 6 years' duration. Though only mild-to-moderate as bunions go, it was extremely painful. She was interested in all options, including surgery. Of interest, she'd also suffered arthritic pain of her left knee for the previous 20 years and had undergone surgery that did not help.

Yvette's exam showed a Limb Length Discrepancy, with her left leg being shorter. She had Equinus on the left side and severe nerve sensitivity on the right side. I gave her lifts to use in her left shoes, and she returned to the office a week later. The severe bunion pain, present for 6 years, was gone. The left knee pain, present for 20 years, was also gone. The left Achilles tendon was no longer tight, and the nerve sensitivity on the right side had disappeared. In her situation, the right foot pain had been the result of nerve hypersensitivity coming from her PseudoStenosis, making a minor bunion very painful. The left knee pain was actually caused by the biomechanical changes and stress caused by the shorter leg. In this situation, we were able to kill two birds with one simple, very inexpensive, and rapidly working stone (or rather, lift).

Incidentally, I felt that this was great medical care—but an accountant that I spoke to afterward suggested that in the future I should do the foot surgery first. I am pretty sure he was kidding!

Yvette B's interview is available on our web site, WalkingWellAgain.com.

Update: Yvette did come in a year later noting that she again had some discomfort in both areas. I replaced lifts that had flattened, which may have been part of the problem. However, she certainly had a bunion and some knee arthritis, and those conditions may also need treatment. Sometimes improvement is only partial or temporary, and additional treatment is required.

4. **Sudden change in overall arthritis pain may be from SS/PS.**

This is especially true if the increase in symptoms is not accompanied by change in appearance. If a person has increased pain in multiple joints, and there are local changes such as redness or swelling that could be seen with an inflammatory arthritis such as gout or Rheumatoid Arthritis, then it makes sense to attribute the increased symptoms to the local changes.

If, however, a person is very active, has a minor injury, a major injury such as a fall or auto accident, or simply has an increased arthritic pain profile in more than one area but without signs of inflammation, the worsening is likely due to spinal nerve involvement. One would not expect multiple areas to have sudden changes in degeneration simultaneously. However, the presence of symptomatic (and now activated) SS/PS can cause exacerbation of symptoms in multiple areas. Once activated, the SS/PS can maintain the symptoms at a much higher level than previously present, and this situation may persist until the SS/PS is addressed.

Throughout this book, I stress that symptoms of SS/PS can be expected to improve in 1–3 days of proper treatment. In this situation, the reverse is demonstrated. In just 1 day, multiple areas may

become more symptomatic. I have seen many such situations in which such diffuse arthritic pain was quickly relieved by Positional Testing or Mechanical Testing.

5. **Many people have arthritis pain with or without visible changes in the joint, due to mechanical stress caused by imperfect body mechanics. This stress may be labeled a "Deforming Force." These stresses are often the same mechanical problems that could give rise to PseudoStenosis, even if the back is not involved. A PseudoStenosis factor can therefore do any of the following:**

a) cause direct pain by way of mechanical stress, arthritis, or tendonitis in the foot or leg

b) cause symptoms indirectly by giving rise to spinal nerve irritation that mimics or exacerbates arthritis symptoms

c) cause problems both ways

Thus, treating a biomechanical problem—even one that is far removed from the painful joint—with Mechanical Testing may also relieve arthritis symptoms that are actually caused by local inflammation, if that local inflammation is aggravated by stress caused by faulty mechanics in other places of the extremity. This improvement can occur in as few as 1–3 days, even if the symptoms have been present for many years. **By removing the Deforming Force that caused the problem in the first place, one can often reduce pain, even if there is already a local deformity present.**

6. **A mechanical stress (Deforming Force) that can cause PseudoStenosis can also prevent healing in areas of arthritis that were caused by direct injury. Though the stress had nothing to do with the beginning of the problem, it may act to prevent healing.**

StoryTime: Anthony S, a construction worker, fell out of a tree. As a result, he developed back pain, leg pain, and neuropathic pain that was attributed to neuropathy caused by his diabetes. All of this compelled him to sit down after standing or walking for only a few minutes, and it left him with poor balance. A physically strong person who was motivated to work, he went through months of physical therapy, medication, and epidural and trigger-point injections. Each intervention provided incomplete relief that lasted only a few days. He eventually had to go on disability and still had no relief of his symptoms after more than 4 years.

At Anthony's initial visit, my exam suggested PseudoStenosis as a possible contributing factor. He had a Limb Length Discrepancy with asymmetric Equinus, a stable foot type, and an asymmetric First Interspace Fine Sign. Indirect measurement and the Iliac Crest Pain Resolution Sign suggested a ⅜-inch difference. There was no loss of sensitivity to light touch, shown by his Loss of Protective Sensation (LOPS) score of "0," although his vibration sensitivity was elevated.

I provided ⅜-inch lifts and eagerly awaited his next visit. I was disappointed. He reported a moderate improvement in ability to stand and walk but no significant change in chronic back and leg pain. The asymmetric Equinus, nerve sensitivity, and hip sensitivity were unchanged.

Further discussion revealed that Anthony stayed at home most of the time and often did not wear shoes—which meant that he usually walked with no lift! I strapped his foot and attached the appropriate lift. Though he had an appointment to return in 3 days, I did not see him for a week. When he came in, he brought great news. All of his back, leg, and neuropathic pain had vanished—within 3 days. He removed the strap but used shoes (with the lift!) at all times, even in the house. At that exam, there was no Achilles tightness, and all of his nerve sensitivity was gone.

There are two major lessons to be learned here. **First, one must be firm about compliance,** whether it involves a lift, a walker, Adjunct Measures, orthotics, or braces. Strict relief of the mechanical imbalance is often needed at least temporarily, and must be rigorously encouraged.

Second is point number six, above: **the initial cause of the problem may not be the cause of failure to improve.** There is no question that the fall was the precipitating factor of Anthony's problems. But the 4 years of failure to improve appear to have been caused by the spinal misalignment caused by the

Limb Length Discrepancy. It is essential to understand that **the initiating cause of the problem may not be the factor preventing improvement.** In such cases, all possible causes of PseudoStenosis must be considered.

Anthony's interview, in both English and Farsi, is available on WalkingWellAgain.com.

Two Essential Clarifications/Disclaimers

First, different conditions have different likelihoods of success with the approaches presented in this book. While I believe that good-to-excellent improvement is seen in some 70% of patients presenting with Spinal Stenosis or PseudoStenosis, the percentage drops to closer to 50% with individuals presenting with either moderate-to-moderately-severe neuropathy or **lower-extremity arthritis.** With arthritis, earlier treatment often brings about better results. Sometimes the degeneration of the joint has gone too far to be helped by anything other than a joint replacement. HOWEVER, I have had many patients with severe arthritis who received enough relief from their pain to avoid surgery. I have also had patients who, having had joint replacement or spinal fusion, continued to experience persistent pain that responded well to these techniques. **I therefore recommend that ALL patients with significant lower-extremity or lumbar spine arthritis be considered for the approaches presented here.**

Second, I want to make sure that I do not receive (or appear to seek) credit for originality when it is not deserved. **The concept of the effect of lower-extremity pathology (such as a short leg or Flat Feet) on other areas (such as an ankle, knee, hip, or spine) is NOT AT ALL ORIGINAL ON MY PART.** Combining this knowledge with insights and approaches regarding Spinal Stenosis and PseudoStenosis and describing how this pattern can affect or mimic some other conditions may be original, but the concept of the effect of the actual arthritis is not. In the appendix of the book, there is a list of articles that report some of the relationships that I present in this chapter and Chapter 19.

To be honest, I am not sure why most standard literature does not stress this link. Articles on this topic have appeared in professional journals. With time, the concepts may be incorporated into standard medical practice. At present, to the best of my knowledge, they have not been.

"Charting" the Possibilities

The following chart provides an overview that may clarify the **overlap and misdiagnosis of arthritis and SS/PS pain**, as there are many possible combinations of arthritis, Spinal Stenosis, and PseudoStenosis. Many other factors could contribute to symptoms, of course, including poor circulation, swelling, stroke, neuropathy, and other medical conditions. The chart is not meant to be all-inclusive, but rather to highlight some of the possibilities.

By offering these different possible combinations, this chart presents opportunities for success. This is especially true if you understand that biomechanically

---

For the very curious

Definitions and Descriptions

Here are some definitions and clinical tidbits that will help some non-clinicians better understand the chart that follows:

1. *Degenerative joint disease (DJD), or Osteoarthritis—also called "wear-and-tear arthritis"—is attributed to the breaking down of structures of the joint due to mechanical imbalance and stress.*

2. *DJD can result from a previous specific injury to a joint (such as a knee injury causing knee arthritis) or from biomechanical problems (e.g., a knee injury that causes a person to walk differently—giving rise to hip arthritis—or either Flat Feet or a short leg—causing foot, ankle, knee, hip, or back arthritis).*

3. *Inflammatory arthritis, such as Rheumatoid Arthritis, can cause the breakdown of a joint that is affected by the inflammation. Fortunately, this is much less common now because of DMARDs: disease-modifying anti-rheumatic drugs. It is important that EVERYONE with inflammatory arthritis have a relationship with a rheumatologist who is expert in these wonderful drugs. The sooner you are evaluated by a rheumatologist so that you can start taking this medicine, the greater the chance of avoiding major arthritic changes and becoming a candidate for surgery.*

4. *Inflammatory arthritis can affect certain joints, such as those in the feet or knees, which can in turn lead to changes in walking. Those walking changes can then cause other joints to break down (DJD), even if they are not directly affected by the inflammatory arthritis.*

5. *The phrase "arthritis and SS" refers to having both an arthritic problem, as defined on the top row of the chart, and also an actual and symptomatic Spinal Stenosis.*

6. *The phrase "arthritis and PS" refers to having both an arthritic problem, as defined on the top row of the chart, and also PseudoStenosis contributing to the symptoms.*

7. *The phrase "arthritis and SS and PS" refers to having arthritis and both Spinal Stenosis and PseudoStenosis.*

8. *By "systemic disease," I refer to one of many medical conditions that can cause joint or muscular pain. These conditions include Lyme disease, inflammatory bowel conditions such as Crohn's disease and ulcerative colitis, and many other conditions best evaluated by a rheumatologist. This chart stresses that while the medical condition may be present, symptoms may be caused or exacerbated by SS/PS.*

9. *Fibromyalgia is a disorder characterized by widespread musculoskeletal pain, often accompanied by fatigue, sleep disruption, memory loss, and mood issues. Researchers believe that Fibromyalgia amplifies painful sensations by affecting the way the brain processes pain signals, as presented on the Mayo Clinic website. I have had many patients who were diagnosed with Fibromyalgia who improved after treatment for SS or PS.*

10. *Sometimes, pain may be initiated by an injury but is either exacerbated or maintained by improper mechanics or by the presence of Spinal Stenosis or PseudoStenosis, as in Anthony S's story above. Even if an injury occurred, it does not mean that this chart cannot still be helpful in providing guidance.*

	DJD from trauma	DJD from biomechanics	Fibromyalgia or systemic disease	Inflammatory arthritis	Inflammatory arthritis and secondary DJD	No arthritis
Arthritis only						
Arthritis and SS						
Arthritis and SS and PS						
Arthritis and PS						
No Arthritis, just SS or PS						

induced arthritis can often be treated biomechanically, and that both Spinal Stenosis and PseudoStenosis can have a tremendous effect on the symptoms. I believe that the information of this rubric should be considered for any patient suffering from arthritis symptoms. Successful use can guide the route to relief for many people, without medication, injections, surgery, or even physical therapy.

Important Questions Regarding Arthritis

The right questions can guide an individual as to how to proceed correctly with the protocols of this book. More importantly, I believe that they should be considered by clinicians treating arthritis, in addition to the other interventions. These questions go beyond the normal Positional History, which is why they are presented in detail here.

1. **If there is degenerative arthritis, is it from an injury?** If the arthritis is local from a direct injury, then direct treatment can provide relief, and might be necessary to provide relief. However, if the pain is quite significant—and especially if it is greater than one would expect from the amount of actual arthritis present—or if it does not improve as expected with treatment, further investigation is indicated.

2. **Is there degenerative arthritis caused by improper biomechanics (i.e., arthritis that developed without any specific injury)?** If the arthritis

is from biomechanical stress, such as Flat Feet or a short leg, then treating the cause can greatly improve the symptoms, even if there is actual local arthritis present. **Limb Length Discrepancy often gives rise to an asymmetric arthritis, where one foot, ankle, knee, hip, or side of the back is much worse or at least different from the other.** Arthritis from symmetrical Flat Feet is usually symmetrical, but it can affect the entire skeletal chain, from feet to knees to back and even to neck, resulting in shoulder pain, jaw pain (TMJ), or headaches.

3. **Is there an inflammatory arthritis such as Rheumatoid Arthritis, Lupus, Ankylosing Spondylitis, or Psoriatic Arthritis?** Inflammatory arthritis, in which the body creates inflammation within a joint, independent of mechanical stress, needs to be treated from a medical standpoint. HOWEVER, the presence of inflammatory arthropathy does not rule out the possibility that mechanical stress, Spinal Stenosis, or PseudoStenosis may be contributing to the overall pathology. IN ADDITION, it is well known that these types of arthritis cause soft-tissue swelling that make a patient more likely to have compression problems of the nerves. SS/PS is just such a problem!

4. **Has the inflammatory arthritis caused actual secondary degenerative changes?** In addition to the symptoms of inflammation, inflammatory arthritis can also cause joint destruction that

persists as a local degenerative joint even after the inflammation has been controlled. An altered gait because of pain or because of a long-term degeneration can cause secondary degenerative changes in joints that were not affected by the inflammatory process.

5. **Is there or is there not true arthritis present,** including changes in soft tissue, bone, or joint structures that can be identified as joint pathology? **Or are there simply symptoms that are diagnosed as arthritis?** Arthritis is a common diagnosis when there is pain of unclear origin. If there are significant symptoms but no significant physical findings, arthritis may not be present. Further investigation for SS or PS is needed.

6. **Is there a positive Positional History? See Chapter 5 for this all-important set of questions. I will review here just two of the most basic ones. First, is there worsening of symptoms with walking? If so, are symptoms relieved by Positional Testing with a grocery cart or walker?** I find that many people suffering from arthritis alone do not receive much benefit from leaning on a walker or cart. They may have increased stability, but usually do not experience great relief of symptoms. Significant improvement would suggest Spinal Stenosis or PseudoStenosis. (If under 5'2", the person may need to rest his or her arms side-to-side on the handle of the grocery cart to get good relief.)

   Second, are symptoms improved when pushing a grocery cart but worse at the checkout counter? If so, this strongly suggests the presence of Spinal Stenosis or PseudoStenosis.

7. **Is there any lower-extremity pathology that could contribute to spine dysfunction, as described in Chapter 12?** PseudoStenosis may be caused by a Limb Length Discrepancy, Flat Feet, or any arthritis or significant dysfunction of the foot, ankle, knee, or hip that affects spine function.

8. **If symptoms suggestive of Spinal Stenosis are present and the spinal imaging is positive, is it nevertheless essential to investigate aggressively the possibility of PseudoStenosis?** Yes. Whether the spine MRI or CT scan is positive or negative for Spinal Stenosis, one should (as described in

Chapter 12) also investigate for PseudoStenosis. After all, just because there is true Spinal Stenosis does not mean that there is no PseudoStenosis component contributing to the problem.

About Fibromyalgia

Fibromyalgia is defined as a disorder characterized by widespread musculoskeletal pain, often including back and leg and arthritic pain, present for at least 3 months. It may be accompanied by fatigue, sleep, mood issues, GI distress and other symptoms.

Fibromyalgia is a disease of exclusion!

*It should only be diagnosed after other possible causes have been ruled out. One therefore should not diagnose Fibromyalgia unless Lumbar and Cervical Stenosis but **especially PseudoStenosis** are considered and treated.*

The clear majority of my patients who presented with spine and lower extremity symptoms diagnosed as from Fibromyalgia had excellent and rapid improvement of those symptoms with the interventions for PseudoStenosis. I therefore present that SS/PS must be excluded before settling on the diagnosis of Fibromyalgia.

StoryTime: Sharon was a woman in her 50s who suffered from long-term back pain, leg pain, and difficulty sleeping because of discomfort and restlessness. She had a long-standing diagnosis of Fibromyalgia. She'd tried orthotics, which had not proved helpful, and had received therapy and medication for known back arthritis and disc disease, without much help. To make a long story short, I found that she had flexible symmetrical Flat Feet, a positive First Interspace Fine Sign, and a moderate response to Positional Testing with a walker. Suspecting that the Flat Feet were causing PseudoStenosis and that the orthotics had not provided adequate change, I applied Unna boots to both of her feet.

Within a few days, Sharon's back pain, leg pain, and difficulty sleeping because of discomfort and restlessness disappeared. I made custom ankle braces for her and hit a home run. Six weeks after she started wearing the braces, her improvement was still maintained. When I called her a year later for the purpose of this book, the same held true. All systems go!

The lesson? Years of symptoms attributed to Fibromyalgia had been caused by Flat Feet that did not respond to orthotics but responded well to custom ankle braces. I believe that, as with so many other conditions, all patients with diagnosed Fibromyalgia who have symptoms involving the back and/or lower extremities should be considered as candidates for the approaches presented in this book.

A video of Sharon's video can be seen on our web set WalkingWellAgain.com.

StoryTime: Patricia C was a 75-year-old woman who came in because of back, leg, and foot pain that had been bothering her for about 8 years. She also had left knee pain, which would temporary improve with steroid injections and then Synvisc injections. Aching was worst in the left lower back and was aggravated by standing and walking. Symptoms persisted even though she took anti-inflammatory medications plus steroids for periodic flare-ups of her Rheumatoid Arthritis. This was complicated by the presence of Lyme disease.

She had a positive Positional History, with symptoms reduced greatly through use of a grocery cart. Examination showed findings consistent with PseudoStenosis caused by Limb Length Discrepancy, including Equinus on the right side, and a positive First Interspace Fine Sign, an increased Q-angle of the knee, and Iliac Crest tenderness all on the left side. It took a ⅛-inch lift under the right heel to make the 2 hips coplanar and eliminate all the left Iliac Crest pain and sensitivity. Considering PseudoStenosis caused by Limb Length Discrepancy, I gave her several lifts.

When she returned a week later, she reported that after 1 day she had had elimination of her back pain as well as foot, leg, and knee pain. She was able to stand for long periods of time and walk long

---

About Physical Therapy

Physical therapy is, for many people, the door to recovery and independence. This assistance is often the difference between independence and dependence, and it is invaluable for so many recovering from surgery, strokes, fractures, and other causes of disability.

For the purpose of discussion, I will divide therapy into two categories. One is the rehabilitation efforts that are so helpful after an acute problem, such as a fracture, a surgery, a stroke, or another possible cause. In no way do the approaches of this book replace that therapy, although they may complement it.

The second category is therapy directed at chronic pain. The pain may be experienced as back, hip, knee, leg, ankle, or foot arthritis. It may be from neck arthritis, or it may be from a diagnosed medical condition such as Fibromyalgia. It may be from painful swollen legs, Peripheral Neuropathy, weakness, or poor balance. Physical therapy for these conditions is frequently helpful, but often does not provide complete or long-term resolution.

*The symptoms addressed in this second category **may** be caused or affected by SS/PS. As such, if the SS/PS is addressed, it is **possible** to have complete and long-term resolution of symptoms without additional therapy. Not guaranteed, but quite possible. I believe that investigation for and treatment of SS/PS should be the first step for most people with the symptoms listed in the prior paragraph, and that traditional physical therapy (as well as other treatments such as medication, injections, or surgery) should be brought in **after** management of SS/PS.*

Physical therapists may be particularly well suited to investigate and treat SS/PS, which they may do independently or in cooperation with a podiatrist, orthopedist, or physiatrist.

There is often great value in combining physical therapy with treatment of SS/PS. Long-term symptoms or disability may lead to deconditioning of the whole body, selective weakness, or alteration of gait, which is often best addressed with expert guidance from a physical therapist.

Three Factors of Arthritic Pain

I consider three factors in understanding arthritic pain, which I want to make sure are clear. Yes, it is much more complicated than this, but I feel that this categorization is eminently practical.

First, there are the symptoms caused by local pathology, including changes in the bones and damaged soft tissues of the joint, or inflammation stemming from systemic arthritis such as gout or rheumatoid arthritis. Treatments including medication, injections, physical therapy, and surgery are not addressed in this book.

*The second factor contributing to pain from arthritis is the presence of a persistent **Deforming Force**. Examples include Limb Length Discrepancy, Flat Feet, or altered gait caused by other pathology that affects the position and forces applied to the arthritic joint. Neutralizing the Deforming Force often provides rapid relief; this is addressed in the next chapter.*

The third aspect is the presence of the nerve sensitivity caused by spinal nerve compression, which can make any arthritic pathology much more painful. This may be caused by primary pathology within the spine such as Spinal Stenosis, or it might be mediated through the spine because of lower-extremity dysfunction, i.e., PseudoStenosis. It is the goal of this chapter to facilitate recognition of that contributing factor.

distances, and she even went to the gym! Examination showed elimination of asymmetric Equinus, nerve sensitivity, hip sensitivity, and all the pain along the left Pes Anserinus.

This is a situation in which symptoms that had been attributed for years to Rheumatoid Arthritis complicated by Lyme disease were caused or at least greatly exacerbated by a Limb Length Discrepancy.

Patricia C's interview at her second visit is available on WalkingWellAgain.com.

StoryTime: This is a complicated story with many lessons, and it is a story that epitomizes the pattern of PseudoStenosis being the cause of extensive symptoms misdiagnosed as a form of arthritis. The fact that the patient is himself a respected physician only magnifies the impact.

Luke was a 42-year-old physician referred to me for treatment of chronic severely sensitive toenails that he was not able to cut himself. For years, trimming his nails was a task that he dreaded.

Dr. Luke had Familial Mediterranean Fever, a genetic auto-inflammatory disease. For decades he had diffuse arthritic pain throughout his feet and legs and spine. The pain in his left ankle, knee, and hip was worse than in the right ones. He had sharp pain, as well as difficulty walking more than a couple of blocks, a difficulty that was even worse going uphill. He had difficulty standing, walked

better pushing a grocery cart, and felt worse at the checkout counter. He had jaw pain that was aggravated with standing and walking and that was much worse going uphill. He acknowledged nighttime leg pain that woke him frequently. Because of Shortness of Breath, he underwent a cardiac evaluation, including a heart catheterization, which demonstrated no pathology. He was unable to bend over to pick things up off the floor and routinely had to ask his children to do so for him, which caused him great distress.

Because of gastrointestinal sensitivity, Dr. Luke was unable to tolerate anti-inflammatory medication. Physical therapy did not provide lasting help.

Physical examination showed many imperfections, including Flat Feet, a positive First Interspace Fine Sign bilaterally, left worse than right. He had Equinus on the right side only, with a mild structural Limb Length Discrepancy identified by indirect measurement. He had pain along his left Pes Anserinus, which is just below the knee, as described in Chapter 6..

Suspecting PseudoStenosis from Limb Length Discrepancy, I provided a ⅛-inch lift for the shorter right leg. Not a home run, but a double! A few days later he reported moderate improvement of the long-term back pain, the inability to stand and walk, the TMJ, and the leg pain at night in bed. He still had limitations from back pain, poor balance and endurance, and pain that was most pronounced in his left ankle, knee, and hip.

Suspecting that his Flat Feet may have been contributing to symptoms, I applied a Low Dye strap on each foot but got no improvement. Positional Testing with a walker did not help. At the next visit, my examination showed severe sensitivity in the left sinus tarsi, which I then injected. Five minutes later, the overall pain in his ankle and entire leg was diminished. At the next visit, he reported having no left knee, hip, or ankle pain, and was able to walk longer distances without pain. He was also able to pick things up from the floor without asking for help.

A few months later, he came in again for me to trim his nails. I was looking forward to this follow-up visit, and I was not disappointed. The symptoms he had suffered for decades were greatly improved. He had rare and only mild back pain, jaw pain, Shortness of Breath, and difficulty standing, walking, and sleeping. No left ankle or knee or hip pain. He was able to pick things up from the ground at will. He was worried that his toenails would be sensitive when cut, but they actually were fine. After decades of dreading that simple procedure, he still had anxiety but no actual tenderness. A year later, all improvement was maintained.

There are four important lessons in this story. First, one must be aware of the many symptoms that are affected by lower-extremity dysfunction. In this case, jaw pain, Shortness of Breath, back pain, difficulty bending over, nighttime symptoms, as well as arthritic pain all improved by treating the feet.

Secondly, there is a powerful imperative to look *beyond the medical diagnosis as a cause of painful symptoms*. Luke had a diagnosis of Familial Mediterranean Fever. For decades, his symptoms were attributed primarily to that condition. In actuality, it was straightforward lower-extremity pathology that was primarily responsible for his many symptoms.

In this book many similar cases are reported in which SS/PS symptoms were attributed to systemic conditions, such as Fibromyalgia, Multiple Sclerosis, Post-polio Syndrome, Crohn's disease,

and Lupus. My position is that **all patients** diagnosed with symptomatic Spinal Stenosis should have an evaluation for PseudoStenosis. Similarly, **all patients** with spinal or lower-extremity arthritic symptoms attributed to a systemic disease should be evaluated for SS/PS. The cause of pain should not be attributed to a systemic disease until the common causes of SS/PS are ruled out. Such an approach could have saved Luke decades of problems.

The third lesson is the need for persistence. After moderate success with my first intervention, I struck out with attempts two and three. With unresolved symptoms, a thorough exam was needed to find the cause of his symptoms. When symptoms persist, one must be willing to redo both the history and the physical exam to try to find the true problem.

The fourth lesson is the need to keep the sinus tarsi in mind. This troubling joint, which may not become problematic until months after an ankle or rear-foot injury, may cause problems for decades, affecting the entire leg up to the spine. I have seen several patients with extensive PseudoStenosis symptoms caused by this problem. A good cortisone injection (deep into the sinus tarsi) often produces immediate and lasting relief. At times, long-term mechanical control with an orthotic, an ankle brace, or even surgery may be needed.

Three Steps to Self-Evaluation

Now that you've been thoroughly prepared, here are three steps to self-evaluation, to decide if YOU might be helped by the Spinal Stenosis / PseudoStenosis protocols. This may also guide you to decide whether you can start to treat yourself or you need reevaluation and help from a doctor.

First, determine whether Spinal Stenosis or PseudoStenosis is causing or worsening your symptoms, either through a Positional History (Chapter 5), through Positional Testing (Chapter 7), or by doing the Grocery Cart Test (end of Chapter 7).

Second, consider checking (or being checked) for nerve sensitivity, including the First Interspace Fine Sign, as described in Chapter 6.

Third, consider whether you have any lower-extremity problem that could be causing PseudoStenosis that may indirectly cause or worsen the lower-extremity arthritis symptoms. The same problem can directly cause arthritis pathology, but that will be addressed in the next chapter.

Let's take these evaluations one at a time.

Positional History and Positional Testing

The first step in investigating possible SS/PS involvement is by taking a Positional History, by performing Positional Testing, or by trying the Grocery Cart Test. The Positional History is presented in great detail in Chapter 5. If in doubt, read that chapter again.

Try Positional Testing to see if it provides good improvement that can be built upon. If you have or can get hold of the proper kind of walker, as described in Chapter 7, do so. If not, the Grocery Cart Test is a quick and readily available substitute. The Grocery Cart Test is actually the first form of Positional Testing I used back in 2001. Take a look at the end of Chapter 7 to brush up on the details of that test.

If there is good improvement with the Grocery Cart Test, this strongly suggests the presence of either Spinal Stenosis or PseudoStenosis.

If there are no signs of PseudoStenosis (see below, or Chapter 12), proceed directly to Positional Testing with a walker (Chapter 7), and use the Adjunct Measures presented in Chapter 8. This protocol alone may provide excellent improvement in your walking ability, as well as relief from pain, all within a matter of 1–3 days. Again, be careful about the height of the walker, avoid hills, and use common sense. The incredible results seen with Positional Testing have been a driving force behind my long-term commitment to this approach—and, of course, to this book.

If you have great results with Positional Testing and transition to Positional Therapy (Chapter 10), it is quite possible that no other intervention will be necessary. If you still have arthritis but much less discomfort or walking limitation, use your judgment as to whether or not to explore any further.

If, however, you note that there is definite potential for a PseudoStenosis component or there is only partial or temporary improvement with Positional Testing

and Positional Therapy, then further exploration is indicated.

The Clue of Nerve Hypersensitivity

The second step—a brief physical exam that includes checking for nerve hypersensitivity—may also be of great value. It is self-evident that people with arthritis usually experience pain in a joint. This is not surprising, as the term "arthritis" actually means "inflammation of a joint". With arthritis, one may also have tendonitis—inflammation of a tendon—or bursitis—inflammation of a bursa, a fluid-filled sac near a joint, which can cause similar symptoms. Any such structure may be quite tender.

However, nerve sensitivity should also be routinely checked. If the nerves in the feet and/or legs are sensitive in many areas, I feel that it is by far most likely that there is a nerve compression syndrome present, most commonly Spinal Stenosis and PseudoStenosis. **Tenderness along specific nerves and a First Interspace Fine Sign, as explained in Chapter 6, strongly suggest the presence of SS/PS.** Depending on the area of spinal nerve compression, nerves may be more sensitive in the feet, legs, or thighs. The sensitivity often corresponds to the areas where the symptoms seem worse. If the nerves are much more sensitive on one side, a Limb Length Discrepancy (structural or functional) is likely. This test not only stimulates a very strong suspicion of SS or PS, but it also allows a patient to track his or her own progress! This is a very valuable test that you can actually do yourself.

If a positive First Interspace Fine Sign or other described nerve sensitivity is present, it strongly suggests an SS/PS involvement that is affecting the symptoms of the arthritis. (This does not mean that other nerve compression problems are not possible, just that they are much less common.)

This observation will be controversial. Some doctors who follow arthritis may note trigger points in the leg or thigh that may be seen with Fibromyalgia or arthritis. I do not claim that trigger points are never a factor. But I feel that the nerve sensitivity that other doctors attribute to an arthritic or other medical condition such as Fibromyalgia are often caused by SS/PS. **I have had well over a thousand patients whose nerve sensitivity improved within a few days by my treating**

for either Spinal Stenosis or PseudoStenosis, with no other intervention for arthritis or neuropathy. I therefore emphasize the value of this specific approach.

Question: If you have taken a Positional History and done Positional Testing, why do you need to check nerve sensitivity? The answer is . . . maybe you do, and maybe you don't. If Positional Testing brings you real relief from your symptoms and you are happy, then I am happy. Nerve sensitivity patterns may not be that important, except of course if you are concerned about a possible Limb Length Discrepancy, in which the sensitivity is most often worse in one of the extremities.

However, bear in mind that not all patients with SS/PS improve with Positional Testing and Mechanical Testing. **If your symptoms do not improve with Positional Testing, you might think that you have ruled out an SS/PS component. Not true.** The presence of nerve sensitivity patterns—like significant lower-back pain or a positive Positional History—suggests a possible SS/PS component. You then require an evaluation for your back, guided by a physician such as a rheumatologist, orthopedist, physiatrist, or neurologist, which may include spinal imaging and epidural injections. You will also need an evaluation by a foot specialist for possible causes of PseudoStenosis. **After all, the techniques shared here, though often diagnostic and even therapeutic, are not infallible.** By all means, see specialists who can investigate other possible causes. If your symptoms persist, seek further help!

Don't Forget PseudoStenosis

The third step is to check for possible causes of PseudoStenosis. Any of them can cause back dysfunction that results in nerve pressure that either leads to or worsens lower-extremity pain. The many causes of PseudoStenosis and the ways to check for them are clearly presented in Chapter 12.

WRAPPING UP

This chapter has stressed the need to recognize and manage the effect of Spinal Stenosis and/or PseudoStenosis on lower-extremity arthritis symptoms. Managing SS/PS can have great benefit even if there is also arthritis present. This alone has reduced arthritis pain in a great many of my patients.

The next chapter deals with some of the biomechanical causes of arthritis, describes how they can directly cause arthritis difficulties, and presents suggestions for treatment that usually do not involve medications, injections, physical therapy, or surgery.

CHAPTER 19

Understanding and Managing Arthritis through the Gift of Biomechanics

In the previous chapter, we dealt with understanding and treating the Spinal Stenosis / PseudoStenosis component of arthritis, which frequently contributes to the overall pain in the lower extremities. This is an essential first step. But what of the actual arthritis that is present?

The Essential Next Step in Managing Degenerative Arthritis

Lower-extremity arthritis symptoms and deformities do not develop in a vacuum. Identifying and treating the mechanical problems that led to development of arthritis can frequently relieve or at least significantly reduce arthritis symptoms, and may also prevent further arthritic development.

I feel strongly that this should be the *next step* in addressing lower-extremity and spinal-arthritis complaints. The possibility that a mechanical problem has caused or may continue to affect the arthritis should not be looked into only after anti-inflammatory drugs, injections, therapy, or even surgery have failed. **Instead, FIRST seek out and treat the potential mechanical causes before any other treatment.**

Standing on the Shoulders of Giants

Patients, family members, clinicians, and researchers—take note. Though this chapter includes some original insights and applications, most of the information I present here has already been reported in medical literature.

I mention this for two reasons. First, I do not wish to appear to falsely seek credit for insights previously reported by other clinicians. There are many people who have worked hard to share this information and who are far more expert in both biomechanics and research than I will ever be. Though I write and have lectured about techniques that apply insights, both original and borrowed, in the field, I would never venture to lecture academically on biomechanics. I am a simple clinician, not a biomechanics researcher.

The second reason is far more important than either ego or reputation. By emphasizing that much of this information can be found in the body of medical literature, I hope that other clinicians will be more willing to make use of the clinical applications that I recommend. To this end, many supportive articles are listed in the appendix of this book.

And to my fellow podiatrists . . . I hope you can look past information that many of you already know and use, in order to get to the original observations and suggestions as well as the reminders that you'll find in this chapter. Bear in mind that this book was written primarily for patients, but it was also intended to be read by non-podiatric clinicians as well as by podiatrists. Most of them will likely not share our appreciation for the extensive role of biomechanical treatment in dealing with arthritic symptoms, as well as with the PseudoStenosis symptoms reported elsewhere in this book. Thanks for your patience as I share what is, for some of you, known information.

Considering the Biomechanical Causes of Arthritis

At the end of the previous chapter, we discussed the steps to take in evaluating possible SS/PS in conjunction with an arthritic condition. After taking a thorough Positional History, trying Positional Testing for primary Spinal Stenosis symptoms, investigating nerve hypersensitivity patterns, and considering PseudoStenosis, you should then proceed to address the biomechanical causes of arthritis.

When I speak of arthritis, I am referring to the **degenerative arthritis** that (usually) begins without the catalyst of a major or moderate injury. **These biomechanical causes are often the same factors that give rise to PseudoStenosis.** I remind you that these mechanical imperfections can create many different problem patterns:

- **Mechanical imperfection can cause the actual arthritic problem**, such as foot, ankle, knee, or hip arthritis, tendonitis, etc. Arthritic pain can be present even without visible or radiological (X-ray) changes.

- Mechanical imperfection, even if only mild, can maintain the stress on an actual arthritic problem and can give rise to any number of unpleasant symptoms. **Many patients in whom arthritis symptoms developed after an injury never improve until lower-extremity biomechanical problems are addressed.**

- Mechanical problems can lead to PseudoStenosis, causing spinal nerve irritation that either mimics symptoms of neuropathy, poor circulation, and arthritic aching, or worsens the symptoms from other problems, such as actual arthritis.

- Mechanical imperfections can cause actual Spinal Stenosis. Although I strongly suspect this to be the case, I am not confident in this hypothesis to state it definitively.

It is essential to understand that mechanical imperfection can either directly cause symptoms in the area of pain by being a *Deforming Force,* or it can indirectly cause symptoms by creating spinal nerve irritation—PseudoStenosis. **Treatment of the mechanical imperfection may thus provide relief of both direct and indirect symptoms of arthritis.**

Let us review the common causes of PseudoStenosis and then proceed to address them from an arthritis viewpoint.

> ### *Common causes of PseudoStenosis*
>
> 1. *Limb Length Discrepancy (LLDx)*
> 2. *A flexible Flat Foot, such as with Functional Hallux Limitus*
> 3. *A rigid or nearly rigid Flat Foot*
> 4. *Equinus, involving a tight Achilles tendon in the back of the legs or limited ankle joint movement for other reasons*
> 5. *An altered walking pattern caused by degenerative or other arthritis*
> 6. *An altered walking pattern caused by a stroke or other nerve problem*
> 7. *An altered walking pattern caused by any lower-extremity pain great enough to make the patient walk differently*
>
> *I am adding a HIGH-ARCHED FOOT to this list for the purposes of arthritis. While I have not personally recognized a High-Arched Foot as causing PseudoStenosis, it can certainly affect either lower-extremity or spine arthritis, so it must be included in this chapter.*

Limb Length Discrepancy (LLDx) as the Cause of Arthritis

There is a long section about Limb Length Discrepancy in Chapter 12. In fact, that section is almost 30 pages long, at least in draft form. In the present chapter, I will touch on some highlights and focus on the problem from an arthritis standpoint, but I will not repeat all important points. I suggest that anyone concerned about lower-extremity arthritis read the entire chapter on PseudoStenosis—or at the very least, the section on Limb Length Discrepancy, which I feel is the most common cause of both PseudoStenosis and lower-extremity arthritis.

To learn—or review—the signs that make you suspect a Limb Length Discrepancy, please refer to Chapter 12. And keep in mind that the presentation may be subtle. How subtle?

StoryTime: My wife has a young cousin in her 20s, whom we see rarely. Before a birthday party, I learned that she had been diagnosed with tendonitis in the foot, which had prevented her from running for 6 months despite anti-inflammatory medication, over-the-counter inserts, and 4 months of physical therapy. Therapy 3 times a week for 4 months is a lot of therapy! Yet she was still unable to run, and her foot continued to feel sore.

At the party, a quick exam showed some things you may be familiar with by now. The pain was in the left foot. Her right shoulder was slightly lower when standing, and her right heel was slightly higher when sitting. Neither difference would have been noticed by someone who was not looking for that exact pattern. When she was standing, her right hip was slightly lower. There was a positive First Interspace Fine Sign on the left side only. The Achilles tendon was somewhat tighter on the right side. And by the way, there was no tenderness along the suspected tendon on the uncomfortable left foot. The pain was actually on the bottom of the first metatarsal cuneiform joint (picture 19.1). There was no tendonitis, but the joint was inflamed—in other words, a localized mechanical arthritis. The shapes of the two feet were the same; neither was flatter than the other.

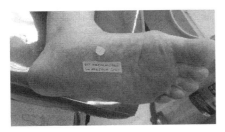

Picture 19.1. The circle identifies the bottom of the first metatarsal cuneiform joint, a common area of mechanically induced tenderness.

I gave her a ⅛-inch lift for the short leg. (I had come prepared.) Four hours later, at the end of the party, the muscle in the back of the shorter right leg was no longer tight! This was a surprise for me, as I normally have to wait a few days to reexamine. She noted that she felt more stable standing—a subtle change.

With no other therapy, she returned to limited running. She reported that even with running, almost all

the tenderness was gone (as long as she remembered to use the lift). Pretty good for a five-dollar lift! (No, I did NOT charge her!)

Reasons to Suspect Limb Length Discrepancy

For many people with arthritic pain and actual arthritis, the signs are obvious if you know how to look for them. Below is a presentation (from Chapter 12) of common differences in the two extremities. Any of these differences may help you suspect the problem so that you may try lifts on your own. (Keep in mind that the lift may not be the only needed intervention.)

The differences shown below suggest a Limb Length Discrepancy. They are, of course, affected by a variety of biomechanical factors, too many to list here. These factors are less likely if the discrepancy is of short duration, as may occur after an injury or surgery. It is important to note that if these factors are *not* found, it does not

How common is Limb Length Discrepancy, and how much discrepancy is important?

One oft-quoted study* reported that 32% of 600 military recruits had a ⅕- to ⅗-inch (5–15 millimeters) difference between the lengths of their legs. In that there was no perceived correlation comparing low-back pain in those with and without that much LLDx, the study presented that this discrepancy is a variation of normal that is not clinically significant.

I strongly disagree with this conclusion, for multiple reasons, two of which are essential to share. First, I observe that even mild LLDx of 2 or 3 millimeters can have a profound effect on symptoms. Second, these were healthy young men whose bodies were strong enough to compensate for the differences, and who had not yet experienced the wear and tear of life. They were men who did not yet have arthritis or spine problems in addition to the Limb Length Discrepancy. The imbalance that was present had not known the cumulative destructive effect of millions of steps taken over a lifetime of walking and working.

Thirty-three years of practical experience with senior citizens tells me otherwise. My practice has had so many patients who appeared to have small **¼-inch, ⅛-inch, or even ¹/₁₆-inch discrepancies,** who were treated with lifts and had excellent relief of symptoms. Not just symptoms that had been bothering them for days or weeks, but symptoms that had been present for years. Follow-up months or even years later showed a maintained improvement, with no other intervention.

Therefore, I believe with all my heart that even small Limb Length Discrepancies should be addressed if there are any symptoms, often before any other treatment is tried. There is nothing quicker, cheaper, or safer. And it is often the last treatment that you will ever need.

Who is right: those who suggest that the discrepancy must be over 3/8 (or even 3/5) of an inch to be a problem, or those who say that smaller differences can have a big effect? I report to you that I have had success with hundreds of patients with just a small lift that often relieved long-term symptoms in a day or two, so you know how I vote. What is important in this situation, however, is YOUR SYMPTOMS. If this is a suspected cause of problems, treat even for small differences, and see how you do. The proof is in the pudding!

*Hellsing, A. L. 1988. "Leg length inequality: A prospective study of young men during their military service." Upsala Journal of Medical Sciences 93 (3): 245–253.

mean that no discrepancy is present. The outstanding signs are more common with a Limb Length Discrepancy that is of long duration and is more than 2 millimeters. My observation is that a small 2-millimeter discrepancy can often cause PseudoStenosis symptoms, but is less likely to cause significant mechanical differences in the two feet.

The following is a list of common but not universal findings for Limb Length Discrepancy. Less frequently, the opposite of the listed finding is true, such as a shorter leg having a flatter foot or worse bunion, or turning out more, which suggests a functional rather than just a structural Limb Length Discrepancy. The patterns listed below are by far more common.

Apart from these physical changes in the extremities, there are a few other suggestive signs.

1. When seated on a podiatry chair with legs extended, one of the patient's heels appears higher than the other.

2. When standing, one of the patient's hip bones is lower than on the other side.

3. The Iliac Crest, the top of the hip joint, is very sensitive.

4. One shoulder is higher than the other. (This may also suggest scoliosis, by itself or with a Limb Length Discrepancy.)

5. One pant leg needs tailoring, or one foot is larger than the other.

6. The outside of shoes, the inside of shoes, and even orthotics wear out unevenly.

7. The patient frequently shifts from side to side when standing, even if only when tired, or the patient finds that standing is often harder than walking.

Again, please read Chapter 12 for a more complete guide on this ESSENTIAL subject.

Longer leg may have some or all of the following symptoms:

1. A more Flat Foot that may become arthritic and develop tendon problems
2. A foot that turns out to the side (away from the body) more when standing
3. A larger bunion
4. A callus in the center of the ball of the foot
5. Hammertoes
6. Swelling along the inside of the ankle if there is tendonitis
7. Greater nerve sensitivity, even if the discrepancy is only 1/16 of an inch (See section on the First Interspace Fine Sign in Chapter 6.)
8. An increased "Q-angle" of the knee with soft tissue swelling, involving tendonitis and bursitis
9. Increased sensitivity of the Pes Anserinus, just below the inside of the knee.
10. Increased arthritis of the knee
11. Arthritis of the hip (although more common on the short leg)

Shorter leg may have some or all of the following symptoms:

1. A less Flat Foot (although it may still be flat)
2. A foot that is likely to be straighter when the person stands or walks
3. A callus or pain on the ball of the foot, behind the baby toe (at the fifth metatarsal base)
4. Hammertoes and, occasionally, dislocated second or third metatarsal phalangeal joints
5. Greater tightness of the Achilles tendon (as will be explained in detail)
6. Limited motion or altered position of the knee or hip, or Genu Recurvatum (backward curve) of the knee (if the leg is shorter by more than about 1/4 of an inch)
7. Greater nerve sensitivity, if the leg is over 1/4 of an inch shorter (See section on the First Interspace Fine Sign in Chapter 6.)
8. Greater wearing-out of the outside of the heel of the shoe on the short side
9. Increased arthritis of the knee, but without the large medial bulge of the increased "Q-angle"
10. Arthritis of the hip (although not uncommon in the long leg)

Isn't It Common for People to Have Legs of Slightly Different Lengths?

Limb Length Discrepancy is an incredibly common problem, as well as a potentially destructive one. After I point out this discrepancy, I am often asked the following question: **isn't it common for people to have legs of slightly different lengths?** My answer is the following: **isn't it common for people to have back pain, lower-extremity arthritis, and difficulty walking?**

Limb Length Discrepancy may give rise to the development of hip arthritis, knee arthritis, and the severe Flat Foot seen with arthritis. For all these problems, ANY intervention for pain may be less effective unless the limb length issue is successfully addressed. **Subtle differences of ¼, ⅛, or even 1⁄16 of an inch have made such a difference for so many of my patients that I feel the need to** *underscore this point* **as strongly as possible.**

Remember, managing care is an art. You need the right diagnosis, the right treatment plan, and good compliance. It calls for active thought, and learning from both failure and success. As you absorb the lessons of this chapter, think things through and keep on thinking about what works and what does not.

About LLDx Treatment and Heel Lifts

Appropriate treatment with a lift can provide rapid improvement for so many symptoms. For most people, there is a distinct improvement within 1–3 days, even if symptoms have been present for years. For others, improvement is appreciated in 1–3 minutes. That is not a typo. There is immediate appreciation of the improved balance and improved symptoms brought on by compensation for the Deforming Force.

Guidance is provided in great detail in Chapter 12, section C, with a 13-point section on treatment tips. Please study that section.

How does arthritis caused by Limb Length Discrepancy present itself? Many of the problems arise from the way the body tries to adapt to or compensate for the length difference.

Effects of a Short Limb on the Foot and Ankle

Let's start with the shorter side, keeping in mind that these are frequent patterns, not hard-and-fast rules.

1. Equinus, involving a tight Achilles tendon

On the shorter leg, the Achilles tendon often presents as being tighter, as the body subconsciously tries to keep itself balanced by pushing down more with the foot of the short leg. This condition can be identified by comparing the range of motion of the two ankles. The technique to use to check this is presented in detail in Chapter 6. **Consistent use of a proper amount of lift often eliminates the Achilles tendon tightness in just a day or two.**

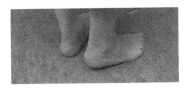

Picture 19.2. In the shorter leg, compensation often involves a tightening of the Achilles tendon. Though the situation is rarely this clear, this picture gives you the idea.

2. Achilles tendonitis with or without a spur in the back of the heel

I have had several patients with chronic pain in the back of the heel, and a Limb Length Discrepancy, and Achilles tendon inflammation or even degeneration where the tendon inserts into the heel bone, who had resolution of pain, swelling, and tightness within a few days of consistently using an appropriate lift.

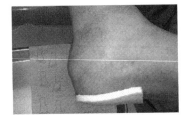

Picture 19.3. An enlargement in the back of the heel that was successfully treated with a lift strapped to the bottom of the heel to reduce the Equinus.

3. Calluses that are not symmetrical

In addition, since the foot is pointed downward, there is more pressure on the ball of the foot in the area behind the baby toe. A painful callus may result, which may not resolve with orthotics or even surgery, as the foot is continually held in a position that maximizes pressure on that area. Sometimes the shorter leg has a higher-arched foot, with calluses behind both the big toe and the baby toe. *I have had patients whose callus in the front part of the foot resolved just by using a heel lift, which reduced the tendency of the foot to contact the ground in an inverted position.*

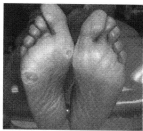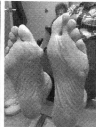

Picture 19.4. Callus on the bottom of the foot under either just the fifth metatarsal head, or, less frequently, under both the first and fifth metatarsal heads, behind the first and baby toes.

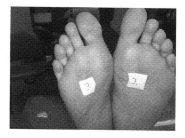

Picture 19.5. A moderate callus beneath the second metatarsal head in the foot of the longer leg, and a severe callus under the third metatarsal head in the foot of the shorter leg. **This person was 18 years old, and had had foot, leg, and back pain for over 5 years, all of which improved in 2 days with use of an appropriate lift.**

In some cases, the tightness of the Achilles tendon does not result in inversion that causes callus behind the baby toe, but rather a callus or just an increased pressure and inflammation on the ball of the foot. This condition is known as "metatarsalgia," which is more commonly seen in a flat pronated foot with an unstable first metatarsal. In this situation there may be a metatarsalgia without any pronation, often with central hammertoes. I have found success with aggressive off-loading of the inflamed joints combined with compensation for the LLDx, as seen in picture 19.6.

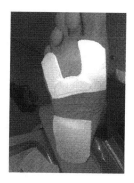

Picture 19.6. Off-loading inflamed forefoot joints in addition to providing lift for Limb Length Discrepancy.

StoryTime: Devorah was a 58-year-old woman who had suffered pain in the ball of her right foot for a very long time. Fifteen years earlier, after conservative care had failed, she had had surgery to fix a large bunion. I was not there, but the concept makes sense and often works. As the bunion gets larger the first metatarsal bone moves higher, and there is increased pressure under the second and third metatarsals. This causes inflammation—metatarsalgia. If orthotics do not work, surgery that puts the first metatarsal into a better position could solve the problem. In her case, it did not.

She had Equinus and a Limb Length Discrepancy, and actually described "landing heavy" on the ball of her foot. At the initial visit, I padded the painful metatarsal phalangeal joints. She had had such padding often before, without help. However, I also padded to compensate for the LLDx. At the next visit, she was better than she had been in years. I padded her shoes, including the lift for the LLDx. At her next visit weeks later, pain was resolved. She still had mild sensitivity at the previously painful joints but was now walking pain free. I padded additional shoes and provided lifts for bedroom slippers.

The lesson? Her metatarsalgia was not caused by the unstable first metatarsal and bunion, but by Equinus that was compensation for LLDx. This is one of dozens of cases I have managed of arthritic pain in the front part of the foot that was only successfully treated by addressing the LLDx.

4. A higher-arched foot (cavus foot)

The shorter limb often has less ankle motion and less pronation, flattening. In other words, it may have a higher-arched foot or perhaps even a High-Arched Foot. Apart from the effect on knee and hip function and arthritis, the high arch gives the foot less flexibility and poorer shock absorption, and makes it predisposed to **developing a stress fracture**.

The inverted position of the foot of the shorter leg can cause increased pressure on the outside of the foot, either in the ball or along the midfoot or even on the heel. **In addition to calluses, these areas of pressure can lead to actual ulcerations and infections in individuals with diabetes or risk factors such as poor circulation or neuropathy.** The inverted position puts greater stress on the outside of the foot. I believe that taking the pressure off the at-risk area poses a real challenge unless you compensate for any Limb Length Discrepancy. **Anyone with pressure, calluses, or ulcers on the outer side of the foot should be checked and double-checked for even a mild Limb Length Discrepancy.**

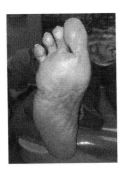

Picture 19.7 In this patient, the callus under the 5th metatarsal head had developed an ulcer and infection that led to amputation of the 5th metatarsal and toe.

5. Hallux Limitus (arthritis of the big toe joint)

Putting more pressure on the ball of the foot may cause increased stress in the big toe joint. I have had a few patients whose arthritic pain in the big toe joint, which was expected to need surgery, resolved with the use of a lift.

6. Tarsal Tunnel Syndrome (a nerve entrapment at the level of the ankle)

A short leg with an inverted ankle can cause pressure on the posterior tibial nerve, causing tarsal tunnel–like symptoms. These include burning, stabbing pain, aching, and numbness that affect part or all of the bottom of the foot. I have had a few patients who were treated with therapy and injections for tarsal tunnel, whose tarsal tunnel symptoms resolved with the use of a lift. (This may also help if there is Tarsal Tunnel Syndrome on the long side.)

7. Ankle sprains

Both the tightness of the Achilles tendon and the more inverted position of the foot lead to a greater likelihood of ankle sprains.

Effects of a Short Limb on the Knee and Above

1. Reduced motion (contracture) of the knee

In a much shorter leg, with a difference of more than ¼ inch, the knee may not extend fully, as a way of bringing the ball of the foot into a more stable position. **This can cause arthritic changes in this knee.** I have had patients with knee contracture (causing limited motion) and arthritic pain, for whom adding a lift for the shorter leg allowed the knee to naturally straighten out without any therapy.

I have even see this with patients whose contracted knee position was attributed to a nerve problem, such as a stroke or Cerebral Palsy. When the proper lift was provided and used, both the ankle and knee motion improved in 1-3 days.

2. Genu Recurvatum (backward curve of the knee)

The shorter leg may develop a Genu Recurvatum deformity, in which the leg curves backward.

I have seen improvement (not resolution) of severe Genu Recurvatum, with both a short leg and severe Achilles tightness, through the use of a lift—strapped to the foot to provide full-time compensation.

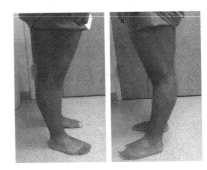

Picture 19.8. Backward curve of the knee known as "Genu Recurvatum." The left leg is shorter and has a greater backward curve. I have at times seen a moderate improvement in this curve after treatment with an appropriate lift.

3. Degenerative arthritis of the knee

In the knee of the longer leg, there is often an increased Q-angle (the angle between the leg bone and the thigh bone), shown in Picture 19.9 The knee of the shorter leg does not show that change, but nevertheless may develop painful arthritis deep within the knee joint, and may also present pain along the outside of the knee. This condition is not diagnostic: it may be caused by problems in the hip as well as problems in the feet.

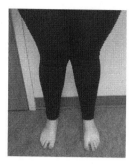

Picture 19.9 In Genu Valgus, with an increased "Q" angle, the knees touch and the feet are separated.

4. Ilio Tibial Band Syndrome

This is a condition affecting the ilio tibial band, a long structure stretching from above the hip joint to just below the knee, on the outside of the thigh. Symptoms include pain and stinging aggravated by activity, and may also include swelling, especially around the outside of the knee. This condition has been associated with both High-Arched Feet and Flat Feet, but it is even more common in people with a Limb Length Discrepancy affecting the shorter side. I have had patients with Ilio Tibial Band Syndrome whose symptoms improved rapidly with use of a lift.

5. Degenerative arthritis of the hip (a very common relationship)

In a shorter leg, the range of hip motion may decrease, and direct hip arthritis may develop. It is reported in medical literature (as well as in my observation) that hip arthritis is significantly more common on the side of the shorter leg. I have had patients with hip arthritis improve with the use of a lift. I have even seen people who had had hip replacements but suffered ongoing symptoms, who improved with the use of a lift for the shorter leg. Sometimes, only ¹⁄₁₆th of an inch is needed for relief, sometimes it may be as much as 1/2 inch or more.

StoryTime: A 73-year-old woman came in with her daughter, and at the end of the visit wanted to talk to me about her own foot. Not an unusual occurrence. She reported right Achilles pain that had been bothering her for several months. Anti-inflammatories had not proved helpful. I took a quick look—a three-minute exam. In addition to a spur in the back of the heel and tenderness with mild swelling at the Achilles tendon insertion, I noted that her right Achilles was tighter, the heel was higher, and the hips were sensitive, suggesting a Limb Length Discrepancy. Also, the nerves in her left foot were much more tender than those in her right foot.

Of course, I asked about other symptoms. She reported fairly severe hip pain that had restricted her activities for over 10 years, with temporary, limited help from physical therapy and anti-inflammatory medication.

I recommended that she use Voltaren gel and ice for the Achilles tendon, but I also told her that because of the Limb Length Discrepancy the Achilles was overly tight, pulling and causing tension at the insertion. I provided her with lifts to help reduce the Achilles tension, and mentioned that this might even help the hip. I (usually) try not to create unrealistic hopes.

One week later, when she came in for an official visit, the pain in her heel was MOSTLY better but the hip pain was COMPLETELY better. She was standing and walking more comfortably than she had in years. The Equinus had resolved, as had the nerve sensitivity. There was still some heel pain; she was doing better but had forgotten to use the ice. But her hip pain had improved in 2 days.

I treated her with a heel lift as well as with ice and some topical anti-inflammatory cream for the right Achilles. When she returned a week later, not only was the heel improved, but her right hip was still better than it had been in years, despite the failure of previous therapy and the anti-inflammatory medicine she'd taken orally. She was able to stand and walk much better and she felt far more balanced. In this situation, the hip arthritis was an incidental finding and improved dramatically with a ⅛-inch lift.

StoryTime: Troy J, a 70-year-old gentleman, came in with a painful growth on the bottom of his left heel. Unsure of its nature, I performed a biopsy. Fortunately, the growth was benign. At the follow-up visit, I took a look at both feet and noted mild mechanical differences and a Limb Length Discrepancy that he was already aware of but did not know was important. The mechanical problems included an asymmetric Equinus and the First Interspace Fine Sign. Upon being questioned, he reported pain in his back and hip spanning the previous 25 years. He had seen multiple orthopedic and spine specialists and had undergone months of physical therapy. He did not experience any persistent relief. Just chronic hip pain, aggravated by limited activity.

I added a ⅜-inch lift to the shoe of the shorter left leg. The following week, he reported that almost all the hip pain was gone, and that he could stand and walk better than he had in years. This improvement was maintained as long as he used the lift . . . which he is still doing 3 years later.

Troy J's interview is available on our web set, WalkingWellAgain.com.

6. Scoliosis

If the leg is even a little shorter than the other, it can cause a change in position in the spine. This can take the form of a pelvic tilt or scoliosis. It is well recognized in medical literature that scoliosis can be secondary to a Limb Length Discrepancy, although the amount of discrepancy needed to cause this is not clear. Pictures demonstrating scoliosis are presented in Chapter 12, and X-rays showing obvious difference between scoliosis with proper lift and scoliosis without proper lift are presented in Chapter 14.

7. Neck or shoulder pain

Patients with even a mild LLDx may tilt their heads slightly when standing or sitting. They also may develop neck or shoulder pain, which often improves rapidly with a lift for Limb Length Discrepancy. I have had dozens of people who had quick resolution of neck or shoulder pain with treatment for LLDx.

StoryTime: Esther K, 22 years old, came in for aching in her arches. She had orthotics but felt they were not that helpful. She reported a limited amount of back and leg discomfort but significant pain in her right shoulder and neck. The exam showed flexible Flat Feet as well as a Limb Length Discrepancy, asymmetric Equinus, and nerve sensitivity.

I thought her orthotics were pretty good, and wondered if the problems were actually caused by the Limb Length Discrepancy. I provided ⅛-inch lifts, either to be attached to her orthotic or to be placed in her bedroom slipper, and I waited a few weeks for her next visit. When I saw her again, Esther reported that all the foot and leg pain was gone, as was her back pain. When I asked about her neck and shoulder pain, she smiled broadly: all the pain had resolved within a few days.

HOWEVER, when a 3-day Jewish holiday arrived and Esther wore only dress flats with no lift, her symptoms returned with a vengeance. After the holiday, she went back to sneakers and orthotics, and the pain disappeared. Another 3-day holiday came the following week, but she had learned her lesson. She used lifts in her dress shoes and had no pain.

I have had several patients with neck pain caused by a Limb Length Discrepancy. For teaching purposes, the sequence of this particular case beautifully showcases the potential for treatment; don't you think?

Esther K's interview is available on our web set, WalkingWellAgain.com.

Effects of a Long Limb on the Foot and Ankle

Let's move on to the longer leg, where arthritic changes are more likely to be clearly visible as well as symptomatic. (Keep in mind that the following presentation is usually true with a structural Limb Length Discrepancy. If the discrepancy is functional, caused by rotation in the pelvis or lower spine, the reverse may be true. The *shorter* leg turns out and flattens more. I believe that pattern is far less common.)

1. Greater pronation, with a flatter foot

When standing, the patient's shorter leg is often straighter, pointing forward, while the longer leg points outward. This asymmetric pronation results in the deformities listed below.

2. A larger and more unstable bunion

This is an enlargement of the bone behind the big toe.

3. A larger and more unstable tailor's bunion

This is an enlargement of the bone behind the baby toe.

4. Bad hammertoes, often involving the second and third toes

5. Hallux Extensus Interphalangeus

In this condition, the big toe points upward in the middle of the toe. This has been extensively reported as being associated with back symptoms, neck pain, TMJ (jaw pain), and headaches, as well as with pain in the foot and leg.

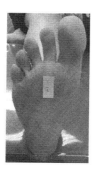

Picture 19.10. Hallux Extensus Interphalangeus.

6. Calluses in the center of the ball of the foot

7. Metatarsalgia

This is an inflammation of joints of the ball of the foot, which are called the "metatarsal phalangeal joints." It can be quite painful and can also lead to hammertoes, overlapping toes, and dislocating joints.

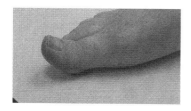

Picture 19.11. Metatarsalgia most often occurs behind the second toe, under the second metatarsal phalangeal joint.

Note: As described above, this may also be seen in the shorter leg if there is tightness of the Achilles but not inversion.

8. Arch pain

This is often associated with sensitivity on the bottom of the arch, in the first metatarsal cuneiform joint.

Especially in the presence of uncontrolled Deforming Force that induces pronation, such as an LLDx or Equinus, this area may cause orthotics to be very uncomfortable.

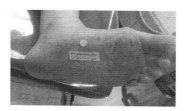

Picture 19.12. The circle identifies the plantar (bottom) aspect of the first metatarsal cuneiform joint.

9. Heel pain

Heel Spur Syndrome (plantar fasciitis) involves pain in the heel and at times in the arch. The pain is worst after arising from inactivity, such as when getting up in the morning or after a meal.

10. Sinus Tarsi Syndrome

The sinus tarsi is a joint on the outside of the back part of the foot, just below the ankle. Inflammation of this area can cause severe pain, usually experienced as if in the ankle, and mistaken for ankle arthritis or pain. It can cause soreness in the lower leg, and is an occasional cause of PseudoStenosis. This area is often greatly aggravated by major or even minor ankle area injury. A pronated foot may also cause this without injury, or may interfere with recovery after an injury.

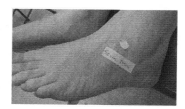

Picture 19.13. The sinus tarsi is located at the circle in the picture; it may be severely sensitive.

Information about Sinus Tarsi Syndrome

I want to call attention to a few important points about Sinus Tarsi Syndrome, an important and often over-looked condition.

1. *Sinus tarsi sensitivity in the longer leg often improves just by using the lift properly under the shorter leg.*

2. *Sinus tarsi sensitivity in the shorter leg is often accompanied by a history of multiple ankle sprains or other injuries. However, the injury can occur many years before the sensitivity is felt, and the patient may live with a diagnosis of "arthritis," not understanding that this problem often improves long term with a single injection.*

3. *Sinus Tarsi Syndrome may affect the leg, hip, or back. I have seen many people who improved in symptoms far away from the foot after this area was injected.*

4. *A recent observation: I have had several patients who could not bend over to pick things up off the floor, who had resolution when I injected the sinus tarsi and addressed the Limb Length Discrepancy. I now ask about that problem. (The chronology of that discovery is presented in a story of Chapter 27 entitled "Fibro-myalgia Resolved in 4 Days (I'll Pick That Up).") In the three months since I made the above observation (June 2015) until the time of this writing, I have seen that pattern at least 10 times. Inability to bend over and pick things up off the floor improves in patients with a Limb Length Discrepancy only after injection for Sinus Tarsi Syndrome. Often the improvement is noted just a few minutes after that injection!*

11. Posterior Tibial Tendonitis

Tendonitis and even degeneration of the posterior tibial tendon involves swelling on the inside of the ankle and can be very painful. It is often associated with development of a more severe Flat Foot.

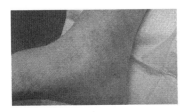

Picture 19.14a

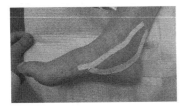

Picture 19.14b. In this picture, there is swelling on the inside of the ankle and on the rear-foot. Picture 19.14b. The tape on the foot demonstrates the course of the tendon and the margins of the swelling.

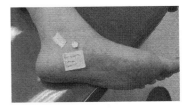

Picture 19.14 c. The small circle marks the site of the tendon insertion into the navicular bone, while the rectangle shows the course of the tendon, without swelling. Swelling and tenderness in this area are often mistaken for symptoms of ankle arthritis or Peripheral Edema.

12. Ankle arthritis

Because of the increased pronation of the longer leg, it is more likely to develop ankle arthritis and rear-foot arthritis.

Effects of a Long Limb--Above the Ankle

What are the effects on the longer leg above the ankle? Let us address the leg, knee, hip, and back. PLEASE keep in mind that I am not presenting original information here, just important insights and applications.

1. Leg cramps or shin splints

These may present as symptoms during or after activities during the day or at night in bed.

2. Knee pain and degenerative arthritis

The longer leg can put many different mechanical strains and pressures on the knee. First of all, the greater pronation causes the lower leg to rotate, putting a direct strain on the knee. Secondly, the longer leg may compensate by not fully extending during either walking or standing. A flexion position of even a few degrees interferes with proper knee function and may cause arthritic pain and, eventually, deformity. Finally, the individual may compensate by holding the leg farther away from the body, with or without a real external rotation, which could put abnormal strain on the knee. Any of these factors can give rise to arthritic pain and changes, and are often helped by simply using a lift when appropriate.

The knee of the longer side often develops an inner angulation, or knock-knee. This is called an "increased Q-angle." It is often present when the knee has significant arthritis, and it could even lead to the need for knee replacement surgery. While use of a lift for the short side will not eliminate the arthritic changes that are already present, it may greatly ameliorate the symptoms by reducing both the PseudoStenosis component and negating the Deforming Force that may have contributed to the development of the problem.

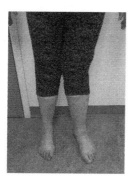

Picture 19.15 An increased "q" angle is shown as the knee bends inward on the left leg.

3. Pes Anserinus sensitivity

The Pes Anserinus is the combined tendon of three muscles that inserts below the knee joint, on the inside section as shown in picture 19.16. Pain is considered to be from either bursitis or tendonitis and may be related to arthritic stress and changes in the medial (inner) area of the knee. I have had at least 100 people with pain in this area who enjoyed quick resolution by treatment

of the length discrepancy. It may be sensitive to pressure when examined, but not something the patient was aware of as a problem area. As such, sensitivity on just one leg is suggestive of LLDx, and may be easy for patients to detect on themselves. This is one of the physical findings presented in Chapter 6.

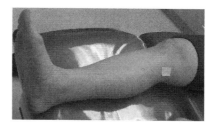

Picture 19.16. The square shows the Pes Anserinus, which is below the knee joint.

StoryTime: Christal E was a woman in her 40s who came into my office to discuss the possibility of surgery for a bunion. She wore Band-Aids to reduce her sensitivity in certain shoes, but otherwise had no complaints. I told her that the bunion did not seem severe enough to justify surgery and was not even tender enough to need an injection. She seemed relieved.

After a quick exam, I asked if she had other problems. She mentioned that she'd been experiencing pain in her right knee for a couple of years and that she'd actually had difficulty with that knee locking up since her preteen years. Yes, she had a short left leg and a sensitive Pes Anserinus on the right side, but no nerve sensitivity that would suggest spinal nerve irritation. I provided lifts for her shoes, and she was strict about use, at least most of the time.

Christal returned to my office a week later and reported that all the right knee pain had disappeared within 2 days. She stood and walked much better. She noted that during the rare times that she stood without the lift, she stood with the long right leg farther from her body or with that knee slightly bent. **She had been subconsciously doing this in compensation for years, perhaps decades, and had only now become aware of it.**

This is a perfect example of arthritic pain in one leg improving immediately upon correcting the Deforming Force. In this case, right knee pain was resolved by using a lift for the left leg. So simple, and so sweet!

Christal's video can be seen on WalkingWellAgain.com.

4. Hip pain

Much less has been written about the hip, and I personally have much less experience in that area. One article I read reported that arthritic pain is twice as likely in the hip of the short leg as in the long-leg hip, and that it was less likely if there was no Limb Length Discrepancy, which I agree with but can add no further observations to. I apologize for being so vague, but I am just being honest. When faced with a case of arthritic pain in the hip, I will compensate for the Limb Length Discrepancy, address any other biomechanical problem that may be present, consider Positional Testing—and hope for the best.

Sometimes, however, hip pain may present differently than as classic hip arthritis. In addition, one must be aware that hip and thigh pain are often associated with spine pathology.

Story Time: Margaret C was a 65-year-old woman who presented for care of an ingrown toenail, but who also reported a tired, achy feeling in her legs that had made walking difficult for a few years—she had an inconsistent one-to-two block maximum. She'd been checked for circulation problems, but both arterial and venous studies had come back perfectly normal. She did not have any back pain and had not been checked for Spinal Stenosis. She noted that she frequently shifted from side to side when standing.

My exam showed an asymmetric Equinus and nerve sensitivity, as well as a mild Limb Length Discrepancy—apparently only ¼ inch or so. I treated it with a ⅛-inch lift and gave her enough lifts for several shoes. I also provided ¼-inch lifts to switch to if she did not see improvement after a few days.

Two weeks later, she was walking a mile without difficulty. The ⅛-inch lift was adequate, and she never switched to the thicker one. All the nerve sensitivity was gone.

In addition, she'd been experiencing burning pain in her thigh, consistent with a condition called **"Meralgia Paresthetica."** That symptom also disappeared, as I have seen it do in several similar patients over the years. The literature also reports that Meralgia Paresthetica is more commonly found in people with a Limb Length Discrepancy.

Margaret's follow-up visit is available on our web set, WalkingWellAgain.com.

An Essential and Often Overlooked Step

The standard of treatment for many foot and leg conditions that are affected by pronation includes medication, therapy, injections, strapping, orthotics, braces, or even surgery. **While symptomatic relief is common with conservative care, I believe that long-term success is far less likely if the Deforming Force is not removed. In these cases, that Deforming Force is the additional pronation force and asymmetry of weight-bearing associated with LLDx.**

At times, use of a heel lift alone is adequate to control the mechanical stress enough to provide relief of symptoms. If the other treatments mentioned above prove necessary, providing adequate lift for the shorter leg will most likely make these interventions much more effective. Without adequate use of a lift mechanical stress will persist, and symptoms are far more likely to recur. At times, surgery may be deemed necessary. Even if the surgery is well executed and successful, there may be either a recurrence of the symptoms or development of new problems if a Deforming Force is still present. **For want of a lift—often only 2 or 3 millimeters, problems may persist or recur indefinitely.**

As a common practice, I will incorporate a lift into an orthotic or brace so that it is automatically present. One must be confident of the long-term need. **I also provide lifts for all sorts of shoes, and even bedroom slippers, to compensate for the discrepancy as much of the time as possible.** At times a good pedorthist is needed to help provide long-term relief, especially if the discrepancy is more than ⅜ of an inch. Further information about long-term management is presented in Chapter 12.

> *People frequently ask me if they should use the lift all the time.*
> *"No," I tell them. "Only when you are awake."*

Iliac Crest Pain Resolution Sign and Functional LLDx

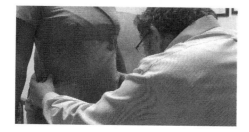

Picture 19.17. Examination of the hip bones.

I want to reiterate two important points. In Chapters 6 and 12, I present the Iliac Crest Pain Resolution sign. With indirect measurement of the Limb Length Discrepancy one will often find that the Iliac Crest, the highest part of the hip joint, is very sensitive. Frequently, the most tender area is on the side of the longer leg. **That tenderness often improves immediately after an appropriate lift is placed under the heel of the shorter leg.** Sensitivity returns when the lift is removed. When the mere use of a lift *immediately* eliminates that tenderness, both the patient and I are amazed. **Most importantly, it encourages the patient to appreciate the potential strong effect of a small lift.** After a few days with proper use of the proper-height lift, the Iliac Crest sensitivity is often resolved even when the person is standing without a lift. Not surprisingly, this often corresponds to resolution of back and hip pain and any other symptoms of PseudoStenosis.

Second, in Chapter 12, I present two possible forms of differing leg lengths: **structural** and **functional**. A functional LLDx is when one leg *appears* to be shorter, but that appearance actually comes about through a rotation or misalignment of the lower-back and pelvic structures. A person may have both a structural *and* a functional LLDx—and even an environmental discrepancy as well. Please check out the relevant sections in Chapter 12 for details on evaluation and consideration.

Even close examination does not always reveal the presence of a functional LLDx. For that reason, it is important to recheck the LLDx at follow-up visits, as the appearance of the LLDx may change. It does not mean that the first measurements were wrong, just that the lower-back mobility may have improved with treatment, and with time one can see a more correct presentation. **It is essential to recheck the pattern.**

In addition, if there are persistent symptoms or unclear signs, consider radiologic evaluation of LLDx, such as with a CT Scanogram. As discussed in Chapter 14, they are often helpful, but not necessarily definitive.

Limb Length Discrepancy and Joint Replacements

Joint replacements are a miracle of modern medicine. "Bone on bone" or severe deformity may make walking painful enough to cripple an otherwise strong person. When the replacement occurs, it can provide great relief. Joint replacement, even with current technology, is a surgery that requires great skill. The results can be life changing.

And yet . . . the process of removing bone and adding an implant may leave behind a new limb length pattern. You may recall my saying that it is no secret that a Limb Length Discrepancy can affect either knee or hip arthritis and may therefore contribute to the need for an implant. Here's a new twist: *after* **an implant, a Limb Length Discrepancy can arise or be exacerbated.** Remember, even a small discrepancy can potentially cause major problems.

Therefore, after knee or hip replacement surgery, be aware that you may have a Limb Length Discrepancy that may cause or exacerbate any of the symptoms described in this book. Even if your surgeon did an excellent job, a small difference may appear immediately or perhaps even develop later. **Therefore, if any back or lower-extremity symptoms become worse after a joint replacement, it is essential to investigate the limb length patterns as well as the status of other mechanical factors.** It's a sad but true fact that solving one problem can give rise to another. But this is a problem that has an easy solution.

If there are any new symptoms—including in the spine, hip, knee, or foot, or symptoms of either neuropathy or poor circulation—following a joint replacement or other major orthopedic surgery, one should double-check for possible Limb Length Discrepancy.

StoryTime: Judith is a good friend of mine from Florida who experienced pain in her right thigh that developed after she had a right hip replacement. Though reassured by the surgeon that the hip was fine, she saw no improvement in the pain after

3 months of intense physical therapy. She could walk or stand for only a few minutes before she had to sit down.

I saw and examined her in New York. Of interest, she had severe sensitivity on palpation of the right femoral nerve, just where her pain was, and she had a short left leg. I happened to have come prepared with lifts, as I'd suspected her problem in advance. The difference seemed to be more than ⅜ of an inch, but she could only tolerate a ¼-inch lift comfortably. But that ¼ inch made a huge difference.

Within a few days, she improved to the point where she was able to walk for more than 30 minutes before she had to stop. She still could not run, and she experienced discomfort if on her feet for a long time, but this was a great improvement over her prior discomfort after just a few minutes of standing or walking.

She also began using the adjuncts to Positional Testing, though never a walker. She had a Scanogram, which demonstrated a ⅜-inch discrepancy, though she still felt comfortable with only the ¼-inch lift.

About 6 weeks later, she emailed me to report that she was walking without limitation, but that the pain returned if she tried walking or running for even a few minutes without a lift. It is obvious that the discrepancy played a major role in her painful symptoms—symptoms that only appeared **after** her hip replacement.

Please understand that this is not at all a case of malpractice. Her hip is fine, and the surgeon did a great surgical job on the arthritic joint he worked with. **It is just that the "minor" accepted discrepancies that can arise after surgery are not really so minor at all. These discrepancies need to be considered and treated.**

There are, of course, many variations of the pattern based upon different structures and capabilities, including neuromuscular function.

StoryTime: A 70-year-old woman came in for treatment of fungus nails. She'd had a stroke, which had slightly affected the right leg, but she had developed contracture (limited motion) of the right knee and hip as well. In addition, she had fallen and broken her neck while trying to access the bathroom. Largely confined to a wheelchair since then, she had done very little walking in the previous 2 years. This woman was only able to stand or walk—with outside support—for a minute at most, and had a feeling of instability that threatened to make her topple over backward.

My exam showed that her right knee was contracted 25 degrees; she could not extend it straight. She also had SEVERE tightness of the right Achilles—about 35 degrees. Her right heel was about 1¼ inches higher than her left (caused in part by the knee contracture). Importantly, despite these two contractures, her muscle strength was active (though weak), much better than it is in many stroke victims who totally lose function of some of their muscles.

Curious as to the effect of the discrepancy and tight muscles on her inability to stand or walk, I attached a ¾-inch piece of felt to her heel and strapped it in place. She stood up holding onto the wheelchair, and then let go. She kept standing, and then bounced on her feet and smiled. The feeling of falling backward had disappeared immediately. It had been caused by the severe tightness of the Achilles—which, in turn, was working to compensate for the Limb Length Discrepancy.

I did not want her to use a rollator walker, as I did not think she was steady enough. Using a standard walker, she began to stand and walk at home in limited amounts with assistance.

When she came back to see me 1 week later, the tightness of the right Achilles had improved from 35 degrees to only 15 degrees. The knee contracture had improved from 25 to 10 degrees. She was able to stand and walk better than she had in over 2 years—just because of the lift that had been added to her shoe.

Unfortunately, when I called her several months later to follow up, she reported that she had made very little use of this improvement. She had not gone for physical therapy as recommended, and she still used the wheelchair outside the house. She had become too comfortable with it.

Back Pain When Sitting, Lying Down, or First Arising

It is a common symptom to have back pain or even pain radiating from the low back into the lower extremities with extensive sitting. How extensive? That varies from person to person. Some sit for a few hours and that is all they can do comfortably, while some can only sit for minutes before they need to shift positions or even stand to try to achieve comfort.

There are many common recommendations written in books and websites about modification of sitting position, chair height, elbow position, pillows, height of the monitor or computer, type of chair, foot rest, and other factors. Far be it from me to discourage you from trying these positions. If you have tried them, I hope that they have helped. I assume, however, that if the problem was truly solved, you would not be concerned and reading this section.

I find two patterns regarding this problem. If the person has problems sitting and there is pain radiating down the leg, it is quite possible that there is a sciatica problem associated with a herniated disc. In such cases, walking may be more comfortable than sitting, and walking symptoms are not necessarily helped by pushing a grocery cart. I have had many patients (between fifteen and twenty) with this pattern who improved by sitting on a pillow or two full time, including when in a car, for several days. Similar to the position induced by *kneeling chairs*, this changes the angle of the back and reduces the pressure on the disc. This is a simple trick worth trying. As with Positional Testing, it should immediately be comfortable and should not increase symptoms. If it increases symptoms, do not do it! If the symptoms persist, see a spine specialist, such as a physiatrist, pain management specialist, orthopedist, or spine surgeon.

The second pattern is addressed in the box below.

> ### Back or Leg Pain When Sitting, and Limb Length Discrepancy
>
> *This essential observation is counterintuitive. One might think that only local back pathology should cause local back arthritis discomfort and referred leg pain when sitting. However, PseudoStenosis is active there as well. The most common culprit is Limb Length Discrepancy, even one as small as 2 or 3 millimeters.*
>
> *Note what I am saying. The pain in the lower back with sitting is frequently relieved by treating PseudoStenosis while standing and walking.*
>
> *I have had over one hundred people with back pain sitting or lying down who had relief within 1–3 days of using a proper lift, proper orthotics, or whatever other intervention was needed for their particular cause of PseudoStenosis.* **It is thus essential that in the absence of clear findings or distinct foot or leg symptoms, aggressive investigation for even a small LLDx be performed.** *Often, the result will be a dramatic resolution of symptoms when sitting, lying down, or first arising in the morning. All from walking in a more balanced manner during the day.*
>
> *For years I have actively solicited details of back and leg symptoms associated with walking, standing, and sleeping. I now include in my questions the presence of symptoms when sitting and first arising. I find that the* **majority** *of people with these problems improve with the techniques presented in this book.*

I hope this very long section on Limb Length Discrepancy has served several purposes. While there is actually more information on this topic in Chapter 12, the present chapter emphasizes the need to be aware of and treat even minor Limb Length Discrepancies for any possibly related arthritic symptoms or deformity of either the low back or lower extremities. I hope this has provided enough information to let you suspect the presence of a Limb Length Discrepancy and to direct treatment accordingly. This seemingly minor problem can, over a span of years, lead to life-changing pain and deformity.

Please, please, please. **Do not try treating yourself or helping a loved one with a Limb Length Discrepancy without first reading Chapter 12 section C, the 13-point section on treatment tips.** Good luck!

The Fascinating World of Flat Feet

In Chapter 12, I shared that Flat Feet could cause spine dysfunction and thus PseudoStenosis. Here, seven chapters later, I still stand by that assertion. But now I'd like to discuss the pathology from an arthritis standpoint.

> *To repeat myself, I do not claim to be a biomechanics expert. I am just a clinician sharing my observations, plus passing on the teachings of many who are far more knowledgeable than I in the world of biomechanics!*

First of all, Flat Feet can cause arthritis in . . . the feet, as well as in places above them. I assume that you are not surprised. Here is a list of common problems.

1. *Bunion deformity*
2. *Tailor's bunion*
3. *Hallux Extensus Interphalangeus*
4. *Hammertoes, often involving the second and third toes*
5. *Calluses in the center of the ball of the foot*
6. *Metatarsalgia*
7. *Arch pain*
8. *Heel pain*
9. *Sinus Tarsi Syndrome*
10. *Posterior Tibial Tendonitis*
11. *Ankle arthritis*
12. *Leg cramps*
13. *Knee pain and arthritis*
14. *Knee tendonitis and bursitis*
15. *Hip pain*
16. *Low-back pain / Spinal Stenosis / PseudoStenosis*

You may have noted that this is a similar list to the one I presented early in this chapter on changes resulting from the flatter foot in the longer leg. The difference is that right now we are dealing with *two* Flat Feet and the problems they may cause in the foot and in ankle function, affecting all the conditions mentioned above.

I will not review the details here. Please review the early part of this chapter to see some of the problem areas with pronation that you may not have known about previously. If your feet hurt, see a podiatrist. Just keep in mind that the pain may be brought on or worsened by either Spinal Stenosis or PseudoStenosis. My apologies if I sound like a broken record; I just want to keep stressing the need to remember this vital point, as it applies to so many different circumstances!

Flat Feet: Recognizing the Problems They MIGHT Cause

Flat Feet can UNQUESTIONABLY, at times, AFFECT KNEE ARTHRITIS. Not so well accepted is the idea that they can also cause back arthritis. **Flat Feet can be associated with neck pain, TMJ, and headaches, according to the well-respected work of Dr. Howard Dananberg and others.** For what my opinion is worth, I agree, and have often seen improvement in these problems (neck pain, TMJ, and headaches) with treatment of the feet.

Why Treat Flat Feet?

BUT WAIT. Lots of people have Flat Feet and no symptoms. They are able to walk or run well with no knee pain or back pain. So why treat Flat Feet at all?

I can offer three reasons: **current symptoms** (of the feet, ankles, legs, knees, back, and occasionally neck and jaw; headaches; and any of the possible symptoms associated with PseudoStenosis presented in this book), **related orthopedic deformity**, and—more subtly—**signs of future problems**.

Let's take these three reasons in reverse order.

The third reason calls for the most professional judgment and, obviously, for integrity as well. If a professional with experience and good judgment regarding feet, legs, and the overall skeletal system looks at the Flat Feet and sees indications of potential problems, treatment should be considered.

What are the kinds of things I look for? First, please understand that the deformities of adulthood do not magically appear at age forty. By that time, deformities are often in the middle stages of mechanical dysfunction as any Deforming Forces have taken their toll over the years. **So if a good clinician looks at the feet (or ankles or knees) and sees early signs of the many problems reported here—he should treat them!** There may never be a way for you to know for certain if this preventative approach was worthwhile. In my opinion, "an ounce of prevention is worth a pound of cure," as long as one does not harm.

Regarding the second reason, if there is already a clearly perceived deformity present, it is important to try to mitigate the Deforming Force. Even if surgical correction is called for, try to prevent a recurrence. And if the deformity is in the knee or spine, controlling the Flat Feet may well be necessary for the long-term success of any treatment, including surgery.

The first reason listed above is the most obvious one for anyone with open eyes: CURRENT SYMPTOMS. **The trick is to recognize the symptoms that can be caused by Flat Feet!**

Symptoms may be caused by direct mechanical stress, and can be felt by pain in the feet, ankles, legs, knees, or back. That covers a lot of ground! Plus, let's not forget PseudoStenosis. Thus, **any of the conditions reported in this book can be associated with Flat Feet**. So back we go to the basic and essential question: when and how should one treat Flat Feet?

Orthotics and Mechanical Testing

I must state here that I do not routinely use inserts, either custom or over-the-counter, for back pain, knee pain, or even foot and ankle pain. *I use them frequently, but not routinely.* I make selective use of these aids. That is a key to success, and to my sleeping better: not routinely selling costly inserts that don't work (especially since my inserts come with a "Goldman Guarantee"). Again, we come back to the same question, phrased differently: how does one decide?

What I do is go back to the concepts presented in Chapter 12—an approach I have used in varying forms for over thirty years. It is not original. It can most likely be improved upon, or it may be used differently, by other more knowledgeable doctors. But it's my book . . . so here goes.

If I feel that the symptoms are possibly being caused, directly or indirectly, by Flat Feet, I simply test to see if mechanical control changes the symptoms. I refer to either Low Dye strapping or use of an Unna boot, as explained in detail in the appendix. It's that simple.

StoryTime: Danielle, aged 33, came into the office with a chief complaint of ankle pain that had been bothering her for about 3 years. However, further discussion revealed that she also had leg pain, knee pain, back pain, and headaches dating back well over 5 years. Anti-inflammatory medicines such as Celebrex, and the pain medication Tramadol, had provided very limited help.

Examination showed that she had a hypermobile Flat Foot with Hallux Extensus Interphalangeus, and a ¼-inch Limb Length Discrepancy. I strapped her up with a Low Dye strap and added a heel lift for her LLDx, and within 3 days the leg pain, back pain, and headaches were completely gone. She was able to walk long distances with only a little ankle pain from the tibial tendonitis, but this was resolved with another week of strapping. Without the straps, just using the lift, most of the symptoms returned in a few days. We therefore made orthotics for her, and she enjoyed long-term resolution of the symptoms that had troubled her for years.

The lesson? I could break into song: the foot bone's connected to the leg bone, the leg bone's connected . . . you get the point. Here was a person with knee and back pain and headaches, all caused by the way her feet functioned. This is the classic "Functional Hallux Limitus" that Dr. Howard Dananberg has written so much about over the years. Orthotics to control her feet completely resolved her symptoms, and I believe that nothing else (other than foot surgery) could have provide that kind of long-term help. I have had dozens of patients with headaches, neck pain, or TMJ whose symptoms resolved with proper mechanical control. Thank you, Dr. Dananberg (and other great teachers of biomechanics)!

Two videos of Danielle—her first visit and a follow-up—are available on WalkingWellAgain.com.

StoryTime: Aaron, 38, came to see me with chronic leg and back pain, in addition to moderate headaches that had troubled him for many years and did not respond to anti-inflammatory medication. A former college athlete who'd suffered a career-ending knee injury, Aaron was resigned to the belief that pain was his long-term lot in life.

My initial exam showed a flexible Flat Foot, including Functional Hallux Limitus. No asymmetry was noted. I strapped his feet and included the modifications of a reverse Morton's extension and a Cluffy wedge. At his follow-up visit a few days later, all symptoms in his legs and back were gone—along with the headaches. Orthotics were the only treatment necessary for this gentleman, and he maintained the improvement in all of his symptoms over the long term. Two of Aaron's interviews can be seen on Walking WellAgain.com.

Strapping the foot properly will usually reduce or eliminate related symptoms in a day or two at most. If that does not work, I often use an Unna boot as a test,

to see if greater mechanical control is helpful. If straps help, orthotics have a great chance of working. If Unna boots help, then braces have a great chance of working. We have demonstrated that altering the foot mechanics alters the symptoms. The question then becomes how to manage that challenge long term.

Both orthotics and braces may require some compromise as to what shoes are worn, but most (though not all) of my patients with severe or even moderate pain have reached the stage of wanting relief so badly that they are not all that particular about their choice of footwear.

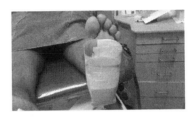

Picture 19.18. Strapping the foot can relieve pain in 1 or 2 days, and is a great test to see if orthotics will work.

If strapping is helpful orthotics are indicated

At times, over-the-counter orthotics can help. I am aware of two companies, ProLab Orthotics and Vasyli Medical, that produce excellent inserts based upon clinical experience and guided by experts in podiatric biomechanics. (I have no business relationship with either lab.) Such inserts may have real clinical value, and could be adequate to relieve symptoms caused by flexible Flat Feet.

However . . . in most cases with symptoms as significant as those described in this book, I recommend custom-built orthotics that are provided through your podiatrist. This is not a place to skimp if you can at all afford it. You can get the inserts with confidence, since the straps have provided such help! It is much easier for me to suggest that my patient spend money after testing by strapping has demonstrated the potential improvement.

When dispensing orthotics I remind patients that although kids get used to orthotics in a day or two, it can take adults several days to accustom themselves to walking with an orthotic. However, orthotics should not be used if they actually hurt.

Please be aware: Orthotic* prescription and construction is an art. If one pair did not work—that is, if they were either uncomfortable or unhelpful—another pair might be much better. If orthotics were expected to work and were either uncomfortable or unhelpful, there should be a second try. Go back to your original provider, especially if that doctor stands behind his or her work. It also might be necessary to try another doctor.

*By orthotics, I mean custom functional foot orthoses, inserts made by a podiatrist or other clinician who thoroughly understands the foot and evaluates yours. I do not mean inserts made from a scan at a shoe store, or those ordered by size. These may be comfortable or even helpful, just as a pair of reading glasses bought off the shelf at a pharmacy might be helpful for some individuals. Yet for individuals with more complex vision problems, these are not nearly as likely to be helpful as glasses made to order by prescription. The same is true with inserts. Buyer, beware!

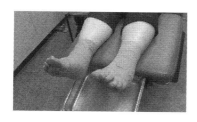

Picture 19.19. Unna boots can relieve pain in 1 or 2 days, and are a great way to test if ankle braces will work. The choice of which method to try is based on the judgment of your clinician.

I hope that those who have read this far have grasped the fact that I am dead set against cookbook medicine. A good history and physical exam can go a long way toward understanding symptoms. This is usually more valuable than any lab test. Hopefully, the younger doctors understand this and do not fall into a pattern of depending on tests, only conducting a thorough history and physical if the tests are inconclusive. After all, regarding the symptoms addressed in

An Editorial to Medicare and Insurance Companies about Orthotics

For what my opinion is worth, I strongly recommend that coverage for orthotics be considered in qualifying cases. Above, I cited three reasons for the use of orthotics: current foot and leg symptoms, current mechanical dysfunction in other areas that can be associated with foot function, and a good clinician's perception of likely future problems.

If there is no interest in preventative medicine, the third reason can be excluded. Excluding the preventative approach will save money in the short run but may cost a great deal more in the long run. Admittedly, prevention covers a broad-ranging spectrum, so it is difficult to argue for blanket preventative coverage. If, however, I generate any sway with this book, I will content myself with highlighting areas where orthotics can do immediate and great good: namely, reasons one and two above.

I have had so many patients—literally thousands—who've found relief of long-term symptoms with orthotics. These symptoms in the feet, legs, knees, or spine could be treated by other means, including physical therapy, injections, and anti-inflammatory medication. However, if the cause of the problem—the foot's mechanical function—is not corrected, then these other approaches are often inadequate. All too often, they turn out to be much more expensive modes of treatment, with poorer long-term outcomes.

A one-month course of physical therapy may cost between $1000 and $2000. A long course of anti-inflammatory medications is much less expensive, but the complications of such medicines can be very costly, especially if there is a need for ongoing medication because the causative problem was never addressed.

I repeat: I am not in favor of cookbook medicine. I do not believe that orthotics should be used routinely for all the symptoms addressed in this book. Many people find tremendous relief with only heel lifts for a Limb Length Discrepancy. Many will not benefit from orthotics at all. **But many others will not see long-term success without controlling the biomechanical cause of problems, either with orthotics or (more expensive) braces.**

If there is good relief of symptoms with strapping, then one can have confidence in LONG-TERM relief with orthotics. One pair of orthotics every year or two, in place of the other treatments, is actually one heck of a bargain. An expense, yes—but a big bargain nevertheless. I hope one day to see broader expansion of coverage for this approach.

Regarding the research that says orthotics do not work for back pain, for example . . . this view **probably** *arises from the practice of cookbook medicine, which one would expect to fail. So many people just need lifts. So many others have pain coming from a primary spine problem. Plus, there are so many variants in orthotics. The best comparison I can make is to the foolishness of evaluating the effectiveness of an antibiotic against all diseases, and not just against select bacterial infections. One does not discount the value of an antibiotic because it does not cure diabetes or a cold. Similarly, orthotics should be evaluated in managing cases where an expert says they may work and an expert has made them.*

Research should be done, but it should focus on the results of good, thoughtful care by competent clinicians who have prior success in dealing with the conditions under evaluation.

this book, tests are rarely conclusive! In the same light, my opinion is that practitioners should not fall prey to studies that conclude that certain therapies (such as orthotics) don't work (e.g., for back pain), **when the treatment was not carried out with the same attention as an excellent clinician would have brought to the job**.

Orthotics have been reported in the literature as not being helpful in treating back pain. **I might agree—if one engages in cookbook medicine.** I do not believe that back pain will always improve with orthotics. **A great many people need only heel lifts for Limb Length Discrepancy, and not orthotics!** People with back pain caused or maintained by a Limb Length Discrepancy may not obtain long-term relief from orthotics—even great orthotics.

But some patients with back pain (and knee pain and leg pain and foot pain and other problems mentioned above) will not get better *without* orthotics or braces.

Given the millions of people who suffer from back arthritis and other forms of arthritis despite aggressive conventional and even surgical care, this seems to be a set of approaches that should be embraced.

I have had patients who underwent extensive medical treatment without obtaining relief, and who saw excellent long-term improvement with orthotics or braces. How to decide? You need good judgment, a high index of suspicion, a good history, and a good clinical exam. PLUS, I must stress the value of Mechanical Testing—strapping or applying an Unna boot—to maximize the frequency of success. At least in my hands.

For clinicians who use this approach, there are important details regarding both strapping and Unna boots in the appendix.

What if orthotics have failed?

You may have tried orthotics before without obtaining relief. You should be aware that there are reasons that orthotics fail or are not comfortable. Often, although not always, success is possible.

Orthotics are often ineffective or uncomfortable when there is something causing a flattening of the foot that has not been controlled. Common causes of this situation are Limb Length Discrepancy, tight muscles in the back of the legs, a curved foot (Metatarsus

Adductus), and a rigid Flat Foot. These conditions often cause the orthotic to hurt in the arch, specifically at the bottom of the first metatarsal cuneiform joint (first MCJt). That spot is often very sensitive, both when the person is wearing orthotics and when external pressure is applied.

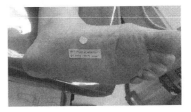

Picture 19.20 The first metatarsal cuneiform joint.

I examine and follow this spot for two reasons. First of all, if the pain is from the nerve only, this spot (as well as other mechanical stress points, such as the sinus tarsi) may not hurt. I then address the spinal nerve irritation and do not necessarily focus on the mechanics of the Flat Foot. If mechanical stress points do hurt, and strapping the foot, using an Unna boot, or even just a lift on the shorter side—diminishes the pain, this provides me with direction as to how I can mechanically treat the problem long term. Obviously, the goal is long-term success.

If that painful spot is still sensitive, I may repeat the strap with some modifications, such as a reverse Morton's extension or a Cluffy wedge.

Such modifications can also be incorporated into orthotics. If they are not helpful and the pronation is severe, I may just proceed with an Unna boot and check again in a few days. If that works, I lean toward using a brace instead of just an orthotic. If the brace is effective, it can often be replaced by an orthotic—at least part time—after months of use.

Remember PseudoStenosis

Remember, a person may have both mechanical/arthritic symptoms and PseudoStenosis, and both contributing factors must be treated. Thus, if the person originally had sensitivity at mechanical stress points and also had nerve sensitivity, after treatment he should be reevaluated to determine what has improved. If the joint still hurts, the mechanical problem has not been solved. If the joint no longer hurts, then both the patient and I recognize success in dealing with the mechanical strain. If there are still symptoms and nerve sensitivity, I strongly consider that PseudoStenosis or Spinal Stenosis may be a contributing factor, as is the focus of Chapters 12 and 18. ***Please*** read those chapters if you have not.

Reminder: the nerve hypersensitivity I refer to is the *invaluable* First Interspace Fine Sign, described in Chapter 6. If there is nerve sensitivity that disappears—as may occur in just a day or two—the patient and I both know that the strap (or other intervention) has accomplished something great. If the nerves are still sensitive, we have more work to do on controlling pressure on the spinal nerves that may be causing leg or foot pain. In such a case, I may add Positional Testing to whatever mechanical treatment we have already applied. (Please see Chapter 7, on Positional Testing.)

Yes, I am oversimplifying!

OF COURSE, I am oversimplifying. These are just a few of the ways that a clinician can evaluate and treat, especially if he gives credence to the original ideas in this book. Care can become much more involved than the picture I have presented, and different doctors use different tools, many of which I could learn from!

I am only providing this information to stress the potential value of using testing techniques for guidance on which symptoms are caused by mechanics and which are caused by Spinal Stenosis or PseudoStenosis, and on how to treat them long-term. Diagnosis is an art that requires evaluation, treatment, and then an objective reevaluation.

Sometimes arthritic foot pain may be too advanced to be treated only mechanically. Injections, medication, therapy, and even surgery are reasonable treatments if the symptoms are significant enough and excellent conservative care is not adequate for the task. **Make sure to follow up with a really good podiatrist or a really good foot and ankle orthopedic specialist.** (If in doubt, get a referral from a trusted clinician.)

More on Knee Arthritis

Clinicians have long known that Flat Feet may be associated with knee arthritis.

Flat Feet can cause several patterns. The tibia, or leg bone, is internally positioned inside the leg. The axis

of ground-reactive pressure in a collapsed Flat Foot is more lateral (on the side of the baby toe, toward the outside of the leg), so that increased pressure is put on the outside section of the knee. There is greater strain on the Anterior Cruciate Ligament, as well as on the ligaments on the medial (inside) side of the knee. Misalignment (think of a car!) may induce pressure between the kneecap and the bone underneath. The story is a lot more complicated than that, but this is the basic scenario for a common cause of knee arthritis, although of course not all knee arthritis is caused in this manner.

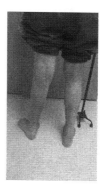

Picture 19.21. A patient with a Flat Foot and increased Q-angle, (a condition in which the knee bulges on the inner side).

There are several points that I'd like to present about knee arthritis.

1. Some patients with knee arthritis can be successfully treated by controlling the feet with lifts, orthotics, braces, or even modified shoes. I test the patient as described above, with a strap or an Unna boot, with or without a lift, as needed. Frequently, arthritic knee pain disappears with proper control of the foot. This sort of Mechanical Testing is quick, *relatively inexpensive*, and safe.

2. When the cause of the knee arthritis is poor functioning of the feet, even knee surgery may not be successful over the long term. If the stress that caused the knee pain is not corrected, the operated-on knee could develop arthritis again, or the joint replacement could fail. The mechanics that cause the knee to have the increased Q-angle shown in picture 19.9 is a powerful Deforming Force that often needs to be treated in order for any knee treatment to succeed. Thus, even if there is knee arthritis present, the mechanics of the foot and ankle need to be considered.

3. Remember—with LLDx, the longer leg often has much worse deformity and pain. For many, it is absolutely necessary to provide length compensation for the shorter leg in order to expect long-term relief of knee problems. Any treatment for the Flat Foot on the longer leg, or of the knee arthritis itself, is much more likely to fail if the height difference is not treated. THIS CANNOT BE EMPHASIZED STRONGLY ENOUGH!

4. In addition, knee arthritis may also be present in the shorter leg. This scenario does not usually produce the same big and sensitive bulge on the inner side of the knee. Rather, the pain may be deep in the knee, or on the outside of it. Knee deformity in the shorter leg is sometimes associated with a contracture (limitation of motion) in the knee, as well as with the usual finding of a tight Achilles tendon. Both the tight Achilles and the knee contracture may improve within days of using the proper lift.

5. The presence of Spinal Stenosis or PseudoStenosis may make the overall condition much, much more painful and therefore resistant to treatment. A positive Positional History (Chapter 5) or the presence of nerve hypersensitivity (Chapter 6) should by now be shouting at you to consider whether PseudoStenosis or Spinal Stenosis may be contributing to the problem. Just as failure to address the shorter leg often dooms any treatment to failure, the same is true of failing to address the spinal nerve involvement.

StoryTime: Gloria, 58, came in for evaluation with complaints of severe back, leg, knee, and foot pain that had been bothering her for years. She'd seen moderate improvement after a total knee replacement on the right side, but less improvement after a replacement on the left side. She could only stand and walk for a few minutes, but she walked much better when pushing a grocery cart. She had hypersensitivity along the nerves in the thigh, leg, and foot. The symptoms in her feet, legs, knees, thighs, and back plagued her in bed each night.

Gloria had moderately severe Flat Feet and no sign of Limb Length Discrepancy. As she was only 5'1", we provided her with a junior walker that was 29 inches high. She was immediately able to walk better, consistent with her experience with a grocery cart. After using the walker for several days, her back pain, foot pain, leg pain, and nerve sensitivity were eliminated. The pain in her knees, however, persisted.

Suspecting that the Flat Foot function was causing knee dysfunction and pain, I applied Unna boots. Within a day, the knee pain was much improved. A week later the Unna boots were removed—and within a few days the knee pain came back. I replaced the Unna boot, and again knee pain resolved. I then casted her for ankle braces for the severe Flat Feet. After they arrived, she enjoyed maintained improvement of the knee pain.

While in Gloria's case the great majority of the overall pain derived from Spinal Stenosis (or possibly PseudoStenosis caused by the Flat Feet), the arthritic pain in her knees was coming from the foot dysfunction caused by her Flat Feet.

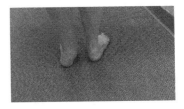

Picture 19.22. Severe Flat Feet.

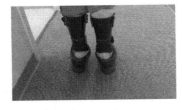

Picture 19.23. Severe Flat Feet whose function is greatly improved with ankle braces. This may be helpful for foot, ankle, knee, and back pain, and also for any symptoms of PseudoStenosis caused by Flat Feet.

Of course, if SS/PS is suspected and positional and mechanical management and basic conservative care are not adequate, **the patient should certainly have a spine evaluation by a physiatrist, orthopedist, or neurosurgeon**. If an MRI is suggestive, epidural injections may provide excellent—though often temporary—help.

If an epidural injection relieves much of the arthritis pain of the hip or knee, then you know that spinal nerve compression is playing a big role in the problem. Remember the story at the beginning of Chapter 18 where an epidural relieved not only neuropathy pain but also the severe sensitivity coming from a hammer-toe? The patient did not need foot surgery, only ongoing care for his stenosis. In the same vein, if an epidural provides good relief for knee arthritic pain, it might be approached in a similar fashion. Discuss this with your doctor.

Back to the ART of management. If the grocery cart or walker does not help but an epidural provides long-term relief, we are all happy. If the epidural provides only temporary relief, the patient should be checked carefully for possible PseudoStenosis. Treating the PseudoStenosis cause may eliminate the mechanical pathology in the back that caused the symptoms to return.

In addition, even if not initially successful, Positional Testing may play a helpful role in preventing recurrence after improvement with an epidural injection. After getting help from the epidural, use the walker and the Adjunct Measures. While these two steps—managing the cause of the PseudoStenosis and then following up with Positional Testing—are not enough to get rid of the symptoms, they may be enough to reduce the mechanical pathology in the back that caused the symptoms to return. Just be sure your walker is properly positioned!

Four final points about knee arthritis

If there is a primary knee arthritis caused by an injury or an inflammatory condition such as Rheumatoid Arthritis, the knee arthritis can also lead to foot, ankle, hip, or spine arthritis by altering the way the person walks. To enjoy real success, it is often essential to treat the initial problem.

Orthopedic joint replacement surgeons usually do a wonderful job when it comes to replacing the knee joint. Failure to resolve symptoms may be due in part to faulty biomechanics, as described above. Please bear in mind, however, that much of the research that supports the need to consider foot mechanics in managing the knee is of relatively recent vintage and is still not universally accepted. One can therefore, in my opinion, judge favorably, and forgive those who opted for surgery without trying these conservative approaches. It is

my hope, however, that everything that has been written about mechanics in the articles on this subject will eventually be recognized and accepted by those who perform joint replacements. To the best of my knowledge, this has not happened yet.

Another form of arthritis in the knee is called "Genu Recurvatum." (See picture 19.7, above.) This is a backward curve of the knee—a hyperextension deformity, which is commonly seen with a tight Achilles tendon. If that is the case, heel lifts can improve standing and walking and can remove the feeling of falling backward that often comes with standing. However, there are many other possible causes. If appropriate heel lifts do not provide magical improvement, I recommend seeing a good physiatrist for evaluation. Braces, injections, or therapy may be helpful.

There are different types of knee arthritis that are affected by biomechanics. A good book on orthotic therapy for foot and leg problems, which contains a separate section on managing knee arthritis, is available. Entitled *Recent Advances in Orthotic Therapy*, written by Paul Scherer, DPM, it is a useful resource for clinicians.

More on Hip Arthritis

Hip arthritis is often brought on by direct injury, such as a fall or an auto accident. However, it can also be brought on by faulty mechanics, though rarely as dramatically or as obviously as with knee arthritis. Hip arthritis can also be affected by spinal nerve compression. To make a positive diagnosis, one must truly be an expert in the hip. I am not such an expert—and yet I have a few valuable points to share.

Articles have been published noting that just as knee arthritis is more common in people with Flat Feet, arthritis of the hip is more likely in a limb that has a higher-arched foot and Equinus (reduced motion in the ankle, often seen with a tight Achilles tendon or muscle). The positions of the bones of the hips are affected by the position of the feet when the person walks, which may cause problems. Another theory is that the combination of the higher-arched foot and the reduced ankle motion reduce the foot's overall ability to absorb impact forces. Greater force is thus transmitted to the hip. I have observed this pattern to affect lower-back arthritis, as it may also affect the hip. I have had many patients whose back or hip pain was reduced by good silicone heel lifts, which absorbed some of the shock of impact.

HOWEVER . . . as you may have noticed from the above section on Limb Length Discrepancy, these two factors—higher-arched feet and Equinus—are also signs that are frequently seen with a shorter leg. Many people have greater knee arthritis in the longer leg, in addition to hip arthritis in the shorter leg. Again, even as little as ¹⁄₁₆ of an inch, less than 2 millimeters, can make a big difference.

(Less frequently, hip arthritis is found in the longer leg. While much more common in the short leg, it is seen in the longer leg of people with an LLDx more often than it is seen in the general population that has no discrepancy.)

Four important points regarding hip pain:

1. If the patient has the associated findings of a tight Achilles and High-Arched Feet (as suggested in published articles), then strict use of silicone heel lifts may be helpful. First of all, they provide improved shock absorption—one factor that is suspected of having an effect on the hip. Second, use of a lift (or a shoe with a bit of a heel) improves the relative motion available in the ankle. Therefore, good silicone lifts used extensively may be helpful.

2. In the early stages of hip arthritis, and even at times later in the disease, use of a lift to balance the Limb Length Discrepancy can provide relief from hip pain. If the shorter leg plays a role in the development of hip arthritis, I suspect that consistent use of the proper lift may prevent progression and the need for surgery.

3. If the Limb Length Discrepancy is recognized only after surgery, keep in mind that there may have been a discrepancy even **before** the surgery! Because the body is very good at compensating—sometimes in ways that are deceptive—the Limb Length Discrepancy may not have been apparent before the surgery. Now that you are walking around with less pain and limitation, the improvement can suddenly highlight a discrepancy that was not apparent before surgery. Alternatively, perhaps there was much arthritic or degenerated bone that had to be removed. Some of that bone may have been resorbed after surgery, as sometimes

occurs with unhealthy bone. The point to grasp is that if you find yourself with a short leg after surgery, it could be because of many different factors that may have been beyond the surgeon's control. The important thing is to bring the matter to the surgeon's or therapist's attention in order to receive guidance and obtain the proper support.

4. Please understand that the hip / sacrum / lower spine area is a very complicated one, and it is often unclear exactly where the pain is coming from. Go back to the Grocery Cart Test and Positional Testing, and if there is good or better improvement with the wheeled support of a cart or walker, I recommend that you use it full time, as described, for 3 days. If you find that you are not only walking much better, but also having a lot less pain, I repeat (for the hundredth time in this book!) that it is likely that either Spinal Stenosis or PseudoStenosis plays a big role in the pain. You must explore these two possibilities.

A Rigid or Nearly Rigid Flat Foot or a High-Arched Foot

A rigid foot, with a far less than normal motion in many of the joints, can be detrimental in a variety of ways. First of all, it can cause pain in the foot and ankle, especially in the sinus tarsi (picture 19.11, above) and posterior tibial tendon areas. In truth, it may affect arthritis of almost any place in the foot or ankle. In addition to local problems, the lack of good shock absorption in a rigid foot prevents the foot from absorbing impact the way it should, with the result that shock is transmitted instead up to the knees, hips, and spine. This is not good. When the foot is incapable of accommodating change in the position of the ground, abnormal stress is transmitted to regions higher up, which in turn can cause misalignment problems that affect the knee, hip, and spine.

A rigid Flat Foot is harder to treat than a flexible one that has normal or even greater than normal motion. Sometimes orthotics or braces with a heel lift can reduce pain or improve position. Extra cushioning can make up for poor shock absorption. Injections or therapy may reduce pain and improve motion. On occasion, surgery is needed. The important thing to consider is the effect of the foot's biomechanical function as part of the overall picture—because even improving the function of the knee or hip may not provide the sought-after long-term relief if the foundation is bad. Professional help is most often needed to help with this foot type.

And of course, if one foot is worse than the other, make sure to address any possible Limb Length Discrepancy.

It is possible to place the rigid High-Arched (cavus) Foot in the same category as the rigid Flat Foot. Although the condition looks quite different, it also presents as a rigid foot that does not absorb shock well, and whose rotational misalignment can sow trouble in the knee, hip, and spine. Custom orthotics may be helpful. Consistent use of good shoes and perhaps silicone heel lifts can greatly facilitate shock absorption. Reconstructive foot and ankle surgery may be needed if all else fails. The rotational misalignment, however, requires good professional care.

* * * * *

Limited Ankle Motion and Arthritis

A tight Achilles or other source of Equinus (with reduced motion in the ankle) has a significant effect on arthritis in many ways. The combination of a short leg with a temporarily tight Achilles, along with greater pressure on the outside of the foot, is one that we have reviewed both in this chapter and in Chapter 12. I hope that oft-painful scenario is clear.

But Equinus can be a troublemaker in other ways as well. If the foot has a propensity to pronate, as it does in a flexible Flat Foot, Equinus can make it pronate quite a bit more and can render the problem difficult to control with orthotics. Frequently, the bottom of the arch has a sensitive spot, the first metatarsal cuneiform joint (picture 19.1), which is very tender if Equinus is present. In fact, the spot may be so sensitive that many orthotics become simply too painful to tolerate.

When a Flat Foot requires reconstructive surgery, there is often value in lengthening a tight Achilles at the same time. There's a much better chance of obtaining long-term relief if this Deforming Force is removed. Also, lengthening a tight Achilles in patients with diabetic ulcers is often helpful. If the tightness is worse on

one ankle than on the other, check for a Limb Length Discrepancy and try lifts *before* resorting to surgery!

Severe Equinus can cause a backward pull on the knee. Do you remember Genu Recurvatum? If the Equinus is very tight on one or both legs, this can be the result.

In addition, Equinus can create a balance problem, in which the person has difficulty standing and feels as if he is about to fall backward. (See Chapter 23, on balance.)

Now let's take a look at an extreme form of Equinus.

After a stroke, a person may have a Drop Foot, characterized by a lack of ability to properly dorsiflex (lift) the foot, accompanied by a moderate or severe, and often rigid, Equinus deformity with a lack of motion at the ankle. This is usually much more severe than the Equinus seen with a Limb Length Discrepancy, although that form I have also seen occasionally severe.

Forced to cope with inadequate motion at the ankle, the body compensates. During the act of walking, the knee may not extend properly when the foot first hits the floor, or again later in the standing phase. There will be a change in the way the hip functions, sometimes resulting in Genu Recurvatum. In short, the lack of normal ankle motion in one ankle can wreak havoc in both the knee and the hip—and thus, the spine—and it can also cause problems in the other foot. Anyone with knee, hip, or spine problems after a stroke may need to have the foot and ankle addressed.

At times, the patient may have an excellent and immediate improvement by adding enough lift under the affected heel to compensate for the severe tightness. Picture 19.24 shows how the lift might look.

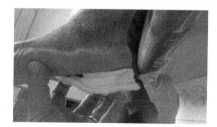

Picture 19.24. Applying 7/8 of an inch of felt to the heel; it will be strapped with a Low Dye strap to secure it.

Usually, the mere use of a lift will provide great improvement in ankle motion if the tightness was caused by a short limb and nothing else. I have also had several patients who had a short leg plus a stroke, and who received moderate relief in this way. With the aid of a lift, their severe Equinus became much milder, leaving them capable of improved walking with a modified brace.

Picture 19.25 shows a brace that may help a Drop Foot if the foot can achieve 90 degrees. Adding the felt can make it more comfortable for a patient who cannot achieve the perpendicular.

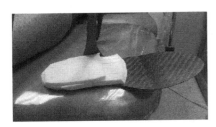

Picture 19.25. Felt added to the top of a brace provided for a Drop Foot. This fills a dual function of both adding lift as needed for a Limb Length Discrepancy, and stabilizing the foot if there is persistent Equinus.

To reduce the tendency to fall backward, if there is Equinus on one side with no Limb Length Discrepancy, it is necessary to provide as much lift in the shoe of the normal foot as was needed in the shoe of the restricted ankle. Otherwise, treatment of the Equinus would end up contributing to an environmental Limb Length Discrepancy.

Similarly, people with Cerebral Palsy involving one leg usually have a Limb Length Discrepancy, with Equinus and shortness of the affected leg, as well as increased pronation and reduced knee extension of the uninvolved leg. It is essential to consider whether a lift is needed for both shoes. Equinus in Cerebral Palsy is addressed in detail in Chapter 12.

If lifts or orthotics or braces do not adequately help, be aware that surgery is a very reasonable consideration for people who develop a rigid Equinus foot after having a stroke. Some surgery involving lengthening of tight tendons can be done under local anesthesia, and can allow the person to stand and walk within a few days. Again, seek a referral to an excellent podiatrist or foot and ankle orthopedist.

Other Causes of Degenerative Arthritis

The next few sections, though important, are much briefer. In my opinion, the conditions they cover are much less common. However, I freely admit that my vantage point is skewed. I am a podiatrist, and although people do come to me for back and neuropathy pain, I still see patients primarily for foot and leg pain. I feel that by far the most common cause of lower-extremity and spine arthritic changes and symptoms is Limb Length Discrepancy, followed by flexible Flat Feet. The following other patterns are much less common in my podiatry practice.

Degenerative and other arthritis can certainly cause problems in secondary areas. For example, if someone fractured his knee or had severe arthritis of the knee, it would affect the function of the bones above the knee (in the hip and spine) and below the knee. There are too many variables to present here. The important takeaway point is the need to address all possible trouble spots or complications from the initial site of the pathology, in order to recognize the impact that the pathology has on other areas.

Improper hip function eliminates the smooth functioning of the spine and can cause spine dysfunction, arthritis, and PseudoStenosis. Similarly, improper knee or foot function can affect the range of motion in the hip and prevent proper spine function. The spine is the place of connection to the extremities, so any lower-extremity dysfunction can cause spine problems by disrupting normal function of the hip. And if the hip has prior problems, it becomes even more susceptible to anything that can further interfere with its normal function. The situation is complicated!

Also—to beat a dead horse—arthritic changes or surgery in the hip may results in a Limb Length Discrepancy. Need I say more? It is not uncommon for someone to have a joint replacement and soon afterward develop "unrelated" problems in another area— problems that are actually caused by the resulting Limb Length Discrepancy. I repeat: it is not malpractice or even a sign of a bad job to be left with uneven extremities after major surgery. The common belief, unfortunately, is that a small discrepancy does not make a significant clinical difference. I hope that this perception changes one day. Until it does, at least anyone who reads this book has the chance to consider my opinion and take action.

Incidentally, these concerns also apply to a patient with an inflammatory arthritis such as Rheumatoid Arthritis. Changing gait patterns can affect other joints. Loss of limb height due to arthritic changes can induce a Limb Length Discrepancy. Treatment of all lower-extremity and spine symptoms should include consideration of these two major points.

Regarding altered walking patterns caused by a stroke or some other nerve problem, there are again too many variables to list here. The most common are the ones described above: the changes with Equinus caused by stroke or Cerebral Palsy, or the changes from damage to a nerve in the back or near the knee after knee replacement surgery. Equinus is the most common culprit behind a host of such problems, but there are others. You will need to consider the mechanics of the lower extremities in dealing with any arthritic problems in the knee, hip, or spine.

I have treated several people who developed a PseudoStenosis phenomenon after a stroke, when an altered gait affected the spine and gave rise to nerve pain. It was assumed that this pain was from the stroke, but Positional Testing for stenosis or Mechanical Testing (such as a brace or a lift) for the local foot dysfunction eliminated the nerve pain previously believed to derive directly from the stroke. Therefore, even if there is another possible cause of the patient's symptoms (in this case, a stroke) it is essential that SS/PS be considered and investigated.

StoryTime: Sheila was a 66-year-old woman who presented with difficulty that began after a stroke 10 weeks prior to her first visit. Fortunately, it did not affect her speech or thinking, but it did affect her left foot and leg. They became weaker, and they tired after walking for 10 minutes. She had difficulty standing, waddled when she tried to carry packages, had a lot of pain in that leg from climbing only one flight of stairs, and had weakness that lasted for 5–10 minutes when she first awoke. One month of physical therapy had not helped.

Physical examination was a bit confusing. A positive First Interspace Fine Sign on the left side, the painful and weak side. The left hip was higher and

more tender, which resolved with a ⅛-inch lift under the right heel, suggesting a shorter right leg. However, she had Equinus on the left leg –10 degrees and Equinus +5 degrees on the right, suggesting a shorter left leg.

In this instance, the tightness of the Achilles tendon was not caused by an LLDx but by the stroke. I did a bilateral Low Dye strap, put a ¼-inch heel lift on the left to compensate for the Equinus caused by the stroke, and put a ⅜-inch heel lift on the right to compensate for what seemed to be a ⅛-inch LLDx.

Home run. By the next day all left leg symptoms were gone. She slept well, stood well, walked much farther, and had absolutely no difficulty going up or down stairs. All nerve and hip sensitivity were completely gone.

Sheila's interview from her follow-up visit is available on WalkingWellAgain.com.

Finally, let's take a look at an altered walking pattern caused by any lower-extremity pain great enough to make the patient walk differently. As a podiatrist, I see this with basic problems that happen to hurt like heck. For example, Sinus Tarsi Syndrome is a very painful condition in the ankle area that can cause a person to dramatically change the way he or she walks—which, in turn, affects other parts of the body. Another example is porokeratoses—excruciating, corn-type lesions on the bottom of the foot.

I have had patients with both of these conditions and others, who complained of diffuse arthritic pain. These individuals might be diagnosed with arthritis or Fibromyalgia if a clinician listened to the symptoms and did not consider the feet. After straightforward treatment, such as injecting inflamed joints, or simply trimming and padding the porokeratoses, several of my patients were then able to walk better, and they saw their other arthritic or PseudoStenosis symptoms disappear.

Thoughts for Patients

Please be aware that despite the length of this chapter, I have only scratched the surface. There are a great many different scenarios and patterns that I have not touched on, and those can be helped by an expert. There are also a great many other ways to approach symptoms. The clinical approaches I've shared have worked well for me, but they are not necessarily better than the approaches used by other doctors.

I hope that this chapter has stimulated your interest in approaching arthritis from a biomechanical standpoint, and that you find a knowledgeable and dedicated clinician willing to work with you from that standpoint.

As always, I invite those who try these approaches to let me know how they do by sending me a note through my website, WalkingWellAgain.com. I look forward to reading your stories, as well as any observations or suggestions. Good luck!

Thoughts for Clinicians

To any researchers or clinicians who are well versed in biomechanics, I apologize if this chapter, which is directed predominantly to patients, has presented some concepts with a simplicity that you may find inadequate. I hope you do not reject ideas presented in this book, which may have value, because of the superficial manner with which the complex field of biomechanics has been presented.

As I've mentioned, there is much in this chapter that is not original. In the appendix, I provide a list of articles that focus on this information. Although controversy exists about many of the details, these articles should offer corroboration to support the concepts I've presented, as well as direction if you choose to do further reading.

I will take this opportunity to make special note of two authors and two books.

Dr. Howard Dananberg is a wonderful author and lecturer on podiatric biomechanics. I have learned much from him, though not enough. The fact that I've presented other approaches should not be taken to mean that I regard myself as anything other than one of his many students in the area of biomechanics.

Dr. Steven Subotnick is a noted author who has written many articles and books on a wide variety of topics related to both podiatric biomechanics and podiatric medicine. His many publications on Limb Length Discrepancy alone should serve as an impetus to anyone treating the musculoskeletal system to always be cognizant of this condition, which may have an effect even when the difference is what others would call minimal.

Dr. Paul Scherer, the podiatrist who founded Pro-Lab Orthotics and who has studied and lectured on biomechanics for some four decades, published *Recent Advances in Orthotic Therapy*. The book is a great tool and reference.

A second book was published in 2011 by Dr. Louis Pack, a podiatrist in Georgia. Its title is *The Arthritis Revolution*. Though not academic, I feel that this book is of real value in stimulating interest in any clinician treating degenerative arthritis, and that it can be helpful for patients seeking help as well. It is quite readable—and inspiring.

Shortness of Breath and Perhaps SS/PS

This chapter is different from the other chapters in Section 3—chapters that addressed conditions that both Spinal Stenosis and PseudoStenosis (**SS/PS**) can both mimic and worsen. Even I, a man preoccupied with SS/PS, do not claim that in the absence of other conditions SS/PS can cause Shortness of Breath (**SOB**). Yet this relationship warrants a chapter because of the role SS/PS may play in limiting activities in individuals suffering from conditions that can cause SOB. If you or a person you care for has restricted activity caused by SOB, the information in this chapter may help improve things. While I do not expect total or nearly total elimination of symptoms, there may be a moderate and rapid improvement.

Some Basic Definitions

Abnormal Shortness of Breath (**Dyspnea**) may be diagnosed when even limited or mild exertion causes heavy breathing. This is in contrast to the more normal SOB that accompanies heavy exertion such as running, long walks or hikes, sports like tennis, or even heavy housework. It is unlikely that the observations shared in this chapter will allow unlimited activity, but they may allow a doubling, tripling, or further multiplying of the time that the person in question can walk or be active. **Specifically, if your SOB occurs with standing or walking, the approaches I describe here may be helpful.** If Shortness of Breath occurs at rest, I am sorry to say that these approaches will likely not help you.

> *It must be made clear that this chapter is not intended for the individual with a new problem of Shortness of Breath. Though many causes for Dyspnea are chronic and stable, some episodes of Dyspnea are acute and dangerous if left untreated. Therefore, any new symptom of Shortness of Breath should be evaluated by your doctor or a specialist AS SOON AS POSSIBLE. This section is designed for the person who experiences Shortness of Breath brought on by limited activity, and who has undergone a thorough medical evaluation of the possible causes.*

Shortness of Breath may be a result of many conditions, though it most likely stems from a problem with the cardiovascular (heart) or pulmonary (lung) systems. The most common causes of SOB are Congestive Heart Failure (CHF) and Chronic Obstructive Pulmonary Disease (COPD). Other possible causes include, but are not limited to, obesity, asthma, pneumonia, sarcoidosis, or other heart or lung problems. Remember, this chapter is not about diagnosing or treating those problems. For that you need care by a qualified clinician.

So what is this chapter about?

Bear with me for one more definition. **Exertional Dyspnea** is Shortness of Breath that occurs when physical activity results in a demand for oxygen or other nutrients that exceeds the capacity of the respiratory system and/or the cardiovascular system to supply. If normal requirements are exceeded, the body tries to increase the available oxygen by increasing respiration. In other words, in Exertional Dyspnea physical activity causes Shortness of Breath. **THIS is the kind of Shortness of Breath that may be helped by the information in this chapter.**

A standard way to address SOB is by improving the efficiency of the cardiovascular or respiratory system. This is the goal of drugs prescribed or therapy provided.

If you have skipped the rest of this book and opened it to the section on Shortness of Breath, you might be a bit lost now. This book focuses greatly on understanding and managing the effect of both Spinal Stenosis and PseudoStenosis on overall symptoms and health. What I have labeled "PseudoStenosis" is the presence of any condition in the lower extremities that causes the spine to function as if there is Spinal Stenosis, often causing symptoms identical to Spinal Stenosis.

A brief guide as to whether you may have either SS or PS is presented below. It is essential to learn, as many people have either SS or PS and do not know it. However, for in-depth understanding and guidance, you will need other chapters, as is directed below.

A Second Way to Help

However, another way to possibly improve the Shortness of Breath would be to increase the body's efficiency by decreasing the demands on the cardiovascular or respiratory system. One method to improve efficiency is to remove any impediment to that efficiency—that is, any factor that unnecessarily adds to the strain on the body.

Both Spinal Stenosis and PseudoStenosis can act as such an impediment, thus affecting Shortness of Breath. While this is not a common problem that I see every week or even every single month, I believe that it is also not a rare one. And it is a problem that often goes unrecognized.

Shortness of Breath and SS/PS: The Overlap of Populations

Since SS and PS are so common within the same senior population that suffers from CHF, COPD, and other causes of Shortness of Breath, **you would expect there to be an overlap of populations**. In other words, you would expect many people with a primary heart or lung condition causing Shortness of Breath to also have SS/PS. And you would be right! **Those individuals suffer from increased energy demands placed upon a system that is already of reduced capacity.** The result is like *adding insult to injury*: a walking capacity that may be far lower than would be the case in the absence of SS/PS. The increased metabolic demands might be caused by the painful symptoms themselves, or perhaps by the effort the patient exerts to try to hold his or her body in the least uncomfortable position while standing or walking, which might not be very easy.

A Review of the Basics

Anyone who has read the entire book until this chapter will likely have developed the insights and instincts needed to recognize and initiate management of SS/PS, understanding six essential tools for recognizing and managing SS/PS:

1. Positional History (Chapter 5)

2. Positional Testing (Chapter 7)

    Combining the above two efforts has a great chance of making it clear that either Spinal Stenosis or PseudoStenosis contributes to the overall condition.

3. Adjunct Measures (Chapter 8)

4. Investigation for PseudoStenosis (Chapter 12)

   With Spinal Stenosis symptoms, even if there is documented Spinal Stenosis, there is always the need for investigation of possible PseudoStenosis.

5. The physical examination (Chapter 6)

6. A detailed understanding of symptoms, guided by the LuSSSExt scale (Chapter 3)

If you are a patient or family member concerned with Shortness of Breath and you have therefore jumped to this chapter, here is a shortened version of the findings of a Positional History. **If they describe the individual in question, there is most likely an SS/PS component, and the person in question can quite likely be helped by the protocols described in the above-mentioned chapters.**

Positional History suggestive of SS/PS componant

1. Symptoms worsen with walking and are not relieved by standing and resting.

2. Symptoms also worsen with standing.

3. Symptoms are relieved by leaning on a support—such as a grocery cart, walker, or counter—or by sitting.

4. There is improved walking ability with a grocery cart but a worsening of symptoms while waiting at the checkout counter.

5. There is increased Shortness of Breath while the person (under 5'2") pushes a grocery cart, or while the person pushes a walker that helps him or her stand straight. This is explained below.

The Invisible 25 Pound Backpack

Let me share with you an allegory. We would expect someone with a medical condition causing Shortness of Breath to have reduced capacity if carrying a heavy load such as a 25-pound backpack. **So too would this person have reduced capacity from the strain of SS/PS . . . only this backpack is not visible.** I now focus on how to recognize and remove that invisible backpack, and how to address *special factors* relating to Shortness of Breath.

In truth, SS/PS symptoms are felt in the back as back pain, or in the lower extremities as neuropathic pain, circulation problems, painful swollen legs, or arthritic pain, as described in Chapters 15–19. They are not symptoms of the lungs or heart or of Shortness of Breath. You might wonder why I am relating the two conditions. It is because, as mentioned above, the SS/PS component may be likened to the invisible 25 pound backpack. **Treating the SS/PS is like removing the backpack.** The medical cause of the Shortness of Breath is still present, but the backpack is gone. **The overall symptoms and walking ability of the individual are improved not by treating the medical condition, as is the standard approach, but by improving the efficiency of the rest of the body by managing SS/PS.** I have had dozens of patients over the years experience such relief. They did not become completely free of Shortness of Breath symptoms, but they became much better.

StoryTime: Irene was an 87-year-old woman who was brought in for evaluation because of difficulty walking and poor balance. She previously had mild improvement with her Shortness of Breath after heart surgery but now, again, could only stand or walk for a few minutes before Shortness of Breath forced her to take a seat.

My exam showed a Limb Length Discrepancy and unilateral Equinus, but also tenderness in the interspaces of both feet. Suspecting both PseudoStenosis and Spinal Stenosis, I treated her for both: a lift for her shorter leg and a walker for Positional Testing.

At Irene's next visit, she had improved quite a bit. There was better stability with standing, and she was now steady with just a cane for short walks. In addition, her daughter took her out to a mall, where Irene was able to walk with her walker for fifteen minutes, sit and rest, and then walk another fifteen minutes.

Managing the SS/PS brought about dramatic improvement in Irene's SOB. She went from being able to walk for just a few minutes to being able to walk for fifteen minutes, simply by removing that "25 pound backpack" that I mentioned earlier.

Irene's follow-up interview is available our web set, WalkingWellAgain.com.

StoryTime: Leatrice C was a 77-year old woman who came in seeking help for a tender toe. She also reported back and leg pain that had made it hard to stand or walk for many years. After walking for one block, about five minutes, she had discomfort and also Shortness of Breath. This problem had gotten progressively worse since she had had a lung removed for lung cancer over 15 years prior.

Physical examination showed the clues I looked for. A short-appearing right leg, with Equinus. Much greater sensitivity on nerves of the left side, and a positive First Interspace Fine Sign. The left Iliac Crest was much higher and was more tender, with a positive Iliac Crest Pain Resolution Sign with only ⅛ of an inch under the right heel. I was optimistic.

Two weeks later, she came in and joked that maybe I had "psyched her out," which I took to mean I had hypnotized her—into relief of pain! She reported that all of her back pain and leg pain resolved in a couple of days, and that she had walked nonstop for 45 minutes the day before. Exam showed elimination of Equinus and both nerve and hip sensitivity. Happy Hips, happy patient.

Leatrice's video is available for viewing our web set, WalkingWellAgain.com.

The lesson? I would agree that the Shortness of Breath she had was in part related to the cancer and lung removal. But once that "25 pound backpack" of painful PseudoStenosis was removed, she clearly had the capacity to be more active than she had been in years. Note the treatment: a ⅛-inch lift. Actually, several lifts, as I gave her enough to wear in all of her right shoes.

Walkers and Shortness of Breath: Three Essential Patterns

Leatrice's and Irene's stories, like most of the information I have mentioned so far, are primarily a recap of the information previously mentioned in this book. I promised earlier to share *special factors* relating to Shortness of Breath. They relate to details about the use of a walker for either Spinal Stenosis or PseudoStenosis, and there are **three essential patterns in how the use of a walker affects Shortness of Breath**.

Pattern 1: Use of a walker (which the patient may need to stand and walk) actually makes the patient have greater Shortness of Breath if the patient has only a short walking distance capability. This can often be reversed quickly.

Pattern 2: Use of a walker (with the person standing upright) helps the patient walk in a stable manner and also helps the patient breathe more easily, especially if the Shortness of Breath is caused by respiratory problems. This walker position is not one I usually recommend, but for people with Shortness of Breath it is often helpful in the absence of active Spinal Stenosis or PseudoStenosis.

Pattern 3: Use of a walker (set to induce proper flexion) makes it *much easier* to walk, and the patient experiences immediate improvement in Shortness of Breath and walking-distance ability, as well as relief of back, leg, or foot pain. Full-time use (Positional Testing) for 10 days provides long-term change, including improvement in Shortness of Breath. The individual is then able to proceed to Positional Therapy, and either stop walker use completely or just uses it for long walks.

Of course, this is a simple and incomplete categorization, as there are many other variables that must be considered. People with PseudoStenosis may benefit from having that condition treated, and that must ALWAYS be considered. The presence of neuropathy, poor circulation, or other arthritis complicates the situation. **However, none of these things prevent there being at least moderate benefit to individuals with both Shortness of Breath and SS/PS.**

Take a look at the three patterns described above as I explain them in reverse order.

Pattern 3: Using a Walker Properly Provides Very Good Improvement

If a person has Spinal Stenosis or PseudoStenosis (SS/PS), using a walker (Positional Testing, Chapter 7) can bring about very good improvement. Why? Walking is a much greater strain when there is back or leg pain, which may increase metabolic demands. It takes extra energy to tolerate pain, as well as to walk in a guarded manner to protect the spine. The comfort that almost always comes IMMEDIATELY with a properly positioned walker often allows a person to walk better IMMEDIATELY. For the right person, Shortness of Breath is improved as soon as he or she uses the walker when walking, and the improvement is maintained as long as the person continues using it.

This is not to say that the person will be able to walk miles again, as is often the case in a patient with only SS/PS and no other medical problems. He or she may be able to double or triple the walking distance quickly but may still be limited by the actual heart or lung problems that are present. However, there can be great improvement in the patient's quality of life with even that limited improvement.

Recall that many people with SS/PS enjoy long-term improvement of their symptoms (in the back or lower extremities) by using the walker for 10 days, after which they may not need the walker anymore, or at least full time. Therefore, people with SS/PS and Shortness of Breath may use the walker for just 10 days and obtain relief, and they may maintain the improvement even after they stop using the walker.

There are three caveats.

• If PseudoStenosis is present, it is advisable to treat it in order to maintain the improvement that was achieved (see Chapters 11 and 12).

• Many people need to use the walker periodically whenever there is a recurrence of spine-mediated pain. If you feel better for weeks or months and then experience a recurrence, don't despair. Just grab the walker and use it for a few days, and see if that brings you back to a higher level of functioning (see Chapter 10).

• The walker is not to be used on hills. A slight incline, either up or down, can negate the value of the walker and make one's Shortness of Breath even worse than it would have been without the walker.

With use of a proper walker, the patient can enjoy increased independence and freedom of motion in two ways. The first is an improvement in walking capability and Shortness of Breath with Positional Testing—that is, the use of a walker. That much is obvious.

There is an additional benefit of using a four-wheeled rollator walker with a drop-down seat. If you still need to periodically sit down, the "chair" is right

there with you! Many people are so limited by SS/PS, and, of course, by Shortness of Breath, that they give up walking entirely. If your symptoms are uncomfortable enough, as they often are, the only relief is to sit. If there is no place to sit, it might be just too hard for some people to sit on the ground and then get up again. A person with these legitimate concerns makes sure never to walk out of range of a seat. The use of a walker with a seat at least allows enough security to be able to walk without fear of being trapped.

Pattern 2: Using a Standard-Height Walker Helps Walking Stability and Breathing

This represents a unique pattern in my use of walkers. I recommend slight lumbar flexion when a patient uses a walker, to reduce spinal nerve compression caused by SS/PS. However, with COPD, sometimes it is fine if the walker is *not* set to induce flexion.

Using a walker can have a benefit specific to COPD patients, in addition to affecting the spine and overall balance. A walker supports the arms, which in turn provide support for the shoulders and rib cage. If breathing is a challenge, supporting the rib cage may make it easier. For this reason, using a walker or a grocery cart in a manner that does not induce flexion may still be helpful.

Because some people without SS or PS may be uncomfortable in a flexion position, it is better for them to stand upright. For these individuals, standing straight while using a walker may be the optimal method.

Picture 20.1 shows what is the optimal position for most people with Spinal Stenosis. For details on walker use, please review Chapter 7.

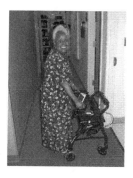

Picture 20.1. This is the normal position for Positional Testing. The person leans slightly forward with the arms straight.

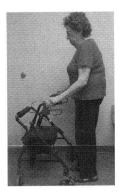

Picture 20.2. This is the standard position if there is no spine-mediated pain. The person stands straight, and there is a bend in the elbows. Using the walker in this way can provide help for a patient that has SOB but no SS/PS.

Pattern 1: Using a Walker Makes Things Worse; How to Reverse That

In contrast to those who find the use of a walker to be neutral—neither helping nor hurting—for SS/PS and SOB, **a walker set to the wrong height may actually make symptoms worse**. People who experience this pattern might mistakenly think that the physical effort of pushing a walker actually is more than they can handle, but this is not true.

The truth is that for individuals with SOB and SS/PS, the handle height of the walker is ABSOLUTELY essential.

If given a walker that induces an erect position, a person with SS/PS will naturally tend to try to open the spine by leaning forward. Leaning forward instinctively feels more comfortable for the spine and legs, even if it is not what the person has been advised to do.

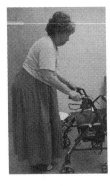

Picture 20.3. This shows a person leaning forward on a walker by bending the arms and shoulders. She attains the correct flexion position, but only by maintaining a challenging and draining position for the arms and shoulders. It's almost like walking around doing a partial push-up!

This position becomes not only uncomfortable, but also very energy draining—and it *may cause Shortness of Breath*. It increases the body's metabolic needs. Recall what I presented earlier in this chapter: *a way to improve Shortness of Breath is to remove any impediment to the body's functioning*. This challenging and draining position is absolutely a major impediment. It may make everyone—the patient, the patient's family, and even the patient's physician—believe that the CHF or COPD is actually worse than it is. In truth, it is not the demands of pushing the walker that are making the patient feel worse, rather the challenge of maintaining a physically difficult position that is draining the patient of his or her functional capacity.

Therefore, with SS/PS and Shortness of Breath, the height of the walker handle must be correct. The person's arms must be straight, the walker should be comfortably close to the body, and the person should lean slightly forward. I have seen many patients who reported Shortness of Breath when walking with a walker—who IMMEDIATELY improved when their walkers were adjusted to the proper position. In addition to improved Shortness of Breath and walking-distance ability, arm and shoulder discomfort disappeared. This transition is as dramatic as any I have seen in my practice. It is both amazing and rewarding to witness this immediate relief.

A Call to Action for Patients and Clinicians

For those suffering from SOB, I strongly recommend that you experiment with the grocery cart or with wheeled walkers whose handles are set at different heights to ascertain your potential improvement. Make sure, however, that you use a *wheeled* walker. If you use a standard folding walker, wheels and skis (slides) are an absolute necessity. This is because a standard folding walker without wheels, or one with wheels in front and only rubber pads in the back, must be lifted to turn or to walk on most surfaces. Lifting and pushing this kind of walker may increase the demands on your system even if the walker is set at the right height.

For clinicians, I strongly suggest that you consider evaluating patients for this potential method of obtaining clinical improvement. Any specialist, including pulmonologists or cardiologists, can keep several walkers of different heights in the office to see if a properly positioned walker will be of value. Another option is to ask the patient to do a formal Grocery Cart Test, as recorded in Chapter 7. It is important to remember that people under approximately 5'2" may not improve with the grocery cart unless they rest their arms on the transverse bar. Otherwise, the hand position does not induce flexion.

Addressing SS/PS symptoms may provide significant improvement for some patients with SOB. I also recommend that the individual in question see a podiatrist, physiatrist, or physical therapist who understands this approach. Managing any aspect of PseudoStenosis, which is almost always done conservatively, may provide the same benefits as Positional Testing with a walker.

StoryTime: John is an 83-year-old man whom I have treated for years for minor podiatry problems. However, he has COPD that got worse over the years, so he needed to use an oxygen tank in order to walk. Carrying the tank, he could only walk for about 5 minutes before he had to stop and sit.

Exam showed no signs of Spinal Stenosis or PseudoStenosis. None. Nevertheless, I encouraged him to do the Grocery Cart Test, and with it he was able to walk much better—for over 15 minutes. He got a walker and was then able to go to the mall with his wife and mostly walk rather than mostly sit. He is quite appreciative of the walker and uses it frequently.

Why? Remember the invisible 25-pound backpack? His backpack was visible! In his case, carrying the oxygen tank was a drain on his functional capacity. With the walker, he simply put the tank into the basket and found that he was able to walk much better.

REVIEW AND SUMMARY

Because I understand that some people will only read or at least begin with a chapter that applies to them, I must emphasize a few points here.

First, it is essential to bear in mind that Positional Testing—full-time use of the walker—is often followed by Positional Therapy, in which full-time or even any use of the walker may not be needed. For those

in whom temporary use of a walker provides relief of the inflammation of the spinal structures and nerves, it is often quite reasonable to reduce or eliminate walker use as long as there is good balance. The improvement in the SOB, obtained with proper use of a walker set at the proper height, may be maintained once use of the walker is over. Perhaps the walker will only be needed for long walks thereafter. Follow the guidelines in the section on Positional Therapy in Chapter 10.

Second, use of a walker is only part of the Positional Testing protocol. There are several other behaviors that contribute to optimal success. Please make use of the information in Chapter 8.

Third, it is valuable to have an evaluation by a good podiatrist or physiatrist familiar with the concepts presented here, to determine possible treatment protocols for any PseudoStenosis that may be affecting physical exertion. Managing PseudoStenosis improves the patient's chances of eventually giving up use of the walker completely.

Let me emphasize that point. **In patients with PseudoStenosis and Shortness of Breath, treating any cause of PseudoStenosis may improve Shortness of Breath.** As with the walker, improvement may be immediate.

I mentioned that some patients with SOB may find benefit in using a standard-height walker—a rarity for me to recommend. The reason is that for some people, such as those with COPD and difficult inspiration (breathing in), the walker's support for their arms provides a frame to improve the stability of the rib cage, making it easier for them to breathe in. For such people who do not have SS/PS, leaning forward to flex the spine provides no benefit. Again, for these patients, a standard-height walker is best.

This is not brain surgery. You may need to experiment to find the best use of this material to suit your individual situation. Please refer to other chapters in this book to understand other concepts as needed.

Please send me a note through my website, WalkingWellAgain.com, if you have success. I'd love to hear from you!

CHAPTER 21

Nighttime Symptoms—Probably Not Restless Leg Syndrome

The Crucial Question

Do you have difficulty sleeping because of aching legs? Is your nighttime rest disturbed by restless legs, leg or foot cramps, or other foot or leg symptoms? Do you find that your back hurts in bed, or that you have back or leg pain when you first wake up and get out of bed?

If the answer to any of the above is yes, it's time to ask yourself the next crucial question: **could these symptoms be related to Spinal Stenosis or Pseudo-Stenosis (SS/PS), or to biomechanical problems of the feet or legs?** This chapter will attempt to guide you in that investigation.

When you're lying in bed at night, your feet and legs should be comfortable. You should not experience any aching, cramping, burning, shooting pain, numbness, or intermittent movement. Such symptoms can rob you not only of your rest, but also of the peace of mind that comes with a good night's sleep.

They actually can cost far more. Studies have shown that successful sleep may play a role in fighting diabetes and even heart disease. Disturbed sleep has been associated with depression and cardiac issues, as well as panic disorders. In 2011, researchers from Johns Hopkins University published a study linking uncontrolled blood pressure to Sleep Apnea, a condition that I address briefly in the next chapter.

As with other conditions addressed in this book, understand that the information in this chapter is primarily for long-term symptoms. New or sudden nighttime symptoms may represent a serious problem with circulation, a spine infection or injury, a medical problem affecting electrolyte levels, a problem with the cardiovascular system, a problem with peripheral circulation, or neuropathy. **If there is any sudden change in sleep patterns, or if the techniques I present here for chronic symptoms are not quickly effective, you should see your primary care provider and consider evaluation by a sleep specialist.**

This chapter focuses on the importance of addressing Spinal Stenosis, PseudoStenosis, and biomechanical problems as they relate to nighttime leg symptoms. I find that well over half of the people whom I see with nighttime leg symptoms improve within days using the approaches I present.

Conventional wisdom says that nighttime leg symptoms are often due to a condition called "Restless Leg Syndrome," or "RLS." RLS is regarded as a condition of unknown cause (idiopathic) which cannot be confirmed by any blood test, though it is reported to be supported by sleep studies. To a very great degree, RLS is a diagnosis of exclusion, usually diagnosed only after other causes of similar symptoms have been ruled out. At the end of this chapter I present a brief background to Restless Leg Syndrome for those interested. First, however, I get to the meat of this chapter.

In opposition to conventional wisdom, I find that for the *majority* of people, either SS/PS or lower-extremity biomechanical pathology is the primary cause of their nighttime foot or leg symptoms. Biomechanical pathology is addressed later in this chapter. Right now, let's focus on our old nemesis, SS/PS and the spine-mediated symptoms that come along with it.

SS/PS as a Possible Culprit

Over the last thirteen years, I have seen more than 300 patients improve from nighttime symptoms that interfered with sleep patterns—after treatment of SS/PS dysfunction. The good news is that many people

For the clinician and the very curious

I initially reported these patterns in 2003, in an article in the **Journal of the American Podiatric Medical Association**. Specifically, nighttime symptoms of aching, burning, shooting sensations, numbness, and discomfort that prevent comfortable sleep were at times part of a syndrome called "Neurogenic Positional Pedal Neuritis," a term I coined to describe the foot manifestations of Spinal Stenosis. Two years later, I reported this pattern in a retrospective study published in an article in **Diabetic Medicine**, the research journal of the British Diabetes Association, in December of 2005. Nocturnal exacerbation of neuropathic symptoms (NENS), previously attributed to Diabetic Neuropathy, was often caused by Spinal Stenosis and often responded well to positional management, including use of a walker during the day and a modified sleep position at night.

The relationship between Spinal Stenosis and sleep-time symptoms was previously reported in the literature as "Vesper's Curse", and was attributed to vein problems associated with Congestive Heart Failure. I observe that this type of problem is much more common than was implied in other articles, and is quite often found in both young and old without any cardiac involvement at all.

with this set of symptoms usually get better within just 1–3 days. This rapid response is expected if the patient is treated with Positional Testing (Chapter 7) and Adjunct Measures (Chapter 8). It may take a few days longer if one treats the suspected PseudoStenosis component first, and only proceeds to Positional Testing for Spinal Stenosis if the first approach proves ineffective.

Although it does take a few days longer, I have found this approach useful in my own practice, as I can easily treat most causes of PseudoStenosis and bring about improvement in a couple of days. In your own home, however, if you do not already have a good relationship with a skilled podiatrist, it might be easier to go straight to Positional Testing with all its adjunctive behaviors, to confirm SS/PS involvement and provide treatment—and wait to investigate any possible PseudoStenosis component until afterward.

In other words, proper use of a walker and a few other behavioral changes can eliminate the nighttime symptoms in a day or two. This is essential to understand. **Changes in daytime activity may completely and quickly eliminate all nighttime symptoms. For other people, modification of sleep position is the key.** Some patients require both nighttime and daytime changes to get the relief they seek.

Why Suspect SS/PS?

Why would one suspect SS /PS as a possible cause of nighttime leg symptoms? Dear reader, if you have read this book straight through, you know to consider a positive Positional History and a good response to Positional Testing, including Adjunct Measures. If you have read this book through, please skip the following box and please forgive me for repeating this information yet another time.

> *If you are a patient or family member concerned with nighttime symptoms and have therefore jumped to this chapter,* here is a shortened version of findings identified by a Positional History. If they describe the individual in question, there is most likely an SS/PS component, and the person in question can quite likely be helped by the protocols described in the earlier chapters.
>
> *1. Symptoms worsen with walking and are not relieved by standing and resting.*
>
> *2. Symptoms worsen with standing.*
>
> *3. Symptoms are relieved by leaning on a support—such as a grocery cart, walker, or counter—or by sitting.*
>
> *4. Walking ability is improved when walking with a grocery cart, but symptoms are worsened while waiting at the checkout counter.*
>
> *5. Symptoms in bed at night are relieved by modifying sleep position, such as putting a pillow under the thighs if sleeping on the back, or between the thighs if sleeping on the side.*

I mentioned above that both daytime and nighttime modifications may be needed to see improvement. However, it is true that modification of only daytime behaviors, including Positional Testing, as described in Chapter 7, and the Adjunct Measures, as described in Chapter 8, may be all that is needed to solve the nighttime symptoms.

Modification of Sleep Position

For some people with nighttime or early morning symptoms of either the low back or the lower extremities, there is often great value in **modifying sleep position**. This may be accomplished by sleeping in a position that affords some spine flexion, such as in a recliner chair. It can also be achieved by using pillows as follows:

1. Place a pillow (or two) under your legs if you sleep on your back.

   If comfortable, it might be helpful to put the pillow(s) under the sheet. This is especially true if you switch over to your side while sleeping and then return to your back. Even after shifting positions, the pillows would still be in place. It is common for people to switch positions during the night. Switching sleep positions is not abnormal!

2. Place a pillow between your thighs if you sleep on your side. Use of a long "body pillow" may be helpful.

3. Place a pillow under your abdomen if you sleep on your stomach.

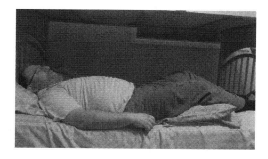

Picture 21.1. THE RIGHT WAY—a pillow under the knees. This position flexes (opens) the spine, relaxes tension on the nerves, and usually reduces SS/PS symptoms.

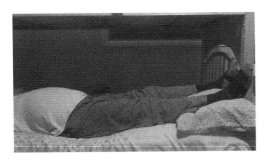

Picture 21.2. THE WRONG WAY—a pillow under the feet or legs. Often recommended to reduce swelling, this position may put more tension on the nerves and make the back or legs more uncomfortable.

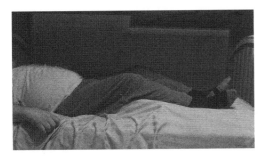

Picture 21.3. For restless sleepers, or for those who turn onto the side and then turn back, a pillow may be placed under the sheet to secure its position.

StoryTime: Catherine was a 72-year-old woman who reported difficulty sleeping for the previous 2 years, due to leg discomfort and frequent shifting of her sleep position from her back to each side. Frequent awakening in the night led to poor-quality sleep. Diagnosed by her internist with Restless Leg Syndrome, she did not tolerate the medications provided. She also experienced leg discomfort when walking more than one block, along with some Shortness of Breath.

My examination showed no asymmetry or biomechanical problems. There was severe sensitivity present in intermetatarsal spaces 2, 3, and 4 bilaterally, and along the tibial and femoral nerves. Catherine reported that her walking improved when she was pushing a grocery cart. Diagnosing likely Spinal Stenosis, I loaned her a walker and had her modify her sleep position, having her use a pillow under her thighs when sleeping on her back and between her thighs when sleeping on her side.

Within 2 days, Catherine's sleep patterns had improved, and she reported better-quality sleep. After

1 week, when I saw her next, she reported elimination of all distal nerve sensitivity except in the third intermetatarsal space bilaterally. This finding was suggestive of Morton's Neuroma, which was not symptomatic and therefore required no treatment. Upon returning the borrowed walker, she had a recurrence of the restless leg symptoms. Catherine acquired an appropriate walker and used it full time initially, and then only for long walks. She enjoyed long-term elimination of her troublesome nighttime symptoms, with no recurrence at her 6-month follow-up visit. This was a clear case of restless leg symptoms that were coming from Spinal Stenosis.

There are two additional lessons to be learned here. The first lesson is what I consider strong support for the effectiveness of the intervention. Some would say that it was mere coincidence that the symptoms improved with use of the walker. They would claim that symptoms come and go in people, and that controlled research is necessary. However, Catherine is just one of dozens of people I have treated who saw dramatic improvement of symptoms with Positional Testing for Spinal Stenosis or Mechanical Testing for PseudoStenosis, who experienced a recurrence of symptoms when the intervention (walker, heel lift, orthotic, brace, or behavior modification) was removed, and who then again had excellent relief when the proper treatment was restarted.

I agree that research is necessary, and have tried repeatedly (so far without success) to have it done properly. Until that time, readers are left with Level Five evidence: that of an expert—or, in my case, of someone who regards himself as something of an expert.

The second lesson to be learned from this story is reflective of a pattern I have seen dozens of times. Individuals who benefit from walker use but never use it full time as recommended, frequently have a rapid recurrence after stopping its use. Other patients who do use the walker full time, even if only for a week, often have long-term resolution of their symptoms even after they stop walker use. Such was the case with Catherine.

StoryTime: Morris D was an 89-year-old man with a primary complaint of burning feet that had made it hard for him to sleep at night for over 10 years. The pain would come within a few minutes of his getting into bed at night, and it woke him up in the middle of the night as well. He'd been told the pain was due to Peripheral Neuropathy of idiopathic (unknown) origin. He did not benefit from or tolerate the prescribed medications. He also had painful legs that often made it hard to stand or walk.

The exam was quick and easy. Morris's circulation seemed fine. There was some mild edema, only in the legs. There was no loss of sensation, either to light touch or to vibration. There was no apparent cause of PseudoStenosis. There was severe sensitivity along the nerves in both legs, with a positive First Interspace Fine Sign. Diagnosing Neurogenic Positional Pedal Neuritis secondary to Spinal Stenosis, I treated him with a walker—classic Positional Testing—along with the Adjunct Measures, including modification of sleep position.

At his next visit 2 weeks later, Morris reported the improvement we'd both been hoping for. There was total elimination of the nighttime pain and elimination of all difficulty walking and standing. After using the walker full time initially as advised, he eventually needed the walker only for longer walks.

For years, Morris had dubbed himself "Dr. Lollipop," visiting sick children in the hospital a few times each week. He reported that it was now much easier for him to go to "work." He never came back to my office after that follow-up visit. He didn't need to. As with many of the patients whose stories are shared in this book, I called him during the writing of these case histories, just to make sure that the advice that had worked so beautifully short term had actually lasted over the long term as well. He was happy to report that there'd been no recurrence of his previous symptoms.

Morris D's interview—a particularly entertaining one, and one of the first that I conducted—is available at WalkingWellAgain.com.

I could present similar stories about relief of nighttime symptoms for each of the conditions causing PseudoStenosis that have been presented. Limb Length Discrepancy and Flat Feet are the two most common culprits. There is no need for many stories repeating the same theme—wonderful improvement in just a day or two. There is only the need for patients, family members, and clinicians to be aware of the patterns suggesting SS/PS contributing to the symptoms, and to have the willingness to investigate.

Extended-Leg Flexion Test . . . Again

I will digress and mention something very important that I explained in Chapter 6, on physical findings. Patients often report that they have neuropathic or other uncomfortable symptoms that are constant or nearly constant. I ask them if they are having them as they are sitting in my podiatry chair, with legs extended straight out as pictured in picture 21.4. If they answer in the affirmative, I reposition them by flexing their knees, and wait just a minute. Immediate improvement of symptoms strongly suggests that the pain is coming from spinal nerve compression, which has been improved by altering position. I have had dozens of people with long-term symptoms who were amazed at the improvement accomplished with such a simple maneuver. I call this the "Extended-Leg Flexion Test." I don't love the name, so if you come up with something better, please let me know via my website, WalkingWellAgain.com.

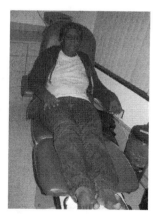

Picture 21.4. The patient's legs are extended, and the patient is symptomatic.

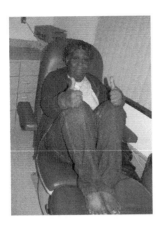

Picture 21.5. The patient's knees are flexed, the spine is thus flexed and opened, and the "neuropathy" symptoms are immediately improved. This strongly suggests the value of positional management, during the day as well as at night.

Sleeping on the Stomach

Sleeping on the stomach is often the worst position for people with Spinal Stenosis or PseudoStenosis, as it leads to a narrowing of the spine. This position can cause greater back pain as well as increased foot and leg symptoms. Some people choose to sleep on their stomach anyway, as this position often reduces Sleep Apnea, a condition addressed in the next chapter. To improve upon this sleep position, **place a pillow side to side under the stomach**, thus flexing and opening up the spine. You will have to experiment with pillow thickness and see what works for you. Sleep Apnea symptoms may also be improved by sleeping partially on the side and partially on the stomach.

Sciatica: Herniated Disc or Limb Length Discrepancy

Some individuals sleep on the stomach because that position eases back pain, sciatica, or other leg symptoms that are associated with a herniated disc. These people often experience improvement of their symptoms with standing or walking, and a worsening of symptoms with sitting. **Sitting on one or two pillows often provides immediate improvement, and full-time use for several days may provide long-term improvement.** If this is the case, use a pillow even in the car!

I have had many patients with sciatica who had moderate-to-severe symptoms caused by Limb Length Discrepancy, who had total resolution of symptoms with the proper use of a lift. Please see the section at the beginning of Chapter 12 that details this problem. Many of these people had severe symptoms lying down, and had improvement after a day or two of using the lift.

If Positional Testing protocols prove effective, nighttime symptoms improve in 1–3 nights. If they do improve, there is little doubt that the pain had been mediated through the spine.

Imperative of a Thorough SS/PS Evaluation

Whether or not the Positional Testing protocol is effective, there should still be an evaluation for possible PseudoStenosis. I have had many patients whose nighttime symptoms were eliminated by their improving lower-extremity mechanical function during the day with lifts, orthotics, braces, or other treatment—so please follow the protocols described in Chapter 12.

If you have had a suggestive Positional History but have had no improvement with either Positional Testing for Spinal Stenosis or Mechanical Testing for PseudoStenosis, then you should be evaluated for Spinal Stenosis. This evaluation may include spinal imaging, as well as treatment such as physical therapy, medication, and possible epidural injections.

If there is no Lumbar Spinal Stenosis, PseudoStenosis, or biomechanical cause of symptoms as described below, then the standard investigations and treatments available for RLS are appropriate. However, the above three patterns should be ruled out first. **Otherwise, a lifetime of unnecessary nighttime symptoms—and perhaps unnecessary medication to control those symptoms—might be the price paid for lack of clarity on this problem.**

Biomechanical (Direct) Causes of Nighttime Symptoms

As in Chapter 19, I want to focus on lower-extremity biomechanics as a direct, rather than indirect, cause of lower-extremity symptoms. By my definition, PseudoStenosis is a condition in which the lower-extremity symptoms are caused by spinal nerve compression and are thus mediated through the spine. The cause of PseudoStenosis is the improper function of the lower extremities, such as is caused when one leg is longer than the other. Thus the biomechanical problems of the feet or legs are the **indirect** cause of the patient's symptoms.

However, it is important to know that the leg symptoms can also be caused **directly** by foot and leg function.

In my opinion, the most common cause of leg aches at night (which may present as leg cramps, but may also include restlessness and aching) is Equinus. The second most common cause is flexible Flat Feet. Treatment for Flat Feet is included in Chapter 12, on PseudoStenosis, and Chapter 19, on arthritis. If you have Flat Feet, I recommend that you read the relevant sections in those chapters and also see a good podiatrist, one who is well versed in biomechanical treatment. Here I will deal in greater detail with the evaluation and treatment of Equinus (which may also be present if you have Flat Feet).

Detailed Presentation of Equinus

Equinus is a condition in which there is inadequate movement in an upward position of the ankle. It is usually caused by a too-tight Achilles tendon complex, most commonly the muscle that crosses both the knee joint and the ankle joint. This condition puts additional strain on the muscles in the back of the leg, which results in symptoms during or after activity during the day or in bed at night.

How tight is tight? Definitions vary, but let us define Equinus as "the inability to lift up (dorsiflex) the foot past the 90-degree right angle like a capital letter *L*." To measure, one should invert the foot slightly, with the knee straight, and bring the foot up as high (toward the knee) as possible.

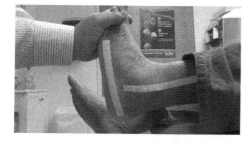

Picture 21.6. Here is a foot at approximately 90 degrees. The strips of tape show the bottom of the foot and the line of the leg.

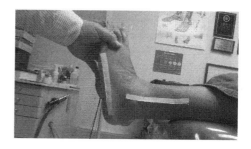

Picture 21.7. Here the foot is about 10 degrees short of perpendicular. The exact measurement is not nearly as important as the awareness that the muscles are tight. This tightness is often best appreciated by the patient when doing the stretching exercises described below!

A brief pause to share a couple of important points about Equinus.

Growing Pains in Children

Equinus is probably the most common cause of "growing pains" in children. Incidentally, growing pains often do not disappear with age. I have had adult and even senior-citizen patients who, after I identified the tight muscles and asked them about leg cramps, acknowledged having had nighttime leg symptoms since they were children. They had a lifetime of symptoms that could often have been resolved with simple stretching exercises.

Just as sad is that the sufferer may compensate for these uncomfortable symptoms by limiting activity. Inactive children (and adults) may not be lazy, but instead may be suffering from leg discomfort caused by activity. **Making an unconscious decision to avoid symptoms, they adopt a sedentary lifestyle that may be associated with childhood obesity.** These kids often watch too much television (or play too many computer games), are exposed to unending commercials about unhealthy food, and snack excessively on them. The combination of these patterns may contribute to our current epidemic of childhood obesity and childhood type 2 diabetes, a relatively new phenomenon.

It is essential to understand that the symptoms of growing pains in children and activity limitation in adults are not merely annoyances. They may constitute life-altering patterns that need to be taken as seriously as possible.

Orthotics and Equinus

Equinus is frequently the cause of discomfort while wearing orthotics. Because Equinus can cause the foot to flatten out as much as possible and an orthotic is firm in the arch, the foot may feel as if it is between a rock and a hard place, with painful pressure in the arch. (The painful point is often the bottom (plantar aspect) of the first metatarsal cuneiform joint, shown in picture 21.8.)

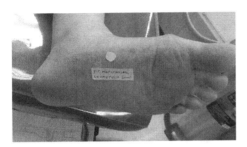

Picture 21.8. This spot is often painful with orthotics if Equinus is present.

This discomfort may be compensated for in several ways.

First, putting a lift underneath the heel of the orthotic may make it immediately more comfortable. Usually, ⅛ or ¼ of an inch is all that is necessary. Wearing this lift may allow the patient to tolerate previously intolerable orthotics. With time, wearing the orthotics may actually help to stretch the patient's tight tendons.

Second, one may use a modified orthotic instead. It can be so soft that it does not put pressure in the arch, though in that case it may not work as well. It can have a deliberately lowered arch to reduce pressure. This type of insert may still be effective, as the function of an orthotic is not the actual arch lift. A plantar fascial groove might be helpful. Using a pronated, flattened orthotic is often better tolerated, although perhaps not as effective. However, as Voltaire is quoted as having said, "The perfect is the enemy of the good." A compromised orthotic that is comfortable is much better than a fully controlling orthotic that hurts too much to wear!

Third, one can stretch as described below, and then the same orthotics may become comfortable.

Stretching Exercises for Equinus

This section addresses different patterns of Equinus and responses to stretching exercises. Need for stretching presupposes that there was not resolution of either unilateral Equinus with lifts, or of bilateral asymmetric Equinus with the taping technique presented in Chapter 12, section F, "Quick Resolution for Bilateral Equinus."

Fortunately, most people with Equinus respond quickly to stretching exercises. Some do not, as will be explained below. Overall, I present six patterns that I recognize, five of which can often be helped easily.

Exercise Instructions:

- *Begin slowly and gently.*
- *Stand barefoot, two or three feet away from the wall with heels flat on the floor and the knees extended straight.*
- *Facing the wall, place hands and elbows on the wall and gently lean forward into the wall with feet pointing straight and knees extended maximally.*
- *Feel the tension in the muscle in the back of the legs. If there is pain (rather than tension), move closer to the wall.*
- *Stretch and hold this position for a count of 30 seconds. Stand and relax for five seconds. Repeat stretching exercise for maximum of five minutes.*
- *Those with flexible flat feet may benefit from the stretch more by angling foot forward about 10 degrees and rotating the leg out so that the arch is elevated during the exercise. This modification may require stretching one achilles tendon at a time.*

THINGS TO REMEMBER:

1. *Stretch to the point of tension, not pain.*
2. *Stretch slowly and gently. Don't bounce.*
3. *If symptoms persist, please discuss this with your clinician, as other things can be done.*

These are the stretching instructions I have used in my office for the past twenty-five-plus years:

Six Common Patterns of Equinus and Response to Stretching

Here are the six patterns:

1. **Pattern 1:** Gentle stretching quickly improves Equinus and ameliorates symptoms. After the nighttime leg cramps resolve, you can reduce stretching to once a day, or even once every other day in most cases. Obviously, if the leg cramps return, you will need to do enough stretching to maintain the improvement. Usually once every day or two is all that is necessary.

2. **Pattern 2:** Even if there is significant tightness in the back of the legs, standard stretching as described above is not effective; it does not bring about a feeling of tension in the back of the legs. This occurs mostly in people who have a very flexible Flat Foot.

   You can tell if you have flexible Flat Feet by looking at your feet while sitting and then while putting some weight on them. You cannot tell by looking at your foot while not putting any weight on it, as the arch is present when the foot is not weight bearing. Here are some pictures that demonstrate this.

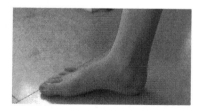

Picture 21.9. This shows a flexible Flat Foot, which has an arch while not weight bearing. This person, who has flexible Flat Feet, appears to have a moderate arch when not weight bearing.

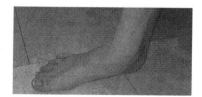

Picture 21.10. This shows a flexible Flat Foot, which flattens out while standing. The foot is not totally flat, but it is flatter than normal.

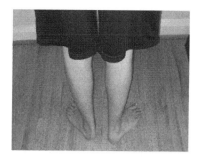

Picture 21.11. From behind, one can see that the feet turn out in this person with flexible Flat Feet. (The feet do not always turn out this much!) With stretching, the same feet may flatten even more. The motion that is attempted with stretching—a gentle pull on the Achilles tendon muscle complex—does not occur, as the foot simply collapses, the rear-foot actually becomes unstable, and the foot does not apply the Achilles tendon tension desired.

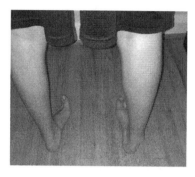

Picture 21.12. The feet have been intentionally turned straight. The legs are rotated out, inverting the feet and creating an artificial arch. If this occurs while you hold your feet in place but rotate your legs out, you have a flexible, and not rigid, Flat Foot. Stretching now is felt in the tight calf muscles, the location of the nighttime leg cramps.

I have used this modification, which I call the "rotational modification," for over twenty-five years. It has helped relieve leg cramps in hundreds of people who otherwise would not have obtained help from stretching. It may take a few tries to get this motion down, or you might need to stretch only one leg at a time. Either way, experiment and see if this modification helps you.

3. **Pattern 3:** Stretching is uncomfortable and aggravates leg or back pain. This pattern often occurs in people who have both Equinus (tight leg muscles) and Spinal Stenosis or PseudoStenosis. When the nerves in the back are inflamed or "activated," stretching in the standard way can irritate them and further activate the symptoms of stenosis. There are two approaches that may allow for success.

First, undertake Positional Testing with a walker and with the Adjunct Measures. After just a few days, the nerves may no longer be sensitive—that is, no longer activated. Positional Testing usually deactivates these inflamed nerves. I usually tell people to wait until they've done a week of Positional Testing before stretching, to make sure those nerves have quieted down sufficiently. I have had many patients who could not stretch initially because of leg or back discomfort, and who were able to stretch comfortably and effectively after Positional Testing.

Second, try stretching in a different manner. As you can see from picture 21.13, the normal way of stretching induces a slight **extension** of the spine in most patients. This poses a problem if you have low-back issues such as Spinal Stenosis or PseudoStenosis.

Another way to stretch might be easier to tolerate (see picture 21.14). Stand farther from the wall, put your hands lower on the wall, and flex—rather than hyperextend—the back. This allows you to put a stretch on the legs but not irritate the low back. This particular stretch is unwieldy and hard to do, but I have had some patients who did not want to use a walker use this approach successfully instead. While I prefer temporary use of the walker, this stretching position is also an option. This stretch can also be used in patients whose SS/PS symptoms do not improve with use of a walker. Keep in mind that if the Flat Feet are flexible, the patient may need the rotational modification.

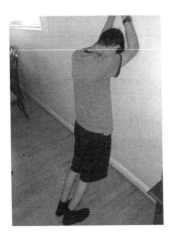

Picture 21.13. This shows a common stretching technique, from a standard distance, which often involves an extension of the spine that can cause discomfort from spine pathology.

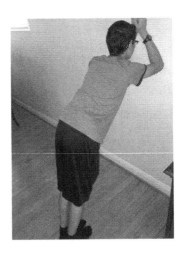

Picture 21.14. Here, the person stands farther away from the wall and flexes the spine, so as not to worsen symptoms from the spine pathology. Rotational modification may be necessary. This stretch may be harder for some people to master, but may also allow people with Spinal Stenosis symptoms to stretch their calf muscles successfully.

4. **Pattern 4:** There is tightness in one leg but not in the other. This unilateral Equinus—tightness on one side and not the other—is commonly associated with a Limb Length Discrepancy, where one leg is longer than the other. The shorter leg is usually the tight one. This condition may be a lifetime situation in which one leg is structurally longer than the other, or it may be secondary to either an injury or a surgery such as joint replacement.

(In some instances the LLDx is not a structural discrepancy but a "functional" one, where for some reason an abnormality in spinal position causes one leg to *function* as though it is longer even though it is not structurally of greater length. In such cases, the shorter leg is often flatter, turned out, and not tight.)

Most of the time, stretching is not necessary with this condition. All that is needed is to wear a lift in the shoe of the structurally shorter leg. Specific guidance is given in Chapter 12. Please review that section in detail. Strict compliance is often necessary. If the patient does not improve as I expect, I actually strap the lift to the foot so that it cannot be removed, and I often see the expected improvement after that. It may seem like overkill, but I stress the need for use of a lift in all the shoes the person wears, including bedroom slippers. Most of the time, unilateral Equinus caused by

Limb Length Discrepancy improves within a few days of wearing an appropriate lift.

5. **Pattern 5:** There is unilateral Equinus that developed because of neurological insult or orthopedic injury. Nerve problems can cause a Drop Foot, a condition in which the muscles in the front of the lower leg become weak or even paralyzed. These nerve problems can include a stroke, an injury to the peroneal nerve (just below the outside of the knee)—which happens occasionally with knee replacement surgery—or an injury to the L4 or L5 nerve root in the lower back. Other causes are systemic neurological conditions, although they more likely affect both legs. With Drop Foot, there is weakness of the muscle in the front of the leg, and often a tightening of the muscles in the back of the leg, causing Equinus.

In my experience, stretching does not usually work well with this type of Equinus, and use of a lift does not eliminate it. However, use of a lift under the heel of the affected leg can make it easier for the person to bear weight on that foot. Under this circumstance, when there is no short leg, adding the lift makes the affected leg longer, so one must add a lift to the heel—or, even better, to the entire sole—of the opposite shoe, in order not to induce a functional Limb Length Discrepancy.

If Equinus is caused by an orthopedic problem, such as a stiff ankle after a fracture or surgery, there is also benefit to having a lift added to both shoes, to keep the person even. A pedorthist can prove helpful in modifying the shoes for long-term help, after the clinician decides what pattern of elevation should be used on each foot.

6. **Pattern 6:** Stretching is simply not effective in relieving the tightness or the nighttime cramping. The person's muscles are tight and he is able to stretch, but there is no improvement of either the tightness or the resulting symptoms. This type of Equinus often cannot be easily relieved.

This pattern is actually much more likely to occur in a person who has an Equinus involving *two* muscles in the Achilles complex: both the gastrocnemius and the soleus. In such cases, the muscle in the back of the leg remains just as tight when the knee is bent as when the knee is straight. Such cases of tightness usually do not improve with stretching.

One may use either heel lifts or shoes with a higher heel at all times to accommodate the tight muscles. If symptoms warrant it, surgical treatment to lengthen the tight Achilles tendon is an option.

SUMMARY

A great many conditions can cause nighttime symptoms. My experience shows that most people with nighttime symptoms have either SS/PS or distinct biomechanical problems. One should certainly consider whether there are daytime symptoms consistent with Spinal Stenosis / PseudoStenosis, such as aching, tired discomfort in the feet, legs, or thighs that is worsened with walking and standing yet quickly relieved by sitting or leaning against something such as a grocery cart, walker, or even baby carriage. If so, a brief trial of Positional Testing, including the Adjunct Measures as described in previous chapters, as well as modification of sleep position, may eliminate all symptoms in a matter of days. **Whether or not the symptoms improve with this approach, the patient should also have a lower-extremity examination to rule out possible causes of PseudoStenosis.**

If tight muscles are the cause of nighttime symptoms, stretching can be very helpful and may need to be done a few times a week, long term, after the symptoms have been resolved.

Only after both SS/PS and biomechanical problems of the feet and legs have been ruled out should a person be diagnosed with Restless Leg Syndrome. Evaluation for these two conditions should be carried out for all patients with nighttime lower-extremity symptoms even if there is another diagnosis, such as one associated with RLS. **(After all, the presence of another condition such as diabetes or poor circulation does not mean that there is no SS/PS or biomechanical problem contributing to the symptoms.)** Otherwise, treatment with medications with possibly significant side effects will be provided in cases where they are not necessarily needed. A good internist or sleep specialist may be able to help you with that evaluation.

Wishing you a good night's sleep!

A Brief Explanation of Restless Leg Syndrome

The above-listed patterns include both primary Restless Leg Syndrome and secondary Restless Leg Syndrome. Secondary RLS means that associated conditions contribute to Restless Leg Syndrome symptoms. These conditions include iron deficiency, low ferritin levels, diabetes, Parkinson's disease, end-stage renal disease, varicose veins, and thyroid problems. Treating these conditions may improve or eliminate symptoms consistent with Restless Leg Syndrome.

There are also other conditions that can cause nighttime leg symptoms that are different from classic Restless Leg Syndrome. These conditions include arterial insufficiency, venous insufficiency, Diabetic or other Peripheral Neuropathy, Fibromyalgia, Spinal Stenosis, PseudoStenosis, electrolyte imbalance, Hypothyroidism, and biomechanical foot problems.

In addition to medication, interventions for Restless Leg Syndrome include lowering one's caffeine and alcohol intake, reducing or eliminate smoking, maintaining good sleep habits (including a regular sleep pattern), getting regular but moderate exercise, and relaxing in a hot bath before bed.

My strong recommendation is this: if you do not get the help you need using the advice you find in this chapter, see a sleep specialist for a thorough evaluation.

Criteria for Restless Leg Syndrome (RLS)

RLS has been clinically defined to include four sets of symptoms, although the diagnosis, especially as seen in private medical practice, may not be limited to individuals with all four sets.

The four are as follows:

1. *A tendency to move the lower limbs in an ongoing and not deliberate or intentional pattern*
2. *Exacerbation of this pattern while resting or sleeping*
3. *Improvement with activity (In other words, intentional movement seems to overpower the unintentional movement.)*
4. *Worsening of symptoms in bed at night*

   Subjectively, the sensation of movement—usually involving the lower legs—while usually unpleasant, is not necessarily painful. Accompanying the restlessness may be aching, cramping, pins and needles, pain, or electric shocks.

CHAPTER 22

Sleep Apnea

In the previous chapter, I review the effect that SS/PS can have on nighttime leg and foot symptoms. Among other things, I mention Sleep Apnea as another problematic nighttime condition. Insofar as it is totally different from the other conditions addressed in this book, I chose to devote a short chapter to this disorder.

Sleep Apnea is not likely to be addressed by most podiatrists—but I feel that it should be a concern for anyone using the approaches presented in this book. It is a common and potentially harmful condition.

A Brief Explanation of Sleep Apnea

Obstructive Sleep Apnea (OSA) is a condition in which the lack of support of the structures in the neck, most often seen in people who are overweight or who have large necks, results in apnea episodes, which are periods of not breathing when in the deepest level of sleep. It is often, but not always, seen in people who are heavy snorers. **An absence of snoring in a person with Sleep Apnea symptoms should not preclude having symptoms investigated.** There are sleep-study centers throughout the country, with physicians specializing in sleep problems. They should be consulted about this condition if you suspect that it is present.

Sleep Apnea is not to be taken lightly. This seemingly innocuous sleep pattern constitutes a dangerous disorder that can worsen an individual's health on many fronts. It is often the cause of uncontrolled hypertension. Even in people not affected medically in a marked manner, OSA interferes with sleep quality and contributes to daytime drowsiness and a lowered quality of life.

Sleep Apnea sufferers may awaken when they stop breathing. Sometimes they wake up with a sense of doom, a pounding heart, or a feeling of having had a nightmare. The physiology of the body reacting to an inadequate oxygen supply is similar to what happens when you hold your breath underwater as long as you can—you experience a panicky feeling before you reach the surface. The difference, however—and this is a big difference—is that the sleeper is often completely unaware of the Sleep Apnea. He or she may go through a cycle of apnea episodes, waking up and going back to sleep numerous times each night—and sometimes numerous times each hour. The person may sleep in bed for many hours but still wake up tired and be inexplicably drowsy during the day.

I cannot overstress the value of having Sleep Apnea identified and treated. Many people try using CPAP machines, and stop because they cannot get used to them. If this is your story, I encourage you to go back to a sleep specialist for a reevaluation of the mask and machine. Newer masks are much easier on the face, and the new machines are quieter and temperature controlled. Some are even self-adjusting, always providing the amount of pressure that the patient needs. CPAP masks and hoses may lose effectiveness with time and may need to be replaced. If you haven't been successful with a CPAP machine in the past, go back and try again. It is worth it!

How Does Sleep Apnea Relate to SS/ PS and Lower-Extremity Symptoms?

People who sleep on their backs usually suffer the most from Sleep Apnea. The soft tissues of the throat block the airway much more easily when assisted by the pull of gravity. Sleeping on your side is preferable, and can be promoted by wearing a special shirt that has an object in the back to make sleeping in that position unpleasant. However, even side sleeping is not the optimum position. Apnea episodes still occur. Some people start on their backs or sides and, because of apnea, gravitate to sleeping on their stomachs. In this position, gravity actually works in their favor, pulling the structures away from the throat and leaving the airway less obstructed.

End of story? Hardly.

When an individual lies on his stomach, the back is placed in a position of increased extension, which reduces the diameter of the central canal and lateral foramen. **This position narrows the spine,** which can not only give rise to local arthritic back pain but can also put pressure on the nerves, causing symptoms in the feet, legs, or thighs. For people with SS/PS in particular, this position may result in increased nighttime symptoms (burning, cramping, tingling, restless legs), or it may keep the nerves inflamed so that it becomes easier to induce these symptoms with walking or standing during the day.

In this situation, the patient is literally caught between a rock and a hard place. Sleeping on the back, on the side, or even in a recliner chair can bring on Sleep Apnea, which in turn interferes with both nighttime sleep and daytime wakefulness. Sleeping on the stomach facilitates Sleep Apnea relief, but can cause nighttime back and extremity symptoms, and may even affect the ability to stand or walk during the day.

What is the solution? Here are the essential steps:

- See a sleep specialist. Go to a sleep lab and get yourself evaluated and treated. The standard treatment, a CPAP machine, is a wonderful, safe tool that helps Sleep Apnea. Getting used to the CPAP can take a while, and you may need to experiment with different masks to find the kind and size you tolerate the best. For many people, adjusting to the machine calls for patience and determination, but the results are worth whatever effort you expend.

- Treat the SS/PS as described in Chapter 21. Once you have the CPAP—or whatever other device your treating physician provides—you may find yourself able to sleep on your back or side again.

- Follow the guidance on sleep positions, and also consider, if necessary, Positional Testing, as described in Chapters 7 and 8. Get evaluated for potential PseudoStenosis, as described in Chapters 11 and 12. Combine an investigation of the source of your symptoms with these straightforward approaches to get the help you need.

StoryTime: Judith N was a 72-year-old woman who came into the office with a chief complaint of severe difficulty at night because of significant aching in her feet and legs that frequently woke her up. Restless legs, coupled with her inability to be comfortable in bed at night, prevented her from using the CPAP that she needed for her Sleep Apnea, and she was frequently tired throughout the day. She also reported difficulty standing and walking due to foot and leg pain.

Judith had a Limb Length Discrepancy and bilateral nerve sensitivity that was consistent with both PseudoStenosis and Spinal Stenosis. I treated both—with a heel lift, Positional Testing, and the Adjunct Measures. Doing so eliminated almost all the difficulty in standing and walking, removed the foot and leg pain, and took away all the restlessness and discomfort in her legs in bed at night. She was then able to use a CPAP and sleep much better.

Judith's interview from her first visit, and another a couple of months later, can be viewed at WalkingWellAgain.com.

Another option, if you cannot obtain or tolerate a CPAP, would be to use a pillow under the stomach positioned from side to side, to open up the spine while sleeping. I have had several patients who successfully used this technique, though many others did not find it comfortable. I reiterate my recommendation that you seek treatment for your Sleep Apnea and do your BEST to adjust to the CPAP.

I wish you a good night's sleep and many wonderful, *healthy* days to follow!

CHAPTER 23

Standing, Balance Problems, Falls, and Near-Falls

In this chapter, I present the need to consider Spinal Stenosis and PseudoStenosis in ALL patients with difficulty standing and with balance problems. I include in this category everyone who has suffered falls, has had near-falls, finds it difficult to stand, or has difficulty walking in a straight line, even if the problem began later in life or after an injury or medical problem. **Spinal Stenosis and PseudoStenosis should always be considered.**

Mechanical Causes of Imbalance

According to the National Institutes of Health web page on balance disorders, *"A balance disorder is a condition that makes you feel unsteady or dizzy as if you are moving, spinning, or floating, even though you are standing still or lying down. Balance disorders can be caused by certain health conditions, medications, or a problem in the inner ear or the brain. Our sense of balance is primarily controlled by a structure in [. . .] the inner ear."*

Please note that I certainly do not disagree with standard medical practice, which aggressively investigates the many possible neurologic, medical, or medication-based causes of poor balance. However, I suggest pursuing another avenue as well.

Many people who have a **balance problem of an unknown cause,** commonly described as an "idiopathic"

condition, actually have a **mechanical imbalance** serving as the unrecognized cause. This mechanical imbalance leads to a "whole-body imbalance," which can result in unsteadiness, difficulty standing, difficulty turning, and a much greater likelihood of falls or near-falls. As you might guess from everything you've read so far, I feel that many people have balance problems that are exacerbated by a mechanical imbalance, **even in cases where there is another known cause**.

A fall can have tragic, even life-threatening consequences. I implore anyone with poor balance to use a walker or cane and obtain the necessary physical therapy to reduce the risk of falls. **However, it is just as important is to find the cause of the unsteadiness and to treat it.**

In my practice, I have found that balance problems are frequently caused by a difficulty in compensating for a mechanical imbalance that is present, **even if the imbalance has been present for a long time**. The reason for this—or at least part of the reason—is that the physiologic changes in strength, endurance, and reaction time that come with aging (or some disease processes) leave us less able to compensate for those imbalances, even if we have been previously compensating for them for years. Age, or a disease process or injury, can be the straw that breaks the camel's back.

PseudoStenosis, Spinal Stenosis, and Peripheral Neuropathy

The problems that can cause difficulty standing and loss of balance are the same problems that can cause PseudoStenosis, or lead to secondary arthritis of the lower extremities. They are as follows:

1. Limb Length Discrepancy

2. A flexible Flat Foot, such as with Functional Hallux Limitus

3. A rigid or semi-rigid Flat Foot

4. Equinus, involving a tight Achilles tendon in the back of the leg or limited ankle joint movement for other reasons

5. An altered walking pattern caused by degenerative or other arthritis

6. An altered walking pattern caused by a stroke or other nerve problem

7. An altered walking pattern caused by any lower-extremity pain great enough to make the patient walk differently

   In addition, there are two large elephants in the room that we will address:

8. Spinal Stenosis

9. Peripheral Neuropathy

Limb Length Discrepancy, New or Old

I find that the most common mechanical cause of balance problems is Limb Length Discrepancy, *even one as small as* ¹⁄₁₆ *of an inch, less than 2 mm.* This discrepancy is frequently, although not always, present since birth. It may be caused by an injury, a surgery such as a knee or hip replacement, or a fracture repair.

I have seen people in their twenties who reported that they've had balance problems their "whole life." This condition often improves in just the minutes that it takes to identify the discrepancy and try using a lift. It is truly amazing how use of a lift can so quickly eliminate symptoms of PseudoStenosis, arthritis, Low-Back Syndrome, as well as a "lifetime" of balance problems. For those young people, what a welcome gift—often with nothing more than a simple ¼-, ⅛-, and sometimes even only ¹⁄₁₆-inch shoe insert.

For older people, however, eliminating unsteadiness is more than just a gift. It's a new lease on life! It can be instantaneous, especially for those who have not had an injury or surgery, but who have gradually noticed increased difficulty in standing, a tendency to slip or almost fall, or a need to lean on something when on their feet.

StoryTime: A 70-year-old man came in for evaluation of balance problems that had developed gradually, starting about 2 years prior to his visit. He was worried about his risk for falls, as he had almost fallen several times. A thorough evaluation by a neurologist identified no problems, and extensive physical therapy brought only mild, temporary improvement.

The patient had had diabetes for 20 years, but the condition had been controlled under the management of a very thorough endocrinologist. He had no complaints of neuropathic symptoms, and my exam showed normal neuropathy parameters and good circulation. What was "off" was a slight Limb Length Discrepancy with his right heel being higher when he was lying down and his right hip and shoulder both being slightly lower when he was standing. His right Achilles tendon was tighter, and that foot was about a quarter of a size smaller than the other. All these factors suggested a mild structural Limb Length Discrepancy. In addition, there was a strong First Interspace Fine Sign in his longer (left) leg.

(If these ideas are new to you because you skipped directly to this chapter, please review Chapter 6, on physical findings, and Chapter 12, on Pseudo-Stenosis.)

I had this gentleman stand on a ¼-inch lift under his right foot, and he immediately smiled, recognizing the improved comfort when standing. His hips and shoulders were almost even now. I put a lift in his right shoe and gave him a supply for all his shoes and sandals. I would like to say that he came back and reported wonderful results the following week, but that didn't happen. The improvement was only moderate. He was a lot better than before, but he was still unstable at times and that worried him.

Further discussion revealed two factors. One: he did not wear bedroom slippers or shoes at home. Two: there had been a day when he did not wear shoes with a lift for the entire day but did a lot of walking. A quick exam showed that he still had a tight Achilles tendon on the shorter leg and nerve sensitivity on the longer leg. Taking no chances, I strapped a felt lift to his shorter leg. Three days later, he walked extensively (miles!) with no instability at all. My exam showed that the Achilles tightness and the nerve sensitivity were gone. It was clear that strict compliance with the lift was needed.

I encouraged him to continue being evaluated by a neurologist well-versed in balance problems and neuropathy, to ensure that there was not another condition present. However, in his case there was no question that the Limb Length Discrepancy played a large role in his balance issues. This is a very common finding in my practice.

StoryTime: A 65-year-old woman came into the office for treatment of an ingrown toenail. She was in a wheelchair, to which she'd been bound almost entirely for the previous 15 months. She had once been an active walker, walking a few miles daily for years. She gradually developed low-back pain that, despite conservative treatment, grew progressively worse, until she could only walk less than a block. Sadly, she developed a flare-up of what was diagnosed as gout, and was hospitalized for several days. After her hospitalization, she could barely walk at all. She spent 10 weeks in a rehabilitation facility, where she built up to walking for a few minutes with physical therapy, a walker, and an ankle brace.

She continued therapy at home for several months with no real change. When home alone, she could stand and walk minimally (fewer than ten steps), and was always afraid of falling backward, which she had nearly done on several occasions. The brace was very uncomfortable.

My examination showed a severe Equinus of approximately –35 degrees on the left and approximately –5 degrees on the right. Her left heel was about 1¼ inches higher than the right. There was also severe interspace and proximal nerve sensitivity.

I applied ⅞ of an inch of felt to her left foot (see picture 23.1) and strapped it in place. She stood up and reported immediate relief from both the pain and the instability. She stood with a walker and walked around the office with no instability. I sent her home with instructions to increase her walking to a few minutes every hour.

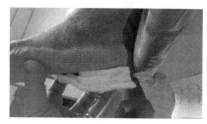

Picture 23.1. 7/8 of an inch of felt attached to the foot to compensate for both Achilles tightness and leg shortness.

At her next visit, the Achilles tightness had reduced from –35 degrees to –15 degrees. No therapy, no surgery—just a lift. She brought in the brace, which was still somewhat uncomfortable with standing after I removed the strap and pad. I then added ⅜ of an inch of felt to the lift (picture 23.2), and it became quite comfortable, since we had compensated for the residual tightness.

I also added the use of an Evenup, a device that adds height to a shoe, which can be easily attached or removed (picture 23.3). She walked comfortably around the office for five minutes. The next time I saw her, she reported having no symptoms.

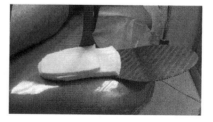

Picture 23.2. Once the ankle Equinus improved, the brace that had been unwearable became comfortable, with 3/8 of an inch of felt lift added to the heel.

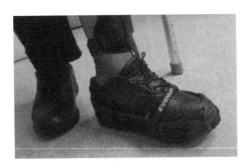

Picture 23.3. Use of an Evenup on the outside of the shoe provided immediate compensation for the Limb Length Discrepancy. This was not comfortable until the Equinus improved by temporary lift application.

I instructed her to use the Evenup at full thickness (2 centimeters, or 0.8 inches) when walking without the brace, and at half thickness (1 centimeter, or 0.4 inches) when using the brace. She did well, and was able to stop using her wheelchair.

Why am I sharing these two stories? They represent two ends of a continuum. One person had mild but disturbing balance problems that developed without any inciting factor. The other person was relegated to a wheelchair, with all therapeutic efforts unsuccessful. Both improved greatly with relatively simple interventions. **Both needed active thinking and follow-up, not just a lift and a send-off. Active follow-up for PseudoStenosis conditions is often necessary for success!**

I am not going to cite similar cases for each of the possible causes for PseudoStenosis, though such stories have occurred often in my practice. Many patients with Flat Feet improve greatly with orthotics or braces (immediately with Mechanical Testing!), just as those with a Limb Length Discrepancy may improve with an appropriate lift. People with foot pain often immediately improve once the cause of pain is addressed. Sometimes instability is the sole problem, but balance issues are often seen in people who have pain or limitation from other problems that are present. In any case, these details of PseudoStenosis should be investigated and treated, often as a first line of treatment.

For details on evaluation and management of LLDx, please read Chapter 12 sections B, C, and D.

* * * * *

Let's shift our focus to three additional conditions: Equinus, Spinal Stenosis, and Peripheral Neuropathy.

Equinus of One or Both Legs

Regarding Equinus, which you'll remember is a lack of adequate motion in the ankle (see Chapters 12, 19 and 21), there is a big difference in Equinus when it is present in one leg and when it is present in both legs. If Equinus is in one leg only, the cause may be that leg being shorter than its mate. One-sided Equinus could also be caused by ankle arthritis resulting from an injury or long-term foot deformity, or it could be caused by a Drop Foot caused by a nerve problem such as stroke, spinal nerve compression, or pathology of the peroneal nerve, which is near the knee. **I have had many patients with Equinus note that they had a tendency to fall backward, in addition to any side-to-side instability.**

If the Equinus is much worse on one side and is caused by a short leg, and the patient has been relegated to using a wheelchair, that shorter leg is usually *obviously* short—e.g., ⅜ of an inch or more. Lining up the heels of a patient's feet will likely show that obvious difference, though one must be sure that the low back is flush against the chair. (This is a clue, but the Iliac Crest alignment resolution, described in Chapters 6 and 12, is a more valid clue.) I have had at least ten patients over the years who came in by wheelchair because of an inability to stand or walk, and who were able to walk decently again in a manner of minutes. In such cases, I strapped the needed amount of felt to the heel of the shorter leg and had the person immediately stand, which they were then able to do, sometimes better than they had in years. In these cases, the lift compensated for two problems: the shortness of the leg, and the tendency of a rigid tight Achilles tendon or arthritic ankle to cause the person to fall backward.

In many instances the discrepancy had been recognized, but the brace or elevator shoe the patient had been given was not comfortable and could not be tolerated because of the Equinus.

Allow me to review a few different scenarios. If the severely tight muscle is caused by the body's subconscious attempt to compensate for a Limb Length Discrepancy, use of a lift will cause the tightness to improve in a matter of days. The shoe and brace may then become more comfortable, as in our story above, but first the tightness must be improved.

This same result may also be accomplished by surgically lengthening the tight muscle, a procedure that often has great value. This surgery may not be necessary in many cases of unilateral Equinus where a lift is used properly first. As mentioned before, please do not be angry at your doctor if such surgery was done. Many of the ideas presented in this book are either original or not well known—which is, of course, the reason for my writing it!

If the lack of adequate ankle motion does not improve with the appropriate lift and surgery has not been done, then a standard shoe elevation will not work. One must use a high enough heel to compensate for the lack of motion, or else the higher shoe will tilt the person backward. In addition, a 90-degree ankle brace will not be comfortable and may cause pressure in the back of the leg, as the foot cannot attain a 90- degree position. In such situations, the brace must be customized to accommodate the improper position of the foot. An off-the-shelf brace, even one provided by a doctor or other provider, cannot do that, unless it is modified as shown in picture 23.2.

Sometimes, one-sided Equinus is not associated with a shorter leg, but rather with arthritis, an Achilles injury, or a nerve problem. A lift for the tighter foot will take away the force that drives the person backward when standing, and that is a good thing. The lift will not improve the ankle motion; it will just compensate for it. However, as you might guess, a lift on that one side will then CAUSE, or REINFORCE, a Limb Length Discrepancy. **In such cases, it is important to provide an equal amount of lift for both sides, so that the Equinus is addressed and the patient can stand balanced. While with the Equinus ankle the lift must be in the heel, on the other side, the lift may involve the entire sole of the shoe.**

The same is true for those patients with tightness in both ankles. Lifts for both shoes can immediately improve balance and take away the force that drives the person backward.

Several scenarios regarding Equinus are possible. The tightness may have been present since youth. Tightness of the Achilles tendon is also a change that can develop with age, and it may be a specific complication seen with diabetes. It also appears to be more common in

women who frequently wear high-heeled shoes, or in men who wear cowboy boots. The question of whether the shoes caused the tightness, or if people chose those shoes because they were more comfortable because of the tightness that already existed, is one of the many things I just don't know. In either case, adding lifts to more practical shoes may be a great help.

However, the problem might be even more complicated. It is possible that the person had a stroke, causing Equinus to affect a leg that already had Equinus caused by a Limb Length Discrepancy. Such a case will require thought, but it will also need experimenting to find the right balance. In many of these cases, long-term success requires cooperation between a physician or podiatrist and a good pedorthotist.

For patients with both **Cerebral Palsy and Equinus**, be aware of the pattern of Limb Length Discrepancy common in Spastic Hemiplegic Cerebral Palsy. This is reported in detail in Chapter 12 Section F.

Spinal Stenosis

What about Spinal Stenosis? I have had dozens of patients over the years who reported poor balance as one of the symptoms that were part of a larger picture, and whom I diagnosed and successfully treated for Spinal Stenosis. These patients experienced immediate improvement of instability with use of a walker, as described in Chapter 7.

This comes as no surprise, since using an external support such as a cane or walker is a primary treatment for balance problems. What may come as a surprise is something that patients cannot usually grasp at the initial visit, and something that I still get a big kick out of: **temporary, proper, full-time use of a walker often provides long-term improvement in symptoms of Spinal Stenosis, including instability (Chapter 10, Positional Therapy).** Back pain, leg pain, and neuropathy symptoms frequently improve in a matter of a few days, and often do not come back for weeks, months, or years. Many of the patients that I described above saw their symptoms, including poor balance, improve dramatically in this way. After stopping walker use, they found, to their delight, that they had regained their "sea legs," the feeling of stability and confidence when standing and walking.

Peripheral Neuropathy

Finally, neuropathy. Please read Chapters 15 and 25 for my take on this topic. If the neuropathic symptoms are caused by Spinal Stenosis or PseudoStenosis, those symptoms—including balance issues—may disappear within just a few days.

Because symptoms of persistent numbness and poor balance MIGHT be caused by Cervical (neck) Stenosis, the patient should be evaluated by a specialist such as a neurologist, physiatrist, or spine surgeon. (Cervical Stenosis often, but not always, also involves symptoms in the hands, such as numbness, weakness, a pattern of dropping objects, and even difficulty buttoning shirts.)

If there is reduced muscle mass or weakness in the thighs, one must consider a Demyelinating Neuropathy, which may be totally reversed with medical treatment. If symptoms involve difficulty walking because of leg weakness, dementia, or incontinence (difficulty controlling urination), then suspect Hydrocephalus—another condition that can be successfully treated. Consulting with a **neurologist or physiatrist is of paramount importance**.

If, however, it is a true Peripheral Neuropathy—which includes Diabetic Neuropathy—that is causing the balance problems, then either Metanx or Anodyne therapy may be helpful. Both treatments are presented in detail in Chapter 25. I have had many patients with balance problems who had neuropathy, who reported improvement with these two treatments. Both have advantages. Anodyne works much faster, but I suspect that Metanx has a greater systemic effect. Discuss these treatment options with your podiatrist, or with another clinician who is familiar with both modalities.

Multiple Causes May Be Present

I must emphasize what this chapter is NOT saying. I am NOT saying that the techniques of this book are adequate for all people with balance problems. It is obvious to any clinician, and I hope to any layperson who has read this book, that commonly, more than one condition contributes to a problem. Even if your symptoms improve with the treatments presented here, if you still suspect that another condition is present, have a good medical evaluation by an appropriate specialist. Finding an additional factor that coexists with the problems I present here can lead to further help.

In addition, physical therapy can provide absolutely wonderful help for people with residual balance problems. It does not work as quickly as the solutions I present above—it often takes a few weeks—but the results are often tremendously valuable. There is no other way to describe it. If the approaches presented here do not work or provide only partial relief, seek further help!

An Imperative: PLEASE Be Honest

Do not give up the use of a cane or walker if you or your loved ones have any concern about residual balance problems. I repeat my plea from Chapter 10:

How tragic it would be for someone who has lived with pain for years and has been limited by Spinal Stenosis to walking short distances, to finally have relief from the pain and regain ability to walk for blocks or miles again—only to fall and break a hip and lose everything gained. In that one fall, that person may lose the chance for an Indian summer, an opportunity to live actively and pain free in his or her senior years. Even more tragic—**in some instances the fall is caused not by poor balance but by pride**.

Refusing to use a walker or a cane when it is needed for stability because of poor balance is a bad, bad choice. Both walker and cane dramatically reduce the risk of falls for many people. If you are at risk for falls and you refrain from using the walker or cane, you put yourself at risk for tragedy

If that fall happens and you lie helpless in bed, that disability will be made many times worse if it is coupled with the awareness that it most likely would have been prevented by using the walker or cane. Your distress will be grievously compounded by the fact that, in cutting short your independence by an avoidable fall, you also ruined or disrupted the lives of those who love you. **If pride, ego, or vanity prevents you from using the support you really need, you are risking your future as well as the future of others in your life.**

There must be an honest evaluation regarding your risk for falling.

Of course, any instability could derive, wholly or in part, from the same problems that can cause PseudoStenosis, so you should be evaluated by a good podiatrist.

If after PseudoStenosis evaluation there is any question about your risk for falling, either in your own evaluation or in the opinion of those who know you well, I strongly recommend that you be referred to a physical therapist for balance training and for evaluation of your need for a walker or cane for long-term use. Your future and the happiness and future of your loved ones may depend upon your being honest with yourself regarding the need for a cane or a walker—and being strict with its use if it is determined that you do need it.

I'd choose quality of life over vanity any day. Wouldn't you?

Inactivity, Chronic Pain, and Depression

This chapter presents no new medical knowledge. Instead, my aim is to reinforce what is already well known and understood, in a way that creates a strong drive for investigating the potential presence of either Spinal Stenosis or PseudoStenosis, with the paths set out in this book.

Chronic Pain and "Learned Helplessness"

There is no question that depression can magnify pain. All too often, people are blamed for their own pain and weakness because they are overweight or inactive. Similarly, pain that is chronic and poorly understood may be at least partially blamed on the fact that the person suffering that pain is depressed. Depression can magnify pain.

The reverse situation is also quite common. **Chronic pain, and the helplessness and inactivity that it engenders, can cause depression.** If pain, inactivity, and the feeling of helplessness are improved, factors that may be contributing to the depression are removed.

Unfortunately, a barrier exists to addressing pain of a non-obvious cause. In addition to the physiologic changes linked to chronic pain, there is also a concept presented by Dr. Martin Seligman called **"learned helplessness."** According to this theory, individuals whose prior efforts at solving their problems were unsuccessful, and who have been advised that no resolution was available, may develop a pattern of acceptance of pain and limitation, along with an overall lack of optimism for improvement. This combination of pain, limited activity, and lack of optimism may result in clinical depression, or at least the appearance of clinical depression.

An essential point of this chapter is that many such people do not take the initiative to discuss the variables that might be affecting their symptoms. As such, it is essential to investigate such symptoms aggressively and then try to treat them.

I have seen many patients with the problems detailed in this book who came in for simple foot care, such as nail problems, corns or calluses, or injuries, and who had the appearance of being depressed. Some had already been diagnosed as clinically depressed and were on antidepressant medication. Typically, they did not share complaints about other foot, leg, or spine problems on the patient history form—a form specifically designed to extract such complaints. At times, they did not share complaints even when I specifically asked about such symptoms, and they denied having symptoms even when I asked if there were any other problems with their feet or legs. After suffering for years with symptoms that had defied treatment, why should they bring them up now? Especially if *learned helplessness* made them feel that nothing they can do will help anyway.

Nevertheless, a quick podiatric exam using the approaches shared in this book, along with a focused discussion, including a specific and sometimes demanding Positional History, frequently led to a provisional diagnosis of Spinal Stenosis, PseudoStenosis, or both, in many of my patients. Rapid improvement of foot, leg, or spine symptoms was sometimes accompanied by an equally rapid improvement of general affect, with the change in symptoms of depression noted by both the patient and his or her family.

Often, the patient's mood is wonderfully different after a day or two of relief from pain. People come in appearing depressed and lethargic because of inactivity and a lack of confidence in the future, and they lighten up considerably when it becomes clear that they can indeed get better and become more active. After a few days, when the pain is either completely or mostly gone and the patient's confidence returns, the depression can greatly improve.

Why is this scenario important enough to warrant an entire chapter of its own? Because patients and the people in their support systems should understand that patients who are inactive MIGHT be inactive because of the discomfort brought on by standing and/or walking. Pain not only robs them of their enjoyment of life, but may also affect their state of depression. As presented in Chapter 2, many such individuals develop a stoic attitude and go through life never mentioning their symptoms. While some embrace life despite symptoms, others give up.

StoryTime: Juanita M was a woman in her 60s who came into the office for evaluation of a possible mass on her toe. The mass turned out to be unimportant. However, further discussion revealed that she'd been suffering with pain in her feet and legs for some 40 years—basically, most of her adult life.

The pain involved her feet, legs, hips, and back, and was so bad that she spent up to fifteen hours a day in bed. She had tried a variety of narcotics, but now used them only occasionally because, as she said, they didn't help much. She indicated that she'd been suffering from depression for years and was taking medication for that—also without much help.

Because of her poor balance, she had fallen many times and had almost fallen far more times. She walked significantly better when pushing a grocery cart, but not completely better. She had severe pain in her feet and legs in bed at night, to the extent that she said the pain was a "10 out of 10" at times, but always at least moderate. No wonder she was depressed!

She had a Limb Length Discrepancy with a unilateral Equinus and a positive First Interspace Fine Sign bilaterally, though much worse on the foot of the longer leg. In her case, the other results of her physical examination were not significant. X-rays did show arthritic changes in her feet, but I did not think they were important.

We treated her with a lift for the shorter leg and with Positional Testing, with all the Adjunct Measures for the Spinal Stenosis. When I saw her again 4 days later, she was a different person! She went from presenting as a depressed individual, consistent with living in chronic pain, to being enthusiastic and happy. She no longer needed to take pain medication. She was not waking up in pain at night. Her hips and legs felt one hundred percent normal. She declared that her overall pain level was a "1 out of 10" without medication, as compared to a "10 out of 10" with medication before. She was stable, she did not feel that there was a balance problem any longer, and she was able to do much more walking.

I offer a word of caution. Most people do not have such severely disabling symptoms. Some do not have such a dramatic turnaround in a few days. For many, the chronic pain and limitation of activity are just part of the package of challenges in life that pull a person down. And yet it can be an important part of the puzzle, and one that is hard to identify, unless you ask specific questions and know how to examine and test. Now, YOU DO!

Juanita's interviews, at her initial visit and then at a second visit just a few days later, are both at WalkingWellAgain.com.

Actively Seeking SS/PS

I present no new information here. I do have, however, a strong suggestion. **I recommend that anyone who is inactive and appears to be depressed (or perhaps merely stoic) be considered for possible Spinal Stenosis or PseudoStenosis.** Observe the patterns of inactivity. **Ask the questions found in the Positional History, and be aggressive about getting detailed answers.** If there is any question about the patient's condition, see that Positional Testing or Mechanical Testing is done as needed. This would be a perfect chance to use the Grocery Cart Test, as it can immediately demonstrate the potential for increased activity without the stigma of using a walker.

Such individuals may need an extra bit of encouragement. After all, many of them have already undergone a great deal of unsuccessful treatment and have been told that there is nothing available to help them.

In my own practice, I find that my ability to describe accurately to patients the symptoms they have been living with (as laid out in the Positional History), and to point out to them areas of extreme sensitivity (i.e., the First Interspace Fine Sign, sensitive Pes Anserinus, and the Iliac Crest Pain Resolution Sign) that they were not even aware of, helps them understand that I have something to share that is different. Something that may actually help. For the caregiver or clinician trying to guide the patient toward a behavior change, these two approaches may have great value.

In addition, in order to get a depressed patient to try a particular strategy, you must project confidence that it is at least possible for him to experience great improvement. If the person does improve, you should shower him with encouragement and explain (truthfully) that there is the possibility of great relief of pain and great increase in overall activity. Guidance should be geared to the patient's individual situation, using the background information provided in the beginning sections of this book.

I have had many patients who were unable to walk even half a block for years, and who slowly built up to walking miles within a few months. The potential is there.

Those who are depressed often feel guilty about past inactivity and dependency. They may have been crippled or limited by chronic pain with no obvious cause. Just as they may not have received sympathy or empathy from others, they themselves may not have understood that there was a real physical condition holding them back. Simply providing a clear explanation of the physical cause of their problem has at times been enough, for some of my patients, to bring about a sense of great emotional relief even before the relief of their symptoms began.

Caregivers and family members must strive to exhibit patience, to understand the effect of chronic pain on the emotions, and to be understanding and empathetic. The potential exists to turn around a patient's ability not only to walk, but also to feel optimistic and to better enjoy life. **Bear in mind, however, that individuals who are depressed and low in energy must often be firmly guided to try even the simplest things.** Every effort, however minimal, looms large. For them, life is like a series of locked doors, confining them to a very circumscribed space. They must be slowly and lovingly led back to a positive frame of mind—one in which they believe that it is possible to actually begin opening some of those doors.

Relief of pain could be the key that unlocks the first of them.

CHAPTER 25

True Diabetic Peripheral Neuropathy: What May Help

Diabetic Peripheral Neuropathy (DPN) is one of the most feared complications of diabetes, and for good reason. It is often, though not always, quite "visible," a complication that the patient is aware of. Many complications of diabetes are silent—meaning that the patient is often not viscerally aware of them. DPN, in contrast, can cause pain that is moderate or even severe, and hard to control.

DPN is also one of the major contributors to foot or leg ulcerations, infections, and amputations. The absence of the warning signal of pain may delay a person's recognizing and therefore treating a problem. Neuropathy may also interfere with the body's healthy and protective response to the danger of minor or major injury or infection, so that things that would otherwise heal normally unfortunately do not. These are valid reasons for the fear of Diabetic Peripheral Neuropathy.

Traditional Wisdom Concurs on Four Points

1. DPN is not a treatable condition. In other words, it is not reversible.

2. One can mask the symptoms of DPN by prescribing medication to block the pain. These medications—which carry some risk of complication—while not usually necessarily able to eliminate the pain, often reduce it, rendering the discomfort

more tolerable. Many people who are put on such medications take them long term, as the medicine blocks the pain but does not deal with the actual disease process.

3. One can try to limit DPN by maintaining good diabetes control.

4. The presence of DPN puts the foot at risk. Therefore, the foot requires additional attention and protection to help the patient avoid the development of ulcers or infections and the need for amputation.

I agree with the last three points listed above. I do *not* agree with the first point. **I believe that many of the symptoms diagnosed as—and at times actually caused by—Diabetic Neuropathy are often reversible.** I will share here the three approaches I have found most effective in my practice. Though not helpful in every case, they are quite frequently at least partially and often entirely effective.

I must begin by saying that I am not an expert on Diabetic Neuropathy. I am merely a clinician who has seen such good treatment results that I feel compelled to share them. Other effective treatments may exist that I do not mention here. Though surgery is touted by some as a cure-all for neuropathy, I rarely recommend surgery for neuropathic symptoms. I have seen too many failures and not a lot of successes. (To be fair, however, this may be because those who've experienced success with surgery do not come to my office seeking additional help.)

Numerous medicines, vitamins, and other treatments have been used in various clinical settings. Some are being used by very respected clinicians. Some are currently undergoing research. Others have been tested and rejected by the National Institutes of Health or other respected research institutes. I am not placing myself in the expert's chair. I only share in this chapter that which I observe to be true from my own experience.

> *Before starting, allow me to voice one criticism. This is something that you may have noticed I virtually never do in this book. My constructive criticism is directed at the way neuropathy treatment is presented. At times, pharmaceutical companies promote their drugs by reporting success in a manner that I feel is too vague. For example, they may claim a 50% improvement in symptoms in 50% of neuropathy sufferers. I feel that this is misleading. They should divide symptoms between those linked to small- and large-fiber neuropathy, and those clinically presented in autonomic neuropathy. Then there should be an identification of which symptoms are likely to improve (and how quickly) and which are not.*
>
> *Both patients and clinicians deserve being guided toward a reasonable expectation as to which symptoms are likely to be helped.*

Checking for SS/PS: A Constant Imperative

The first and very important step is to make sure that the symptoms are really coming from Diabetic Neuropathy. This practice is neither as standard nor as common as one might think, or at least as one might hope for. Protocols presented in this book—protocols that are primarily designed to recognize and manage Spinal Stenosis and PseudoStenosis—are very useful for picking up other conditions as well. This is essential, as Diabetic Neuropathy is a disease of exclusion. In other words, it is only firmly diagnosed if other potential

causes of the symptoms have been ruled out. I believe that this step is not always well executed.

By this time, those who have read this book know the routine. Take an aggressive Positional History. Invoke Positional Testing for possible Spinal Stenosis. Check and manage possible causes of PseudoStenosis. If you skipped directly to this section, go back and read Chapter 15, on neuropathy. **This protocol is of paramount importance for the majority of people who present with diabetes and moderate-to-severe neuropathic symptoms.**

I repeat: the majority. In a study I published in *Diabetic Medicine* in 2004, I reported that over 60% of (ambulatory) people with moderate-to-severe neuropathic symptoms have Spinal Stenosis (I would now include PseudoStenosis) contributing to their symptoms. Most of these patients improved quite well with Positional Testing. If either Mechanical Testing or Positional Testing proves effective, the success clearly demonstrates that at least some of the symptoms were being mediated through the spine. After all, if the symptoms were exclusively from DPN (or any other Peripheral Neuropathy), changing a patient's foot or spine function would not help. If either approach works, follow it to the fullest. I cannot stress this enough. The inherent potential is truly magical, and if improvement occurs, it always happens within just 1–3 days.

> *Today, over 14 years since I did that in-office study, I find the same pattern. Well over 60% of the people who present in my office with moderate-to-severe symptoms attributed to Diabetic Neuropathy have Spinal Stenosis or PseudoStenosis responsible for most or even all of their uncomfortable symptoms.*

It is important to understand that a reevaluation of symptoms and physical findings must take place after each step. Very often, after eliminating the main symptom, other problems become more apparent. For example, both Spinal Stenosis and PseudoStenosis cause severe sensitivity in many of the intermetatarsal spaces. After this sensitivity resolves with a few days of Mechanical or Positional Testing, if the third interspace persists in being sensitive, the cause is most likely a Morton's Neuroma. If there are lingering symptoms that are consistent with neuroma, treating with injections may provide additional relief. Note that because of the sensitivity in many intermetatarsal spaces initially, one could not at that time with certainty make a diagnosis of Morton's Neuroma. Diagnosis only becomes possible after the initial treatment, which eliminates other symptoms and findings. A few follow-up visits will greatly enhance your success, if the doctor uses a step-by-step approach and reevaluates your condition after each visit and intervention.

Recall that numbness—a true loss of sensation—if caused by SS/PS, often improves quickly, but sometimes takes up to 2 weeks to resolve. For numbness, you must be more patient.

If there is no suggestion of Spinal Stenosis or PseudoStenosis, or if after treating the spine-mediated pain through Mechanical Testing or Positional Testing, symptoms such as burning, aching, pins and needles, or numbness remain, then one may treat what is more likely a true Diabetic Peripheral Neuropathy.

True DPN has multiple presentations. I have had by far the greatest success with small-fiber neuropathy symptoms, including numbness, burning, pain, and paresthesia (a pins-and-needles sensation). Much less frequently, my patients appear to have limited improvement with large-fiber symptoms.

Apart from the many medications designed to mask pain, I have two recommendations that may be useful. The first has helped hundreds of my patients, and the second has helped several dozen, and it is what I use most frequently now.

Anodyne Therapy

The approach that has helped hundreds of my patients is Anodyne therapy. This form of physical therapy generates a specific wavelength of infrared light, also known as "Monochromatic Infrared Energy." I began using this therapy in 2001, and much to my delight, this simple physical tool has made me look like a genius, or at least a great doctor, to so many people.

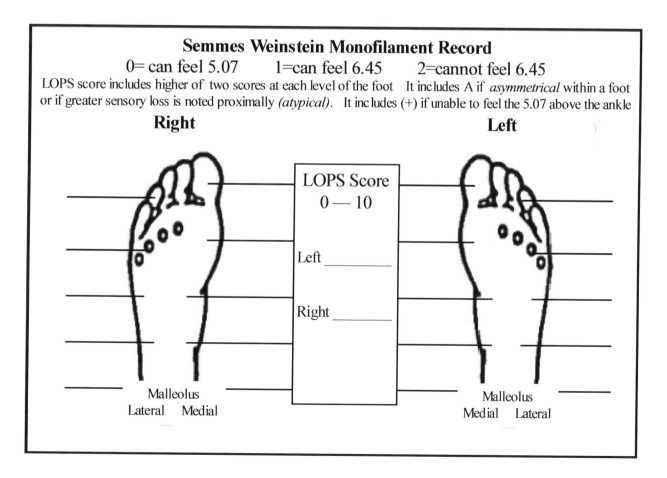

Semmes Weinstein Monofilament Record
0= can feel 5.07   1=can feel 6.45   2=cannot feel 6.45
LOPS score includes higher of two scores at each level of the foot   It includes A if *asymmetrical* within a foot or if greater sensory loss is noted proximally *(atypical)*.   It includes (+) if unable to feel the 5.07 above the ankle

Right   **Left**

LOPS Score
0 — 10

Left _____

Right _____

Malleolus   Malleolus
Lateral   Medial   Medial   Lateral

Picture 25.1. The LOPS record.

This form of physical therapy usually involves placing pads on four places on each foot and leg segment and applying infrared energy for forty minutes at least three times a week. This therapy often improves and even totally eliminates burning, tingling, and loss of sensation. Best of all, I have found that **everyone who improves with this therapy does so within just six sessions**.

As explained in Chapter 2, there is great value in establishing the level of pathology before starting therapy. Both of the following forms can be used before and after treatment for SS/PS and before and after treatment for DPN.

> *My understanding is that Anodyne therapy was originally investigated as a possible treatment to help heal foot ulcers (for which it is indeed often helpful). Many patients reported elimination of their uncomfortable neuropathy symptoms, as well as improved sensation. This is just one of many examples of how an effective treatment was found for a condition for which it was not originally intended.*

Establishing the starting pathology level involves knowing the details of the symptoms as well as establishing the amount of Loss of Protective Sensation (LOPS) present. I use a modification of the LOPS scale that I published in 2003 in an article in the Journal of the American Podiatric Medical Association. (This concept is explained in detail in Chapter 6.) Picture 25.1 shows the LOPS template.

Since we are seeking to eliminate burning and tingling, it is wise to establish what is present before treatment so we can follow improvement. This requires much less detail than does the full LuSSSExt scale presented in Chapter 3. Here is a short set of questions to be answered before and after either Metanx or Anodyne therapy.

This questionnaire is useful in helping you to understand what helps. Numbness, paresthesia (pins-and-needles sensation), discomfort, burning, and what is described as "pain" are often manifestations of small-fiber neuropathy, and they often improve greatly with Anodyne therapy. Of the symptoms of large-fiber neuropathy, the cold feeling in the feet is the one that is occasionally reported as improved. I do not recall success reported by patients regarding the leathery, stiff, cardboard feeling listed in the chart shown in picture 25.2.

Again, establishing the level of your symptoms and loss of sensation both *before* and *after* treatment is of great value—to evaluate your success as well as to help you set up reasonable expectations.

Overall, with 10 severe, and 1 mild, how would you rate the following symptoms in your feet?				
	Severe	Moderate	Mild	None
Numbness	10 9 8	7 6 5 4	3 2 1	0
Paresthesia (pins & needles)	10 9 8	7 6 5 4	3 2 1	0
Discomfort	10 9 8	7 6 5 4	3 2 1	0
Burning	10 9 8	7 6 5 4	3 2 1	0
Pain	10 9 8	7 6 5 4	3 2 1	0
Cold Feeling	10 9 8	7 6 5 4	3 2 1	0
Leather / Cardboard / Stiff	10 9 8	7 6 5 4	3 2 1	0
Other _____	10 9 8	7 6 5 4	3 2 1	0

Picture 25.2. Neuropathic symptoms questionnaire.

Another way for a patient to test efficacy of the therapy would be to do therapy on one foot only every day for a week, and then compare the two feet. If one is less numb or less uncomfortable, it will be clear.

In my experience, all of the patients who improve with Anodyne therapy do so within six sessions carried out over the course of one or two weeks. Those who are helped initially may continue to improve with additional sessions done regularly for a total of twelve–eighteen sessions. However, if good improvement is not seen after six sessions, my experience says that you should forgo this treatment, assuming that you have ruled out Spinal Stenosis or PseudoStenosis first. If SS/PS is present, the improvement obtained with Anodyne may be masked by the symptoms of SS/PS.

Long-term success and the need for further Anodyne therapy are inconsistent. I have had patients who underwent Anodyne therapy who then had a recurrence of their symptoms within a few weeks of stopping the treatment. Others maintained improvement for years, and only came back for additional therapy years later. Today, with inexpensive Anodyne home units available, patients may just buy a unit on their own and use it periodically.

An Anodyne home unit can be purchased directly from the manufacturer with no prescription needed. It costs only about $500, much less than the $2000 home units that were all that were available up until a few years ago. It"s not a small price to pay, but it's absolutely worth it if it works. With the relative confidence of success, the company provides a one-month money-back guarantee. Because of the guarantee, this is a no-risk proposition!

I do not recommend Anodyne therapy casually. I have used it for over thirteen years and have seen hundreds of patients enjoy marked improvement of their neuropathy symptoms. They began to experience less burning or tingling, along with improved sensation. I believe that I have seen good and consistent results with this therapy because I have learned how to select those patients who are likely to benefit by it. Much of this success comes from first treating Spinal Stenosis and PseudoStenosis, as well as other conditions that can cause nerve symptoms, and only then considering Anodyne therapy. For all patients with possible Peripheral Neuropathy—diabetic or non-diabetic—the Positional History, Positional Testing, and Mechanical Testing are essential to cull out many spine-mediated symptoms.

StoryTime: Lillie was a woman in her 60s who had been diagnosed with diabetes more than 2 decades before she first visited my office. She presented with symptoms that made walking, standing, and sleeping difficult. Leg and back pain came with standing and walking. At night, burning, tingling, and numbness in her feet were problematic. She walked better when pushing a grocery cart.

Exam showed bilateral nerve sensitivity, although the nerves in her feet were not as sensitive as the nerves in her legs and thighs. She had a LOPS score of "7 (22111)" on both feet, with no asymmetry.

Considering Spinal Stenosis in addition to Diabetic Neuropathy, I prescribed a walker and told her about the Adjunct Measures, which she used. A week later, she was only a little better. She could not use the walker. I had prescribed a 28-inch-handle junior rollator. The durable medical equipment dealer tried to fit the bill with a walker that did not have holes to allow the handle to go down that low, so he drilled new holes. Unfortunately, the holes were too low. The handles were 27 inches high and caused Lillie a lot of pain! I spoke to the dealer, who then drilled new holes at 28 and 29 inches, and she then did great. All of her back and leg pain disappeared, and within 2 weeks she was able to walk literally for miles.

Despite the improvements with Positional Testing, Lillie still had uncomfortable nighttime symptoms and residual numbness. With Positional Testing, her LOPS score had reduced from "7 (22111)" to "3 (21000)." We added Anodyne therapy. After six sessions, almost all of her nighttime burning and tingling had resolved. Another six sessions—and we met our goal of one hundred percent relief of symptoms. She was now able to feel the 4.07 monofilament in every place that was tested. **Please note that when she'd begun she could not feel even 60 grams of pressure. Now she could feel one gram of pressure.** A year later, all of her neuropathy improvement was maintained.

The lesson? In many people, both SS/PS and Diabetic Neuropathy are present. Both must be addressed to achieve great improvement. As in hundreds of my patients with small-fiber neuropathy over the years, Anodyne was just what the doctor ordered.

Canary in the Coal Mine

NOTE that the possible global effect of Metanx is not a concept that has been promoted by the manufacturer, to the best of my knowledge. This is only my conjecture, which may perhaps be investigated in the future. I believe that following the peripheral symptoms of DPN is akin to the "canary in the coal mine."

Before sensors were invented to detect toxic gases in coal mines, coal miners would bring a caged canary into the mine with them. The bird would become distressed or would even die before the conditions reached a level that was unsafe or toxic for the miners, and thus it would serve as an early warning system. This system was used in England until the 1980s.

Similarly, I use the success of Metanx in the foot as a way of judging if the other anatomic areas of neuropathy might be helped as well. If the feet improve, then **perhaps** *the product will also be helpful in other areas.*

For this reason I do not initially provide Anodyne therapy for my patients with Diabetic Neuropathy, despite the fact that it works more quickly. Once I used Anodyne therapy, I would lose the ability to follow my patient's loss of sensation and symptoms in order to ascertain if the Metanx was working.

This is a potential area of research that might bear fruit in the evaluation of neuropathy. If the improvement of **Peripheral Neuropathy** *with Metanx, which can be documented easily, can be matched with the improvement of* **other presentations of neuropathy**, *the idea of the foot as the "canary in the coal mine" could prove of great value. However, now it is just a theory that I have no way of supporting.*

Metanx: A Prescription Medical Food

The next treatment that I recommend, and the one with which I usually now start after addressing SS/PS, is a vitamin supplement called Metanx.

Metanx, made by Pamlab, is a prescription formulation that is listed as a "medical food." It contains three vitamins that are reported to be in the usable (that is, biologically active) form that some diabetics (and others who suffer from Peripheral Neuropathy) are not able to derive from standard vitamins. Included are L-methylfolate (vitamin B_9), methylcobalamin (vitamin B_{12}), and pyridoxal 5'-phosphate (vitamin B_6). It is thus a vitamin B supplement, although one with **patented, different versions of the vitamins** other brands contain. **It has been reported to help patients with symptoms of Diabetic Peripheral Neuropathy as well as with other Peripheral Neuropathy problems.**

You may remember from Chapter 6 my explanation of a relatively new nerve test known as the Intra-epidermal Nerve Fiber Biopsy. The doctor takes a biopsy of a very small piece of skin, and a laboratory, using special tools, evaluates the small nerve fibers in several ways. Metanx has been studied in this way, and it has been reported that Metanx improved the number and quality of nerves in the skin of patients with small-fiber neuropathy. I have reviewed the literature; if it is true, it is an impressive improvement.

I include the reference to Metanx because I am convinced that there is merit to the claims. I have prescribed Metanx and have heard well over one hundred patients sing its praises over the past few years. They report reduced levels of pain and uncomfortable sensations. Many of them have had great improvement in their LOPS scores, which corroborates the improvement they reported. Based upon the patient reports and my own examination of those patients, I can recommend this as a good vitamin to try. Contact your primary care provider or podiatrist, as a prescription is required.

For those who decide to try Metanx, I suggest that you first make the thorough evaluation described above, both of physical presentation and of specific symptoms, so that you may accurately appreciate the improvement and potential value of this supplement.

Of all the treatments I regularly employ, Metanx is the slowest. While some patients report improvement within 2–4 weeks, most are confident of the improvement only after 1–2 months. Pamlab, the manufacturer, recommends a full three-month trial before deciding on its value. If you are also taking Metformin (Glucophage), a common medication for diabetic patients, it is reported that it may take up to 6 months to see optimal results. Fortunately, there is limited financial risk: an online company offers a money-back guarantee on sales of Metanx through their website. In addition, cost for Metanx is now being covered by some insurance companies, but you must of course check with your provider or your pharmacist to determine insurance coverage.

When Do I Use Metanx and When Do I Use Anodyne?

You may wonder why I usually begin to treat Diabetic Neuropathy with Metanx, which can take months to get improvement, when Anodyne therapy works so much faster. Good question.

As mentioned above, I truly like Anodyne as a therapy. However, it has limitations. While it can improve neuropathic pain, improve sensation, and even help ulcers heal, its effect is completely local. In other words, it affects only the feet and legs, and not the rest of the body, to the best of my knowledge.

Metanx, on the other hand, also frequently improves neuropathic pain and improves sensation associated with small-fiber neuropathy. I do not know if it can help ulcers heal. However, it has **a potentially global effect** on the rest of the body. Diabetic Neuropathy affects so many organ systems in the body. **If a vitamin can improve nerve function in the nerves in the feet, I consider that it is quite possible that it may also improve nerve function elsewhere.**

In case you were wondering, I still use Anodyne therapy, usually for one of four reasons.

- Some patients have had such success with Anodyne in the past that they simply do not want to change.

- For diagnostic purposes, because of rapid improvement, Anodyne excels.

- Some patients cannot afford Metanx, so I either provide them with Anodyne therapy in my office or lend them a home Anodyne unit. This may now be less important, in that insurance coverage for Metanx is now getting much more positive.

- Finally, I have had a few patients who did not improve with Metanx but did get better with Anodyne therapy performed afterward.

SUMMARY

All patients with diabetes and symptoms of neuropathy should be thoroughly evaluated for Spinal Stenosis and PseudoStenosis, since these conditions so often contribute to neuropathic symptoms. Those with persistent small-fiber neuropathy symptoms are often helped by either Anodyne or Metanx.

If these approaches do not prove effective for you, it is essential to follow up with a good neurologist or physiatrist. There are, after all, many types of neuropathy, as well as other conditions that can cause neuropathic symptoms in the feet or legs. If you need further help, I recommend that you seek it—aggressively.

CHAPTER 26

Sports Again: Tennis, Golf, Swimming, and Treadmill

This chapter presents scenarios more likely relevant to patients with Spinal Stenosis than to those with PseudoStenosis. Many patients with PseudoStenosis have relief of symptoms with less restrictions on their activities, and no longer require the lumbar flexion addressed in this chapter.

As the title of this book implies, there is great value in walking. Walking is a key to independence, to maintaining good health, and to getting the most from the beautiful opportunities we can enjoy in this world. This book highlights ways for you to get rid of the pain and limitation that curtail your movement, so that you can make the most out of life and become a person who is Walking Well Again.

There are many forms of exercise that are just as effective as walking for maintaining or improving health, and that are often, for many people, a lot more fun. There's nothing like having another good reason to get out of bed in the morning! Over the years, I've made certain observations associated with some common forms of exercise. I'd like to share them with you now, in a manner a bit more casual than that of the rest of this book.

Tennis Anyone?

What would you think of this situation? Using his walker, a man walks the few blocks from his condominium to the local tennis court. He takes out a tennis racket, warms up, hits a few serves, and then plays a match. Not a game, not a set, but a match—a few sets. There are a couple of minutes of sitting with a cold drink between sets, but otherwise he plays vigorous tennis for well over an hour. He is sweating but smiling. After a well-deserved rest and another cold drink to help him recover from the heat, he slips the racket back into his walker and starts back home.

Is this some crazy person looking for sympathy by showing up with a walker? Is he hoping to get three serves instead of two per point? To use the doubles part of the court on his opponent's side? Perhaps he is a shill, looking to find someone willing to bet on a game of tennis with a guy who needs a walker?

Maybe there's a different reason. Perhaps he is a person who understands the disease of Spinal Stenosis and is willing to use all possible tools to engage life fully despite his condition.

Me, I vote for the latter. Here is a man who understands what is going on and is committed to enjoying life despite an imperfect situation.

Not all sports accommodations are as dramatic as the tennis match I've just described. That is a heck of a scenario—but it is also a real one. I had several patients in Florida who used a walker for walks of more than a block or two, but who still found that they could play tennis or golf or could swim quite capably.

Obvious questions arise. "How does a guy who needs a walker play tennis so well?" And "Why does a guy who plays tennis so well need a walker?" I'd like to focus on the second question, as it allows us to address many situations with a single explanation.

Our tennis player above has Spinal Stenosis. If you are reading this and you are a person with stenosis, this will all make sense to you in a few minutes. In fact, it will be one of those "aha!" moments.

Keep in mind that different activities place the spine in different positions. Walking takes place in an erect position. Using the walker in a manner consistent with positional management induces a slight flexion. To take the case of our tennis player, there will be a few minutes between points when he is standing straight, as a walking person normally does. However, there will be many times during the game when his knees are bent and his spine flexed, similar to the position of leaning on a walker.

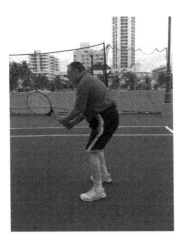

Picture 26.1. While waiting to hit a ball, a tennis player may flex at the lumbar spine.

All of these moments in a game of tennis have our player flexing the spine. For many people who cannot walk a block or two without flexion and who thus need to use a walker to walk comfortably, the amount of time spent flexing during a tennis game is enough to keep them comfortable, without stenosis-induced symptoms. They can be without external support as they play, because the positions of tennis are comfortable for a patient with SS/PS. I have had several patients who, before they came to see me, could not walk without pain but could play tennis. Some of them felt that the surface of the tennis court must have been softer, which protected them from leg and foot pain, but they all eventually grasped the effect of position on SS/PS

symptoms, and the benefit of seeking, or at least using, positions of comfort within the game.

Here is the bottom line: patients who persist in having SS/PS symptoms despite treatment, who still frequently need a walker to cover a few blocks, may be able to play tennis without difficulty. Amazing, and true.

There may, however, be some restrictions. Serves and overhead smashes, if executed the way Jimmy Connors did, require a hyperextension of the spine. I do not recommend that, as it could quickly exacerbate inflammation of the spine and pain in the spine and legs.

I have a personal story to share about tennis. My father, Albert Goldman, may he rest in peace, had a detached retina and took medical retirement when he was about fifty-seven years old. That was when he learned how to play the guitar—and tennis. He was a former soldier of the Army Air Corps from World War II, who went in as a buck private and came out a sergeant, serving as a radio operator in a bomber. He garnered many medals and, thank G-d, few injuries. (For anyone interested in an intimate look at the life of such Army Air Corps heroes during World War II, I recommend the book *The Wild Blue*, by Steven Ambrose, a portrait of the experiences of George McGovern and his crew.) Dear Old Dad was, by nature and by training, a persistent fellow, so age did not deter him from learning what he wanted to learn. Within a few years he learned to play the guitar well enough to entertain himself and others, and tennis well enough to give me a good game on the tennis court.

Although he eventually recovered enough to return to work for several more years, he unfortunately developed additional eye trouble that robbed him of almost all the vision in his right eye. Doctors told him that without the necessary depth perception, he would not be able to play tennis anymore. He thanked them for their advice . . . and went on to play tennis for several more years. He could not hit a high backhand (as his head had to be turned to the side in a way that was totally dependent on his left eye), and he did not play quite as aggressively as before. However, he compensated enough to have a lot of fun on the courts, especially since I became quite good at avoiding the high backhand shots.

This is not only a fond memory but also a lesson to me—and to you—from Dear Old Dad from beyond the grave. *Doing what you enjoy at a lower level is better than giving it up completely.* For many people who love tennis, there is certainly hope. My advice is to go gentle on the courts, to rest periodically, and not to try to hit the ball quite as hard anymore. If you do go back to the game, rally for a long time before playing competitively, no matter how good you once were. Do a lot of gentle stretching of both the upper and lower body before and after each session. Seek physical therapy for guidance as to exactly what you can and cannot do.

Remember, if you find that playing causes your symptoms to get worse, it is time to stop and get help.

How about Golf?

I'm glad you asked! As with tennis, I have had many patients tell me that golfing is easier than walking. They think it must be the soft grass compared to hard concrete pavement. These people are partly right, but mostly wrong.

Sure—soft surfaces may be easier on the back and legs than hard surfaces. In retrospect, however, some of these patients acknowledge that walking in grassy parks is no better than walking on the sidewalk. So back we go to body position.

Consider a golfer's stance as he addresses the ball. He stands in a flexed position for a moment or two before every shot. Also, while waiting for another player to hit, he may lean on a club.

Both positions put him in a flexion position which, even if he holds it for just 10, 20, or 30 seconds, might open up the spine enough to prevent symptoms from developing.

In addition, using the Professor Position can make the waiting perfectly comfortable. Holding the club behind your back and stretching gently as you take that position may make you look more like Tom Watson than a college professor!

Combined with the use of a golf cart, these positions, especially if understood and used intentionally, might be all that are necessary to allow someone to golf long past his or her ability to walk miles, or even blocks.

The same concerns raised about the tennis player apply equally to the golf pro. Here are three warnings:

- Don't try to kill the ball. Making a full rotation of the spine in either tennis or golf offers you a greater chance of aggravating your spine. Don't pull back all the way, and don't try to maximize the follow-through in a way that can stress your lower back. This may be especially true if you've had surgery, or if you have instability in your back. Check with your spine specialist before you play. Give up the shot that requires maximum effort, and use a more measured and limited effort instead of going for broke.

- *Stretch.* If you have questions about what stretches to do, see a physical therapist who deals with athletes to obtain guidance on the stretching. Once you have grasped and practiced the stretches, do them daily as part of your morning routine and then again both before and after playing. This will bring you to maximum limberness before the game and prevent you from tightening up too much afterward.

- Stay in shape. Make sure to keep yourself in good enough shape not to be exhausted by golf or tennis. When you're tired, you're more likely to hurt yourself. To keep up your cardiovascular conditioning, walk as part of your normal life routine as best you can (following the suggestions in the section on positional management), or walk on a treadmill. Perhaps you could use a stationary bicycle—something along the lines of a Schwinn Airdyne—to provide you with upper-body as well as lower-body exercise. Lift light weights at the gym, or take a low-impact aerobics class led by a teacher who knows how not to aggravate the spine in a patient with your condition. Perhaps get into the pool for some water exercises or swimming.

If you have any questions about your ability to get back in the game, especially if you've been out for a while, take a few lessons with a teacher who understands the distinct challenges facing older athletes. See a physical therapist who has experience with older athletes. In this situation, an ounce of prevention is certainly worth a pound of cure.

In the Swimming Pool

A swimming pool is a great tool for helping a person get back in shape. For those who have been sick or weak, the ability to move comfortably without the stress of bearing one's full body weight allows a return to activity that might not be accomplished outside a pool. Water exercise, including swimming, is great for restoring flexibility and full range of motion. Doing such exercises as part of a pool physical therapy program has great value during rehabilitation.

(I am writing this chapter with the assumption that the patient is capable of independent activity without help. Despite that independence, however, it is probably always best to swim either with a buddy or a lifeguard present, for safety reasons. No explanation needed.)

Many people with Spinal Stenosis report that they can no longer swim comfortably. Here is a potential key to resume swimming:

For some of my patients, it was the full extension of the spine—which many people do in order to breathe when swimming—that aggravated their Spinal Stenosis. Whether swimming freestyle or doing the breaststroke, lifting your head out of the pool, or at least rotating your neck or body, is necessary for breathing. While a perfect style would allow you to rotate your body sufficiently without hyperextension, not too many people swim like Johnny Weissmuller.

The key is simple—as simple as the proper use of the walker. Use a SNORKEL and a MASK, or goggles. These apparatuses allow you to swim with your spine comfortably flexed, without any of the strain that comes with overextension. Actual swimming, with all the benefits of cardiac conditioning and the gentle exercising of so many muscle groups, can be easily done again. All you have to do is get used to the snorkel and mask, which may require some practice in the pool. Afterward, you may be able to swim for exercise or pleasure, even on those days when your back is not perfect, because this modified exercise may not aggravate your spine.

I recommend that you get a good snorkel and mask and have it set up for you by someone who can help. There are even versions of both masks and goggles with prescription lenses, which will make it easier for you to see well enough while you swim.

Remember how to get to Carnegie Hall? Practice. Wear the snorkel and mask at home and during your first few times in the pool. Practice without expecting too much if you have not used them before. Even use them, at the start, when doing the wonderful exercise of walking in a pool. Once you're comfortable with them, the pool can become a great friend, as you glide on the water without the back or leg strain that previously threatened to turn a pleasurable and beneficial activity into a painful one. Walkers on the ground, snorkels in the water: two keys to getting rid of that unnecessary spinal pain.

Of course, as with all activities, use common sense. Increase your activity slowly. Remember, you're in this for the long haul, and it may take weeks or even months to be as active as you used to be. But if you make all these changes slowly, a month or two from now you may be doing things you have not done in 10 or 20 years. Enjoy every minute!

I hope that these thoughts will soon help you *walk, golf, play tennis, and swim well again*. (That's too bulky to use as a title, though.)

Walking Well . . . on a Treadmill

The treadmill is a great tool for walking. Just like with the walker or grocery cart, you can lean on it and seek a flexion position that can open up the spine and relieve symptoms. Many people can walk miles on a treadmill but less than a block without wheeled support.

Keep in mind that even if the treadmill eliminates your SS/PS symptoms, you still need to increase your activity level gradually. You need to overcome the pain from the spine, but you also need to overcome the deconditioning that may have developed over the years.

Some shorter people have difficulty using a treadmill just as they may have limited improvement with a grocery cart or a standard walker. The standard position does not induce them to lean forward, the maneuver that opens up a spine with either Spinal Stenosis or PseudoStenosis. These individuals might benefit from standing farther back on the platform and leaning with their arms farther forward; this could help them get relief.

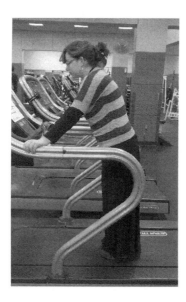

A treadmill with multiple handle position heights could better accommodate people of different heights. I hope to help make such a device available in the future. You may check my website, WalkingWellAgain.com, for any updates.

Picture 26.2. An individual at 5'3" stands straight with her arms bent on a treadmill and must hold her arms far forward in order to get even mild lumbar flexion.

Final Encouragement and Final Thoughts

More Stories and Lessons Learned

Over the years, I've amassed a great many stories from cases that are too complex to neatly fit into a single chapter, or from cases that point toward important lessons. Some involve repetition of evaluation and advice. These are often interesting cases, which can be learned from. For those readers who have not found answers thus far in this book—and I hope there are not too many of you—you may discover valuable clues in the stories I am about to present. For clinicians interested in the thought processes of an old-timer obsessed with conservative management of pain, they may also be of interest.

The ability to clearly understand the case histories presented in this chapter will be based on an understanding of the concepts in this book. Reading these stories "cold" may give you insight and encouragement, but not the kind of help you might get if you read the rest of the book first.

In preparing the stories for this book, I drew primarily upon the people whom I video-interviewed in my office over the past 2 years. Since I had not seen many of them in a long time, I called most of them to make sure they were still doing well. The great majority of them were. A few found the improvement only temporary and did not return for a follow-up visit. That was a mistake, as the care often requires thoughtful tweaking, so I invited them back. A few had simply slipped into old patterns and were not willing to make the effort to change.

Change, of course, is hard, but it's certainly worth the effort, especially when the prize is nothing less than regaining one's ability to truly enjoy life.

The majority of these patients were doing much better and were greatly appreciative. Most of them have been interviewed, and the interviews are available for viewing at WalkingWellAgain.com. A few interesting case histories came from a list of patients I had amassed previously. No interviews are available for those people, but their stories are worth sharing.

Reality Check

Before I get to these case histories—all of which are accurate representations of individuals I have treated—let me present a "reality check," and outline a few hypothetical stories that reflect a different reality:

1. Patient came in for burning feet, and none of the approaches I tried were helpful. Patient was referred to neurologist.

2. Patient had difficulty walking because of leg pain. Grocery cart was somewhat helpful, but walker and mechanical control of feet did not provide relief. MRI confirmed severe Lumbar Spinal Stenosis. Patient was referred to physiatrist for evaluation and management.

3. Patient came in for numbness, poor balance, limited walking, and difficulty buttoning clothes. No help with Positional or Mechanical Testing. MRI of neck showed Cervical Stenosis, so patient was referred to physiatrist for evaluation and management.

4. Patient had painful arthritic knees and back pain. Limb Length Discrepancy was found, but lifts did not prove helpful. He had flexible Flat Feet, but strapping and Unna boots did not remove symptoms. Positional Testing was not effective in eliminating back and knee pain. Patient was referred to spine specialist for management.

5. Patient came in for painful swollen ankle. Conservative treatment, including lift for short limb and brace for Flat Foot with tendonitis, did not provide adequate long-term help. Medication and physical therapy did not help. Patient was referred to foot and ankle surgeon for surgical management.

6. Patient noted difficulty standing, and had apparent Limb Length Discrepancy. Examination showed that discrepancy was functional, not structural, so patient was referred for treatment of the spine.

7. Patient presented for an unrelated problem. Physical examination showed Flat Feet, and a Limb Length Discrepancy. The patient, in his 70's, had no symptoms of evidence of secondary deformity. No treatment was done, other than to caution of the presence of the identified problems and to advise to return for evaluation if any of the common symptoms associated with PseudoStenosis developed.

These hypothetical stories are representative of the *lack* of success I experience on a weekly basis. I present these scenarios at the beginning of this chapter to reinforce what I've said all along. While many people get help with the approaches presented in this book, not everyone does. I claim "only" about a 70% success rate with Spinal Stenosis and PseudoStenosis patients, and closer to a 50% success rate with patients with many other conditions. I share the following histories in order to present new insights and encouragement, but not to convey a guarantee.

Now, on to some great stories and the lessons that can be learned from them.

StoryTime: Creating Problems

Eva J was an 84-year-old woman with spine trouble **that had begun almost 30 years prior, after an automobile accident.** Moderate back and left leg pain had gradually improved over the years, until they had become just an annoyance. Then, 4 years before her first visit to my office, she began experiencing an aching, tingling sensation in her left leg, aggravated by standing, walking, and sleeping.

Eva had a hammertoe and a painful corn on her left foot, and she decided to make more space in her shoe by removing the shoe insert. Thus, she created an *environmental* Limb Length Discrepancy on top of the real structural discrepancy that was already present. I trimmed the corn and she went back into shoes with balanced inserts, but these provided only moderate help. A few days later, I added a lift for the structural Limb Length Discrepancy, and Eva was soon floating on cloud nine. Four years of leg discomfort had disappeared within days!

StoryTime: Small Differences Make a Big Difference

Concetta K, 63, had a complicated medical history. She presented with left leg pain and inability to stand or walk for more than a few minutes at a time for the past 4 years. She had previously been given a motorized wheelchair. She had a lift for a Limb Length Discrepancy, but it was only a ¼-inch lift, while the discrepancy was more than ½ inch. I switched her to a ½-inch lift, which helped her stand better, though she was still in pain. Then I had her use a walker at a height calculated to induce flexion, and she walked around for several minutes without any pain.

Considering both Spinal Stenosis and PseudoStenosis, I loaned her a walker. (Her insurance would not cover one, since she'd recently received a motorized wheelchair.) Concetta did great! She returned the wheelchair, obtained a walker, and continued to enjoy relief from pain. She could then walk several blocks, for the first time in 4 years.

The lessons? First of all, it is crucial to get the correct lift height. Small differences can make a big difference. Second, success often requires multiple treatments. Third, just because someone has been put in a wheelchair, that does not mean they need to stay there. She'd had extensive medication and therapy that had not helped, while the proper lift and walker worked beautifully for her.

Concetta's interview is available at WalkingWellAgain.com.

StoryTime: Post-polio Syndrome Was NOT the Problem

Edward K, aged 67, came in with a complaint of left foot pain that had been bothering him for a month. After my physical exam and a few pointed questions, he acknowledged that he also had left knee pain that had interfered with his standing and walking for decades. The knee pain was attributed to Post-polio Syndrome, which had caused him problems since his teens.

I wondered if the two symptoms might be related. Edward's left leg was shorter than the right by about ⅜ of an inch, and he had Equinus of –15 degrees in the left leg only. He had pain in the ball of his foot, with sensitivity in the third metatarsal phalangeal joint, behind the third toe.

I strapped up his foot, adding a pad to take pressure off the ball of the foot, and gave him a ¼-inch lift for the shorter leg. HOME RUN. A week later, the ball of the foot was almost all better, and the knee was all better. Indirect examination again suggested a discrepancy. I modified his shoes with the pad and lift and gave him extra lifts.

I did not see him again, as he had instructions to come back only if necessary. When I came across his interview while writing this chapter, I gave him a call. Both Edward and my spy (i.e., his wife) said that he was doing fine. There had been no recurrence of the knee pain at all.

The lesson? Years of knee pain attributed to Post-polio Syndrome were actually caused by a Limb Length Discrepancy. I have had a few other patients with symptoms attributed to Post-polio Syndrome who had conditions that were treatable with positional or mechanical management. Not enough to warrant an entire chapter, but certainly enough to warrant a story or two.

StoryTime: Such Sensitive Nails!

Nancy W was a 57-year-old woman brought in by a caregiver for treatment of very long and uncomfortable fungus nails. For years, she resisted having them cut because they were so sensitive, and the drill used by a podiatrist to reduce and smooth the nails was always so uncomfortable. At her initial visit, I noted the sensitivity by the way she resisted and winced at my efforts.

She also had long-term difficulty walking and standing because of back, leg, and foot discomfort, and only obtained relief with sitting. With a symmetrical positive First Interspace Fine Sign and no evidence of PseudoStenosis, this seemed a classic case of Spinal Stenosis. Fortunately, she responded well to Positional Testing and Positional Therapy. She was able to increase her activities and had minimal pain.

The next time she came in, things were different. She was anxious, but after I trimmed the first few nails, she did not resist or wince, once she perceived that the procedure was not painful as it had been in years past. She had no sensitivity to the use of a drill on her nails. Fortunately, this improvement persisted the next few times she came back for nail care.

The lesson? Nancy had for many years resisted having her nails cut because the procedure was so uncomfortable. Once the Spinal Stenosis was controlled, her nails were no more sensitive than anyone else's. This reflects a pattern I have seen often. In people with SS/PS, nails or corns or arthritic changes in the foot may hurt much more than would be normal for the pathology present. I believe that anyone with pain out of proportion should be checked for SS/PS, even if the concern is something as benign as thick and sensitive toenails.

StoryTime: Ehlers-Danlos Syndrome Is Not the Cause

Simcha was a 17-year-old young man who came for evaluation of chronic discomfort that had limited him for as long as he could remember. He could only walk for a block or two before he had to stop because of pain in his legs and feet. Standing was always uncomfortable, and he had a tendency to shift from side to side. He had discomfort in his back and neck and shoulders. Physical therapy had always provided limited help.

He was told his symptoms were associated with Ehlers-Danlos syndrome (EDS). EDS is a disorder of the connective tissue of the body, resulting in joint hypermobility, skin extensibility, and fragility of the soft tissue. There are 6 major types of EDS. He had been referred by a family whose children had EDS, whom I had previously treated.

Not surprisingly, he had severe Flat Feet, with a presentation consistent with hypermobility of the joints, a characteristic of EDS. However, he also had 4 signs of Limb Length Discrepancy, including asymmetric Equinus of -15 degrees on the left, and greater nerve sensitivity, hip sensitivity, and Pes Anserinus sensitivity on the right. It took only ⅛ of an inch to make the hips balanced and eliminate the hip sensitivity. I provided him with lifts.

Three days later, he returned with good news. He felt ninety-five percent better. Neck pain, shoulder pain, leg pain, and back pain were all gone. He had mild aching in the feet. He had been able to walk several blocks without difficulty. My examination showed elimination of the 4 signs of LLDx listed above. He still had Flat Feet and some discomfort in the first metatarsal cuneiform joint and in the sinus tarsi, but that was all. He was elated. I provided more lifts, and we decided to incorporate that lift into the orthotics ordered.

The lesson? Like Rheumatoid Arthritis or Diabetic Neuropathy or Lymphedema, this misdiagnosis was a reasonable mistake. Since EDS causes hypermobility and instability in so many joints, one could logically diagnose EDS as the cause of symptoms. In this case, however, symptoms were greatly affected by LLDx. Were the symptoms worse because of EDS, or because of Flat Feet? I don't know. But he definitely needed orthotics.

However, since I have had improvement in every one of the (less than 10) individuals I have treated with both EDS and arthritis symptoms, please add this condition to the list of those that require a thorough evaluation for both biomechanical problems and SS/PS whenever there are symptoms that could *possibly* be related.

An interview from Simcha's second visit is available on WalkingWellAgain.com.

StoryTime: Ticklish 9-year-olds, not just 90-year-olds!

Meir is a 9-year-old boy who was brought in by his mom with a chief concern of aching in the feet and legs that had been bothering him for a couple of years and was aggravated by activity. Both Mom and two of his siblings had Flat Feet that caused symptoms that responded well to orthotics, so she assumed that Meir did too, and that orthotics would solve his problem.

One problem. His foot structure was quite normal, with no pronation problem present. He did, however, have 4 signs suggesting a Limb Length Discrepancy, including asymmetric Equinus, nerve sensitivity, Pes Anserinus sensitivity, and a positive Iliac Crest Pain Resolution Sign from placing ⅛ of an inch of felt under the short right leg. I dispensed lifts.

At the next visit, he and his mom reported success in eliminating symptoms just a day after the first visit. Exam showed elimination of the 4 signs, and indirect exam again suggested a mild LLDx. We provided lifts for long-term management, understanding that orthotics were not necessary.

The lessons? First, the obvious: not all family members have the same problems, although in truth, many do. Second, I have shared many stories about rapid improvement in 80- and 90-year-old people, but perhaps not enough stories about 9-year-old children to stress the point. I have lots of youngsters in my practice who have a rapid improvement with strapping and then orthotics. As most podiatrists and many other specialists know, most "growing pains" can be resolved just by improving the biomechanics of the youngster with stretching exercises and often with orthotics. However, many who get imperfect resolution also need to have the Limb Length Discrepancy addressed, and many others only need the LLDx addressed. Meir's was one of those cases. I hope this story serves as a good reminder that even youngsters should be checked for LLDx as part of an initial evaluation.

The last point is something mentioned previously in the book, but perhaps it is too easy to miss. The Iliac Crest sensitivity reported as pain or discomfort in adults is often reported as ticklishness in children. I therefore regard ticklishness in the hip area as a sign of likely LLDx, and I often see complete resolution of the ticklishness immediately with a lift, and days later, when the nerves are no longer sensitive, even when standing without the lift. One more thing to consider that I hope will eventually be researched.

StoryTime: Painful Injection to the Rescue of a Preteen

Janice was a 12-year-old girl who came in for treatment of a painful ingrown toenail. She was apprehensive, since previous injections in her foot had been very painful. She hated the ingrown toenail, but she did not want an injection.

I must confess: I often missed this kind of opportunity in the first 30 years of practice. However, this time, I recognized the clue and did investigate. When questioned, she admitted that her legs and feet hurt with sports or extensive walking, something that was not written on her questionairre. She did not have Flat Feet, but she did have mild Equinus on the right side and a positive First Interspace Fine Sign on the left. My exam revealed a Limb Length Discrepancy. Standing, she had sensitivity to palpation of the left hip, which disappeared with use of a ⅛-inch lift under the right foot.

Appreciating the possible effect of PseudoStenosis on her pain with both the ingrown nail and prior injections, I delayed treatment for a few days while she used a lift full time. At the next visit, the nail was much less sensitive, as were the nerves. Still apprehensive, she let me inject her and tolerated it quite well, noting that the injection was much less painful than it had been in the past. For anyone still skeptical about the concept of PseudoStenosis, please note: a lift under the shorter right leg reduced the toenail sensitivity of the left first toe.

We can derive two lessons from Janice's story. First, the history of pain out of proportion should be a sign to check for SS/PS. This includes individuals, young and old, who report excessive sensitivity to foot injections. Most injections given on the top of the foot do not hurt that much, so when they do, it is cause for suspicion.

Second, the expansion of the population that should be considered is important. I wish I could tell you that I check every single child who comes in for nonmechanical problems, such as warts or ingrown toenails, for causes of PS as well, but I can't. I try to do that with all adults. The truth is, however, that the more I look, the more I find! Many children with knee or back or even neck or headache symptoms have PseudoStenosis conditions, usually Limb Length Discrepancy or Flat Feet. With treatment they see improvement in symptoms in areas far above the feet. One simply has to take the time to question and investigate!

StoryTime: Multiple Sclerosis, but Not Mission Impossible

If you think some of these stories are incredible, wait until you read this one. I have trouble believing it myself, but fortunately have four interviews to back me up.

Willie K was a 90-year-old man who came to the office for the first time in a motorized wheelchair, accompanied by his girlfriend. From his appearance, you could see he had once been very strong, but for the past decade he had only been able to walk thirty to sixty feet before being halted by back, leg, and foot pain. Though he'd already had some long-term symptoms, things had taken a decided turn for the worse when he had been diagnosed with Multiple Sclerosis about 10 years earlier. He used a walker at home, but its use provided limited help, as his neck and shoulders had become very painful. He'd previously had fusion in his neck.

I am not an expert in Multiple Sclerosis. I never have been and never will be. I simply examined him from a podiatry standpoint, using some of the insights presented in this book.

Willie had, among other things, a Limb Length Discrepancy, with his left leg being about ⅜ of an inch shorter than his right, and with a severe –30-degree Equinus on the left side only. The nerves in the right foot and leg were very painful, with a positive First Interspace Fine Sign. He was unstable when standing, but that instability improved when I added ⅜ of an inch of lift to his left shoe. Willie had moderate strength in his hands but stated that when he walked short distances in his house with his current walker, there was significant pain in his shoulders and upper arms. He indicated that the walker I had him try, which induced a slight lumbar flexion, was much more comfortable for him, both for walking and with regard to the pain in his shoulders and upper arms. He noted the walker handle height so that he could adjust the walker he had at home.

Five days later, he reported a moderate improvement in his symptoms. He had much less aching in his arms and shoulders with a walker set at the correct height. He was able to increase his activities and, using a walker, could now take a bag of trash out to a garbage chute on the same floor of his building. Willie was now walking up to 200 feet, up from a maximum of 60.

Despite the improvement, he was still experiencing a great deal of aching in his legs at night, a problem we had not discussed at his initial visit. I advised him about modifying his sleep position. He also noted that his right foot was dragging. I had focused so much on his tight left ankle at the first visit that I did not appreciate that there was a moderate weakness of the lifting muscles (dorsiflexors) of the right ankle. I therefore put him into an ankle brace, to hold his foot at a 90-degree position.

Two weeks later, he was walking 400 feet twice a day. The ankle brace on the right foot and the heel lift for his shorter left leg had eliminated his instability and poor balance. All the arm and shoulder discomfort was gone, as well as was most of the back and leg pain. He still had neck pain, primarily at night in bed, and I told him to follow up with his internist about getting a neck brace, medication patches such as Flector or Lidoderm, or a physical medicine examination.

At his next visit 6 weeks after the first, Willie was able to walk 2 blocks at a time—a total of 1000 feet. He still had to follow up with another specialist regarding his neck.

Then Willie terrified me. Proud of his progress, he wanted to show me that he could try walking without a walker because his balance was so good! I reacted vehemently, indicating that I was firmly against the idea. I told him in the strongest possible terms that I did not want him to try getting around without a walker—even using a cane—until he'd had extensive therapy and evaluation regarding his balance by a physical therapist. I was so emphatic about his never walking without the walker that both he and his girlfriend agreed that he wouldn't try.

For the purpose of this write-up, I called Willie 3 months later, and he was still doing well. After 10 years of minimal walking, he was now able to walk as much as 2 blocks at a time, with only mild and tolerable discomfort.

The lesson? Here was a 90-year-old man with Multiple Sclerosis, bound to a wheelchair for 10 years. Seems like an impossible task, right? The trick is to see the straightforward pathology, sequentially address it, and see what happens. You might be surprised. In this case, I certainly was!

Entertaining interviews from four of Willie's visits can be seen on WalkingWellAgain.com.

StoryTime: Another MS Success Story

Darren S, 42, had severe walking limitations attributed to Multiple Sclerosis. He had been using a wheelchair since he was a teenager and was unable to walk more than half a block with a walker. The worst of the pain centered in his left ankle.

As many of you will guess by now, his history and exam suggested Spinal Stenosis. Did you know that Spinal Stenosis has been reported to cause symptoms in people in their twenties? In Darren's case, it may have been present even earlier.

A walker set to the proper height provided him with moderate help. He could walk a couple of blocks but still had fairly severe pain in the area of his left ankle. By his next visit, however, Positional Testing had eliminated all the diffuse nerve sensitivity. What was left was severe sensitivity in the sinus tarsi. I injected this with cortisone and advised him to use the walker as much as possible.

A month later, his left ankle no longer hurt and he was able to walk 8 whole blocks. He went from using a wheelchair for over 20 years—to walking over half a mile with a walker! The picture wasn't perfect. Darren still had MS, and his legs still got tired if he walked without the walker. Overall, though, there was quite an improvement.

Again, this is another MS success story, if one accepts less-than-perfect results as success. I do. I aim for perfect results, but I am pleased with good results if that is all I can get.

StoryTime: First Do No Harm

Irwin was a 93-year-old man who came in for treatment of foot pain. He had a painful callus, and was disappointed with a podiatrist who did nothing but trim it, because the pain had come back quickly. He was looking for a second opinion.

The callus was under the fifth metatarsal head on the left foot only. Perhaps you remember that this pattern suggests that the left leg is shorter. He did have Equinus on the left, but he had no nerve sensitivity, nor did he have arthritis pain of the feet, knees, hips, or back. No balance problems. Indirect examination suggested a 3-millimeter LLDx. He walked well, sat well, and slept well. This World War II veteran was spry and active.

Regarding his chief complaint, the callus, I trimmed it, and did provide longer relief by padding the removable inserts in some of his shoes. Otherwise, no other treatment was indicated. I certainly was not going to provide lifts for his LLDx. He was doing great, so why change the way he walked?

The lesson? I have had many people at all stages of life—from 5 years old to over 90—with problems caused by LLDx. I standardly check with the points provided in this book. I treat the LLDx whenever there is potential benefit. And yet this man is the answer to a question: does an LLDx always cause significant problems? The answer is no. Especially in older people who are doing well and for whom treatment is no longer considered for "prevention," one must take into account the potential benefits and potential problems of treatment.

In Irwin's case, I did him a favor. I did not treat his LLDx. I have made this decision many times; I just wanted to make sure this was expressed clearly, so I did it in a story.

StoryTime: Back to Basics

Abigail O, 50, was a nurse who originally hailed from Nigeria. She came to my office with a chief complaint of right heel pain that had been bothering her for 6 months. She also reported pain in her knees and back, aggravated by standing and walking, dating back more than 5 years. She had received anti-inflammatory medicine, therapy, and injections for her knees, without significant help.

To make a long story short, Abigail had Flat Feet on both sides, as well as a Limb Length Discrepancy. I strapped her with a Low Dye strap and included a heel lift. Within a few days, she had elimination of all foot, leg, knee, and back pain, including the severe symptoms that had been troubling her for several years. Use of the lift alone was much less helpful. I had orthotics made for her, and she regained improvement of all symptoms. Months later, she was still feeling fine.

Three of Abigail's interviews can be seen on WalkingWellAgain.com.

The lesson? Back to basics. Mechanical treatment of Flat Feet can eliminate symptoms of PseudoStenosis as well as mechanically induced foot or leg pain. Mechanical Testing with strapping or Unna boots is a great way to quickly determine if this treatment approach will likely work.

StoryTime: It Might Be in the Leg

Michael was a 56-year-old man who presented with moderate pain that gradually got worse in the front of his right leg and foot. He also had back pain and difficulty sitting. An MRI of his back showed a herniated disc, which improved symptomatically with sitting on a pillow. Herniated discs often become asymptomatic on their own over several weeks, so the pillow simply provided comfort.

His leg pain persisted. There was severe sensitivity where a nerve (the superficial peroneal nerve) came toward the leg surface. Suspecting a local nerve entrapment, I injected him with cortisone, which provided moderate relief, only for a number of days.

I did not see Michael professionally for a few months, as his internist was convinced the leg symptoms were from the back, and took over. A couple of months later there was a turnaround. His doctor showed me the report of the MRI of his leg, which showed a benign nerve tumor involving the nerve I had originally suspected. Michael had surgery to remove the tumor, and after a few months was ninety percent pain free.

The lesson? Even if there is a spine or spine-mediated nerve problem, there can still be a problem in the foot or leg. When there are nerve problems at multiple levels it may be called a "double crush syndrome." In addition to the very real spine problem, this gentleman also had a nerve tumor in his leg. Especially in a person who does not respond as expected to treatment, one must check for all the likely or even unlikely causes.

StoryTime: Even in Young Adults, It Might Not Be the Leg

I am sorry that I cannot remember this person's name, but this is too good a story to pass up. She was a 25-year-old woman I saw in Boca Raton, Florida, about twelve years ago. When her husband asked me to see her, she had pain in both legs that had bothered her for several months. She had seen a clinician who had ordered both oral medication and physical therapy, both of which did not help. MRI scans of the legs were normal. The patient was in both physical and emotional distress.

She had a positive Positional History, and she had sensitivity along the nerves in her legs and thighs. (I have been using that pattern as a clue for a long time!) Strongly suspecting congenital Spinal Stenosis, which usually only becomes symptomatic in the third decade, I ordered an MRI of her spine. She tried Positional Testing with a walker, which did not help at all. The MRI was positive and showed fairly severe congenital Spinal Stenosis, which responded temporarily to epidural injections and then responded well to spine surgery.

Two important lessons. First, congenital Spinal Stenosis can occur in young people, just as PseudoStenosis can. One must keep in mind that even in young people, foot and leg symptoms may be coming from primary spine problems, as well as from biomechanical problems of the feet or legs.

The second point to focus on is the fact that I would consider this a successful case. Although the treatment I provided did not help her, the proper testing and diagnosis directed her to the practice of a clinician that could help her. That is success. Podiatrists who find conditions in their patients that they themselves cannot help, and who then direct the patients to the proper specialists, are providing a great service. Other specialists who recognize the possible PseudoStenosis etiology of the many conditions listed in this book, who refer to a qualified and thoughtful podiatrist for evaluation, are providing a great service. As long as the team effort provides good long-term relief by addressing the cause of problems, all members of the team can claim success.

StoryTime: A Happy Ending

Sandra was a 19-year-old woman who came in to see me for aching in her right leg and thigh. She had evidence of Limb Length Discrepancy—Equinus and nerve sensitivity in the right leg,—and no evidence of other pathology. Convinced that a ⅜-inch discrepancy was causing the problem, I started her with some ¼-inch lifts and asked her to follow up in a week. She did not.

A few months later she came in, greatly upset. She had followed up with a specialist who was convinced that the pain was coming from her spine. He therefore ordered an MRI, which was negative. He provided anti-inflammatory medication, which did not help. When she returned to see me, her thigh was so painful that she could barely walk on it. She had lost her insurance and could not have any therapy. To make matters worse, she was scheduled to get married in three weeks and was seriously thinking of canceling the wedding.

My examination again suggested LLDx and sensitive nerves, but also something else. She was thin enough for me to be able to feel her thigh bone, the femur, and it was extremely sensitive. Considering stress fracture of that bone, I put her on crutches and sent her to an orthopedist. Again, she did not follow up with me. I always wondered what happened.

A year later, she returned, six months pregnant. The crutches had done the trick; she had had adequate relief of pain and had gotten married. During this return visit, she again had symptoms of an LLDx, but now was willing to be compliant. After all, she was walking for two ...

The lesson? You may remember from Chapter 19 that the shorter limb is far more likely to have hip arthritis develop in it. In fact, I have had dozens of patients with degenerative arthritis of the hip report excellent improvement with the appropriate lift. Keep in mind that the shorter limb also carries an increased risk of certain types of stress fractures, as seemed to occur in Sandra. Such problems, which appear to occur for no reason, often have a reason that is not recognized.

StoryTime: Post Traumatic PseudoStenosis

Chante S is a 37-year-old woman who came in because of poor balance that had been a major problem for about a year. However, her overall foot, leg, and back pain had gotten so bad that she had become disabled from working for years, with all symptoms beginning after she was in an automobile accident 12 years prior. Fracture of her right leg required multiple surgeries, and she was not able to walk on it without a brace for a year and a half. When she began walking she developed an overall body arthritis that had gotten worse with time. She had been getting ongoing orthopedic and physical therapy management for over 10 years. She had tried medications, including narcotics and Tramadol, but they had only provided moderate help, and the side effects were such that she had decided to stop them and simply live with the pain and inactivity. Of interest, she had had over 10 courses of physical therapy. Not 10 sessions, but 10 courses of physical therapy, each of which involve approximately 12 sessions. She had had multiple X-rays of her legs and an MRI of her back, which identified some arthritis.

In addition to poor balance and severe difficulty with walking and standing, she also had aching in her back and legs after sitting for a long time and while lying in bed.

She did have a positive Positional History, was able to walk significantly better pushing a grocery cart, and had a positive Checkout Counter Sign. Physical examination showed an asymmetric Equinus; she was 10 degrees short of 90 in the right leg, the one that had been injured. She had a positive First Interspace Fine Sign that was moderate on the right but absolutely severe on the left. Severe tibial and femoral nerve sensitivity were much worse on the left side. Her left foot was flatter, and she had tenderness in the sinus tarsi and the plantar aspect of the first metatarsal cuneiform joint. Her left Iliac Crest was higher and quite painful; ¼ of an inch of lift underneath the right heel made the hips coplanar and eliminated all hip sensitivity.

I strapped her with a ¼-inch lift underneath the right heel, and within a day she felt dramatically better. She indicated that there was 70% relief of the back pain and leg pain; she was able to stand and walk much better. There was elimination of the arthritic pain in the knee. She was able to sit better and sleep better.

Examination showed she still had moderate discomfort in the sinus tarsi and the plantar aspect of the left first metatarsal cuneiform joint, suggesting that there were still mechanically induced symptoms, with this flatter left foot. I therefore repeated the strap for the right foot, and also added a strap with a reverse Morton's extension for the left foot. At follow-up 3 days later, she reported relief of almost all of her pain.

The lessons? First, this is just another of many cases in this book in which the diffuse arthritic symptoms that developed after a fracture were actually caused by PseudoStenosis, not arthritis. Improving the way she walked, helping her Walk Well Again, eliminated the severe, diffuse, and long-term arthritis symptoms.

The second lesson is the reminder of the need to address multiple contributing factors to PseudoStenosis. Heel lifts were helpful but not adequate for her, nor would orthotics without compensation for the LLDx have been adequate. Addressing both Flat Feet and LLDx was necessary for a successful result.

Interviews from her first, second, and third visits are available on WalkingWellAgain.com.

StoryTime: Fibromyalgia Was PseudoStenosis

Theresa H was a 57-year-old woman who came in for treatment of uncomfortable toenails. Further discussion revealed that she had been suffering from foot, leg, knee, hip, and back pain for over 30 years, diagnosed at age 25 as having arthritis, and then in her early 50s as also having Fibromyalgia.

She could walk at most 1 block before being stopped by pain. She walked better pushing a grocery cart and had a positive Checkout Counter Sign. Pain was almost always relieved by sitting or leaning, but she also had back and leg pain with extensive sitting, and uncomfortable stiffness when she first arose in the morning. She had Equinus on the right side and a flatter foot on the left. The Iliac Crest Pain Resolution Sign showed with a 3⁄16-of-an-inch (5-millimeter) lift under the shorter right leg. She had tenderness in the sinus tarsi and the plantar aspect of the first metatarsal cuneiform joint of the long left extremity, and pain along the inside of the knee, a sensitive Pes Anserinus. If these areas are not clear to you, review Chapters 6 and 19 please.

I was unsure of the answers to a few questions. Were all of her long-term problems caused by PseudoStenosis, and was it just LLDx or was it also her moderate Flat Foot deformity? Would lifts be enough, or did she also need orthotic control? Was there a primary Spinal Stenosis component that I should treat with Positional Testing? Were her toenails painful because of SS/PS, or because of a separate issue?

She was appreciative of the depth of the investigation and gave me a "blank check." Not of money, but of time—she was willing for me to experiment as I chose. I provided her with several 5-millimeter lifts for her right shoes, and did no other treatment. I explained that I would do additional treatment if she still had symptoms.

Five days later, great news. The foot, leg, knee, hip, and back pain that she had suffered for over 30 years was over 90% gone. She could stand and walk well—for many blocks without pain. She no longer had stiffness or pain when sitting or first getting up. Balance was better. Exam showed elimination of the Equinus, nerve sensitivity, and even joint sensitivity. All from 5-millimeter lifts.

She was not all better; the toenails still hurt. I injected the toes and removed the borders, which at least temporarily solved the problem. I told her to continue with the lifts and follow up in 2 weeks.

Two weeks later, she had maintained improvement. She had gone out walking in a mall for over 2 hours nonstop, experiencing only minimal right hip pain, likely caused by the compression of the felt lift in the shoe she used.

This story conveys a few lessons. First, in this case, 30 years of arthritis pain were actually caused by a Limb Length Discrepancy. Not only did back arthritis symptoms and sensitivity disappear, but so did the areas of sensitivity in her feet caused by biomechanical stress. I had thought she would probably need orthotics. I was wrong.

Her 5-year diagnosis of Fibromyalgia was not correct. Remember, Fibromyalgia is a diagnosis of exclusion, which means that other possible conditions must be excluded first, including Lumbar Spinal Stenosis, Cervical Stenosis, as well as all common etiologies of PseudoStenosis. I have seen over 50 people with long term disability attributed to Fibromyalgia who had total or at least very good improvement with treatment for SS/PS.

This is another example supporting my position that the proper diagnosis can often only be made with thorough clinical evaluation and management. For people with arthritic pain, I find that testing, including spinal imaging, a CT Scanogram, nerve tests, circulation tests, and blood tests are often unnecessary and are sometimes misleading. Quite frequently, the best results are derived from combining a thorough history and physical examination with thoughtful treatment, especially when combined with the cooperation of a flexible and compliant patient.

An interview of Theresa H, a flexible, compliant, and very happy patient, can be seen on WalkingWellAgain.com.

StoryTime: Surgery Scheduling Cancelled

Alma E was 73 years old when she came to my office with a chief complaint of foot numbness of a few years' duration, and a secondary complaint of severe ankle pain dating back about 6 months. She'd also had leg pain and low-back pain for several years caused by spinal arthritis, a Spondylolisthesis that was due for surgical scheduling two weeks later. Her many symptoms had received only mild temporary help with oral medication, physical therapy, and epidural injections of cortisone.

My exam showed a severely sensitive left sinus tarsi, below the ankle, moderate Equinus of the shorter right leg, and mild loss of sensation. She had a positive First Interspace Fine Sign—much worse in her longer leg—and moderate Flat Feet. At the initial visit, I injected the sinus tarsi, strapped both feet, and included a lift for the shorter right leg. I must say that I enjoyed her return visit 4 days later. The ankle pain was gone, as were the numbness, back pain, and leg pain. I was not sure if she would need just a lift or also orthotics, so I gave her the lifts and waited.

At a follow-up visit almost 16 weeks later, we were still waiting for the back and leg pain to come back! She returned to work teaching at a community college and was very happy. At least temporarily, her surgery was cancelled.

Two of Alma's videos are available at WalkingWellAgain.com.

StoryTime: Fibromyalgia Resolved in 4 Days ("I'll Pick That Up!")

Yael Q was a woman in her 40s who had had progressive arthritic symptoms for over 15 years. With all other diagnostic tests negative, she was diagnosed 8 years prior with Fibromyalgia. No medicine or therapy provided significant help. She had back and leg pain when standing, walking, sleeping, and sitting. Raising children, she just put up with symptoms, as she really had no choice.

A quick exam showed classic signs of a Limb Length Discrepancy. On the right side she had a tight right Achilles, while on the left side she had a positive First Interspace Fine Sign, a sensitive Pes Anserinus, and a very sensitive Iliac Crest. She also had a severely sensitive sinus tarsi on the left foot only.

I used ³⁄₁₆ of an inch for her shorter right leg, and in 2 days she reported being about 45% better. Her sensitive areas and tight tendon were all moderately better, not completely better. In addition, the sinus tarsi still hurt like . . . heck.

Suspecting the need for additional lift, I switched the height of her lift to ¼ of an inch. Suspecting the sinus tarsi as a contributing factor (which I mentioned at the first visit), I injected her with a steroid injection.

Only 2 days later she reported wonderful relief of pain. She had been extremely active the day before, much more that she could have been in years past. Minimal pain. She walked, stood, slept, and sat without difficulty. Yes, she was happy. You can see it in her video!

I cut some additional felt lifts for her to take home, and one fell on the ground. She immediately got up and said, "Now I can pick that up!" She did, and reported that she had not been able to pick things up for years. Even when she had worked as an X-ray technologist, she had asked her patients to pick anything up that fell. Hence the second name for this story.

When she said that, bells went off in my head. A couple of years earlier, a man in his 40's with chronic pain had said the same thing—that he had been unable to pick things up for years but after treatment had no problem. Of interest, that person was also misdiagnosed as having arthritic pain from a systemic condition, in his case Familial Mediterranean Fever. He also had relief only when I injected him for his Sinus Tarsi Syndrome. It is most likely just a coincidence, but such observations are sometimes the beginning of something learned.

This addition is inserted in the final stages before publication. This is actually a pattern that I have now recognized over 25 times in the last year. Inability to bend over and pick things off of the floor has improved in patients with a limb length discrepancy only after injection for sinus tarsi syndrome. Often the improvement is noted just a few minutes after that injection!

Enjoy Yael Q's enthusiastic video on WalkingWellAgain.com.

StoryTime: Post-wedding Blues

Yael is the same person mentioned in the story above. It is several weeks later, and she has a new story, one that she did not mind being published. It involves a rare time in which I got upset, though I did not mention it until the following visit.

Yael had a recurrence of fairly severe pain, and, understanding my perception that the pain was mediated through the spine, she went to a spine specialist. A spinal X-ray showed arthritis, so the specialist ordered an MRI and physical therapy. Her pain improved within a few days, and she saw me for a scheduled follow-up. When I heard that she had a recurrence and did not come back to me, I was a bit indignant, at least inside of my head. I did not want to show it.

Why, after such magnificent improvement, did she have recurrence? Note the name of the story! Discussion revealed that she had gone to a wedding and danced up a storm—in shoes without a lift! Just as getting better can be a very quick process, so can getting worse. We discussed strict compliance, which she agreed to make a priority. I gave her extra lifts for her glove compartment, not wanting to take any chances.

A month later, she came in for a follow-up visit and said she wondered why she was even there. Having been strict with use of the lift, she had no significant symptoms. A little backache if on her feet extensively, but all other symptoms mentioned at the beginning of the previous story were gone. She said she was so much better that she decided against having an MRI, and the physical therapist observed that she was so much better that therapy was not really needed.

At that visit, I revealed to her that I had previously felt upset that after such wonderful improvement with my treatment she did not follow up with me immediately when there was recurrence. I hope that it was primarily concern that she might get unneeded treatment, but to be honest there may have been some unhealthy ego involved as well. Do not forget: doctors are only human!

The lesson? For a person with a vulnerable back and a Limb Length Discrepancy, extensive activity can bring back symptoms severely—and rapidly. Kind of like a person with a vulnerable back (or hip or knee or ankle) dancing up a storm wearing only one shoe. Not a good idea. I wager that she will not do it again.

StoryTime: Double-Check!

Rebecca was a 73-year-old woman who came to the office for evaluation of foot and leg pain that she had been living with for a very long time. She'd been diagnosed as having Multiple Sclerosis about 7 years earlier but felt in retrospect that her MS symptoms had possibly been present for 30 years and were never diagnosed as such. Of interest, 18 years previously she'd had a right hip replacement that had succeeded in relieving her right hip pain. However, she had very poor balance after that. She had a Limb Length Discrepancy, but although she used a lift for the shorter left leg, she told me that she'd nevertheless fallen more than a thousand times over the course of the previous 18 years.

She walked much better pushing a grocery cart. Without the cart, she was only able to walk for five or ten minutes at a stretch. That had been the case for many years. She had nerve sensitivity that was much worse on the left side, and a very tight Achilles tendon on the right side.

Those of you who were paying attention will have noted that this pattern suggests a Limb Length Discrepancy with the RIGHT leg being shorter, not the left. Indeed, that was the case. However, for many years she'd been using a lift on the left side. In her situation she had a *structural* Limb Length Discrepancy (either by birth or caused by the hip surgery) and an *environmental* Limb Length Discrepancy caused by using a lift on the wrong side. No wonder she had such poor balance and so many falls!

We shifted the lift to the proper side, and she immediately stood better. Just 2 days later, Rebecca's Equinus was eliminated, along with the nerve sensitivity and the feeling of poor balance. She was able to walk much better after only 2 days of being properly balanced. There was still some limitation and she still did better with a grocery cart, so I also instituted Positional Testing.

The lesson? Again, the devil is in the details. With something as important as a Limb Length Discrepancy, one must check and double-check. Note that in the instruction section on managing a Limb Length Discrepancy in Chapter 12, I advise to double-check to see that the perceived difference is still there after a couple of weeks—and then again down the road.

StoryTime: A Parkinson's Parable

Leo had had balance problems for 2 years, attributed to progression of his Parkinson's disease, which had been identified almost 10 years earlier. A few months before his visit to my office, he developed right foot pain underneath the first metatarsal head, which had a thin callus but was obviously dropped lower than the other bones.

He had an LLDx, with Equinus on the left and a higher hip on the right. Uncharacteristically, his arch was higher in the longer leg, the right one. (I find that the longer foot is more likely to have a flatter foot, but it's not always that way!) I relieved the foot pain by applying padding to relieve pressure, and I compensated for the LLDx with the appropriate lift.

A few days later, the foot pain was gone, as was the balance problem. He no longer had to hold onto the wall or a chair as he walked in his apartment, nor did he feel that he needed the cane outside the apartment, although I advised him to continue to use the cane for stability. His feeling of instability disappeared the first day of use of the lift.

Please note that I am not saying that Leo did not have Parkinson's disease. What I am saying is that his LLDx contributed to the balance challenge, and addressing it helped control that challenge. I believe that with aging or with this disease, Leo was no longer able to adequately compensate for the LLDx. Once the need to do that was removed by use of the lift, he improved greatly.

There are two main lessons. This story reinforces the lesson of Chapter 23—that all patients with balance challenges should be evaluated for SS/PS even if they have other conditions that are known to cause such problems. In addition, it is a reminder that the asymmetric patterns of LLDx are usually classic, but not always. Do not let an unusual presentation interfere with good medical care!

StoryTime: Medicine's Loss is Psychology's Gain

Dr. Christina T, a woman in her 30s, came in for an ingrown nail. (It's amazing how many stories start that way!)

She reported more than a decade of foot, leg, and back pain so severe that she had to stop attending medical school. Conventional treatment with medication and therapy provided only moderate, temporary relief. When epidural injections were found to provide excellent but only temporary help, surgery was recommended. She chose not to have the surgery and instead became a psychologist, a less physically demanding profession.

My exam showed Flat Feet and a Limb Length Discrepancy, asymmetric Equinus, and nerve sensitivity. She had tried multiple pairs of orthotics, and not only had they not helped—they were actually quite painful. I assumed she might need orthotics or even a brace because of her Flat Feet. I was wrong.

Instead of strapping her, I simply provided ¼-inch lifts for her shoes. That was that. She returned a couple of weeks later and reported that all of her pain was gone. Indirect examination again suggested LLDx. Her feet, legs, and back were absolutely fine. She still had some Achilles tightness in both legs, so I had her stretch. Having been inactive for so many years, she began exercising on a treadmill. We discussed the option of ordering orthotics if she felt that they were necessary.

Christina never came back. Ten months later, while reviewing case histories for this book, I called her and we chatted. She had not returned to my office because she had not needed to. All of her foot, leg, and back symptoms had maintained their improvement, and she was strict about using the lifts.

The lessons? The back surgeon recommended surgery because there had been good, temporary improvement with epidural injections. I believe that surgery would NOT have worked, since the main problem—a shorter leg—was not addressed. I agree that good improvement with epidural injections is an indication that the pain is being mediated through inflamed spinal nerves, but that does not mean that the spine is the primary problem. Christina's is a classic case of PseudoStenosis. I think it is quite common.

I want to mention one more thing. Christina had corns that had bothered her for years. They were mild but quite sensitive. I did not treat the corns, and at the next visit they were no longer sensitive. This is an example of how SS/PS can make everything in the feet more sensitive. In other circumstances, and certainly in my own practice many years ago, surgery would have been performed. Here, with just a lift, the corns were no longer a problem.

Interviews of Dr. Christina's only two visits are available at WalkingWellAgain.com.

StoryTime: Crohn's Disease Falsely Accused (The Level Is Essential, #1)

This case is complicated and simple at the same time. Urmila W was a woman in her 50s who presented with severe pain with her feet and legs that she'd had for about 6 years, which limited her walking to a maximum of half a block and caused her pain every night in bed. She'd suffered for over 35 years from Crohn's disease, an inflammatory bowel disease that can also cause arthritis symptoms. About 6 years prior to seeing me, she'd begun having a great deal of difficulty standing and walking. She'd been told that the problems were secondary to her Crohn's disease. Diabetes developed later, as did anxiety and depression.

Let's make a long story short. My exam suggested Spinal Stenosis, but not PseudoStenosis. There was severe sensitivity in intermetatarsal spaces two, three, and four, and along the tibial and femoral nerves bilaterally. She saw immediate improvement in her walking when using a walker set at 31 inches. I advised her of the Adjunct Measures, which provided moderate nighttime improvement within days.

Several days later, she obtained a walker that was only moderately helpful. She could then walk a full block before the onset of pain. The situation was not terrible, but it was certainly not good.

On her first return visit, Urmila did not bring the walker. I requested that she do so. She brought it at her next visit, and lo and behold, the walker was set a little too high. Upon obtaining a 31-inch walker, she immediately improved. She was able to walk all the way around the block—four blocks in total—with absolutely no pain. As you may not be surprised to hear, her mood improved tremendously, a common finding when chronic pain and forced inactivity are resolved.

In Urmila's case, we have two lessons. The first is the misdiagnosis of Spinal Stenosis symptoms as stemming from Crohn's disease. In my opinion, EVERY patient with lower-extremity symptoms that cause difficulty walking should be considered for SS/PS, even if there is another possible cause. Use of the Positional History facilitates questioning. Once suspected, it's so easy to test for, and then so easy to treat in the majority of cases.

Second is the importance of walker handle height. Her initial walker was set at 32 inches—just 1 inch off her optimum height. However, there was a huge difference when she got a different walker set at 31 inches. Believe me: I had to do a lot of explaining to the durable medical equipment dealer when I asked that it be replaced, as the adjustable model that he provided had a minimum handle height of 32 inches. When I explained the details, he replaced it with a junior rollator that would go down to the needed 31-inch handle height.

The number one cause of failure of Positional Testing is having a walker set at the wrong height. After fourteen years of doing this, I still do not claim to always get it right. I consider readjusting a patient's walker if a trial of 2–3 days does not provide expected help. Remember, if the walker is not set at the right height—even if it is just a little bit off—many patients will simply not get the benefits that they otherwise could. Taking the time to establish the proper walker height is worth the effort. It can be life changing!

Urmila W's interview is available on WalkingWellAgain.com.

StoryTime: Lyme Disease Falsely Accused (The Level Is Essential, #2)

Rosalyn D was a 76-year-old woman who came in referred by a friend. She reported long-term, disabling symptoms, including severe leg pain with walking, hip and knee pain, and back pain. She had poor balance and had fallen several times. Using a walker improved her stability, but she still had persistent back and extremity pain, and she also had arm and shoulder discomfort when using the walker. Even with the walker she could only go about half a block with a lot of pain, and she had a lot of symptoms thereafter. She did somewhat better pushing a grocery cart and had a positive Checkout Counter Sign. She had pain in her feet and legs every night, and she had difficulty standing, often shifting from side to side. Epidural injections for known Spinal Stenosis provided very short-term and limited help.

Her long-term diagnoses were Lyme disease and Spinal Stenosis. She took Tramadol and Cymbalta for pain and depression.

Her exam was almost but not quite classic. Indirect examination suggested a right leg shorter by ³⁄₁₆ of an inch, with asymmetric Equinus. She had nerve sensitivity bilaterally, but it was greater on the right. Recall that sensitivity is usually greater on the longer leg but does occasionally occur on the short leg, being more likely if the short leg is more than (about) 5 millimeters shorter. She had a larger bunion and a sensitive Pes Anserinus on the left. She had a positive Iliac Crest Pain Resolution Sign with the lift on the right side.

She is about 5'3", and she was using a walker set at 35 inches. She walked leaning forward, with her arms bent as if doing a partial pushup, which explained the arm and shoulder pain. I lowered her walker to its minimum height, 32 inches, which was somewhat more comfortable for her. This was not, however, the position needed for classic Positional Testing.

I chose to treat only the PseudoStenosis component from LLDx first, strapping a ³⁄₁₆-of-an-inch lift to her right leg. The next week she came in very happy, noting that she was about 70% better, her first relief in years. She was standing, walking, and sleeping a lot better, with significantly less pain. When I later pressed for details, she said she felt best the first few days, but in truth had regressed a bit after that.

When I examined her, I found only partial improvement in the signs of LLDx, including Equinus, nerve sensitivity, and Iliac Crest pain. When she stood while wearing the strap, one additional ³⁄₁₆-inch lift eliminated residual Iliac Crest pain. I considered that I had undertreated the LLDx, and I resolved to use a slightly thicker lift—a ¼-inch one.

I then removed her strap and found it wet and compressed. She admitted to taking a shower with a plastic bag covering the strap; the bag leaked, and her foot (and strap and lift) got soaked. Putting two and two together, she noted that her symptoms regressed after the shower, which I feel occurred because her felt lift compressed after getting wet. I repeated indirect examination for LLDx and again concluded that ³⁄₁₆ of an inch was optimal.

I provided several appropriate lifts, and I also loaned her a walker of the appropriate height for her, 30 inches. At her next appointment, she reported nearly complete relief. She was able to walk and sleep without pain, but she had only walked up to one block. She did not have pain getting up from a seated position, and her balance was fine. Exam showed elimination of Equinus, nerve sensitivity, and knee and hip sensitivity. A few weeks later, she was able to walk two blocks without difficulty, and she was living with no significant pain.

The lessons? First, Lyme disease was falsely accused. I have only had a few cases similar to this one, but they have been enough to conclude that Lyme disease is another of the systemic conditions in which the SS/PS component must be considered as a possible contributing factor to symptoms.

The second lesson is that Mechanical Testing for PseudoStenosis or Positional Testing for Spinal Stenosis can prove far more effective than epidural injections, like it did in this case and in many others.

The third is a lesson repeated many times in this book, but this time it has a different twist. Just as the walker height should be exact and the walker should be used full time initially to obtain relief, so should heel lifts be exact and used full time initially. If the height is just a millimeter or two off, improvement may not be optimal. VERY frequently, I have to add a small amount after the first visit to get maximum improvement. I often give extra lift to the patients to add on their own, but I find that they often wait for me to do it when they come in.

In Rosalyn's case, however, loss of lift height caused by the immersion in water was detrimental. The lesson: the straps and lifts used must be kept dry until the follow-up visit, which is ideally within 3–4 days, and should be within the week. I know that the felt lifts may compress, especially in heavy or extremely active people, but it seems that the compression gets much worse after immersion in water, and that can skew the results. Both patients and clinicians need to pay attention to these important details, as indeed, *the level is essential*.

Enjoy Rosalyn's delightful interview on WalkingWellAgain.com.

StoryTime: Mix-ups Mandate Follow-ups

Thelma was an 88-year-old woman who came in because of difficulty walking. She had had diabetes for 10 years, and she had had a stroke 5 years earlier. Since that time, she had had poor balance, knee and hip pain, and classic neurogenic claudication. She could walk or stand for only a few minutes before she had to sit or lean against something, and she walked much better pushing a grocery cart.

She had signs of LLDx, including Equinus, a positive First Interspace Fine Sign, and sensitivity at the Pes Anserinus and the Iliac Crest. She reported being a lot better with a ⅛-inch lift under her short leg, so I provided several lifts for her shoes. At the next visit, she reported moderate improvement in balance and knee pain, and she could walk or stand for several minutes. She still had some Equinus, nerve sensitivity, and Pes Anserinus sensitivity. I felt that I had not given enough lift, so I gave her several ¹⁄₁₆-inch lifts for her other shoes.

At the next visit, she was worse. No surprise. She had gotten a bit confused. She was wearing a shoe with only a ¹⁄₁₆-inch lift, not quite remembering all the instructions. All signs of LLDx were back with a vengeance. I modified her current shoe to contain a lift of ³⁄₁₆ of an inch, and I had her wear it all the time.

At the next visit 2 days later, all Equinus, nerve sensitivity, hip pain, and balance difficulty were gone. She could stand or walk for over 15 minutes. The knee was mostly better, but not all better. At my request, she brought in all of her shoes, and my staff padded each one appropriately, as there had been different heights in each shoe because of the confusion.

I won't go into the details, but the next day I had a patient come in because of recurrence of back and leg pain that had previously resolved with a lift. When I examined her shoes, there was no lift. Spring had come, and since she had been doing so well she had forgotten to put lifts in her springtime shoes. After one week, she was back to square one. When I put the lift into her shoe, she smiled as she noted the immediate improvement. She promised to remember.

Two stories share one lesson. When dealing with LLDx, follow-up evaluations are essential.

StoryTime: PseudoStenosis and Sitting

Sylvia W is a 49-year-old woman who presented for a thorough diabetic foot examination, as is recommended by the American Diabetes Association to be done at least yearly for all individuals with diabetes. Fortunately, she had great circulation and nerve function, and was at low risk for any complications. Good news.

Further discussion revealed that she could usually walk several blocks before she had to sit. However, she had difficulty sitting for a long time, often fidgeting and changing her position or getting up to walk. She also had restlessness when sleeping and often woke up with back or leg discomfort. She often felt stiff in the legs for several minutes after getting up from sitting or sleeping.

She had Equinus on the right side and a positive First Interspace Fine Sign on the left. When not weight bearing, her right foot was a little higher than the left. Her left hip was higher than the right, and it was quite tender. Hips became symmetrical and all sensitivity resolved with a ³⁄₁₆-inch lift under the right heel.

Suspecting a 5-millimeter LLDx, I put a ³⁄₁₆-of-an-inch lift under her right heel and applied a Low Dye strap to hold it in place. She indicated it was comfortable.

At her 1-week follow-up, she reported great news. Within a day all the back discomfort had resolved. She could sit and lie down without limitation. All stiffness was resolved. She was able to walk longer distances, although she had not considered that a problem before. My exam showed elimination of Equinus, nerve sensitivity, and Iliac Crest pain, even without a lift. Indirect measurement again suggested a 5-millimeter LLDx. I provided her with lifts for all shoes, and we discussed getting additional lifts as needed.

The lesson? Compensating for the LLDx, which only has a direct effect on standing or walking, may allow quick resolution of the inflammation of the spinal structures that cause symptoms while sitting. Between lifts, orthotics, and braces, I have noted dozens of patients who had relief of difficulty sitting in the past few years. To be honest, I did not recognize that pattern until a few years ago. I guess you can teach an old doc new tricks!

Sylvia W's interview at her follow-up visit is available on WalkingWellAgain.com.

StoryTime: Pregnancy Pain

Rochel was a 37-year-old woman who presented with burning pain in her feet that had been present for 5 months, since the last trimester of pregnancy. This involved pain when she first got up in the morning and any time she stood or walked for a few minutes. It started in the heels and extended along the arch. She had moderate back pain during that time. She walked better pushing a grocery cart and felt worse at the checkout counter.

She had asymmetric Equinus, asymmetric nerve sensitivity, and asymmetric Iliac Crest height and sensitivity, which improved with ¹⁄₁₆-inch lifts under the left heel. Diagnosing Neurogenic Positional Pedal Neuritis secondary to PseudoStenosis, I provided ¹⁄₁₆-inch lifts for all her left shoes. Within 1 day, all burning pain was gone. At the next visit, the Equinus and nerve and hip sensitivity were all resolved.

The lesson? In this book there have been many stories about accidents or surgery bringing on pain that improved with management of PseudoStenosis. Add pregnancy to the list of conditions that may induce PseudoStenosis symptoms that may be reversed with straightforward podiatric care.

StoryTime: My Walker Readjustment Record

David is a 70-year-old man whom I met in an unusual way. I was at a rest stop in Delaware with my family, returning from a trip to Philadelphia, when I saw a man with a walker walking with great difficulty, stopping to sit every 50 feet. Suspecting Spinal Stenosis, I approached him and explained that adjusting his walker might provide great help. He was grateful, although my first attempt provided little help. As I was readjusting the walker his wife appeared, and after I explained what I was doing and why, she informed me that David had an appointment to see me in two days. We all celebrated when the next adjustment induced the position that allowed him to immediately walk pain free. It was one of those "aha!" moments. He later told me that if the Almighty wants your pain to disappear at a rest stop in Delaware, that is when it will happen! He did well for many months.

With a lot of arthritis, he was referred for physical therapy. The next time I saw him he was doing worse, as the therapist had raised the walker to the level that is recommended in classic literature. He stood taller, but walked with much more pain. I readjusted the walker, and the pain disappeared.

This happened at least another three times. Once, when the walker was raised, he developed such pain in his legs that his primary doctor ordered MRI of his legs. Whenever the walker was raised, he had greater difficulty with back pain, leg pain, and walking. He knew what level was best, but it was hard to argue with other physicians or therapists who adjusted his walker.

The lessons? It is a nice story, one that I get to laugh about when he comes in. But the real lesson is that the most effective walker height should be comfortable, as described in detail in Chapter 7. If there is increased discomfort or restriction with using a walker, it should be adjusted. Those who become confident with the direction provided in this book should not hesitate to stand up for the patient's right to lean forward!

StoryTime: Assess and Experiment!

Barbara was a woman in her 60s who had suffered chronic pain involving her knees and back, pain that was aggravated by standing and walking, for many years. Therapy and injections had provided no long-term help. Knee replacement surgery had been recommended, but she chose to avoid that surgery. Some long-term neck and shoulder pain had been resolved with physical therapy. When standing, she often shifted from side to side, and she experienced nighttime pain in her right leg on an average of three or four times a week. She had fractured her right ankle years before.

Examination showed an asymmetric Equinus of about −15 degrees on the left and 0 degrees on the right. She had a positive First Interspace Fine Sign, much worse on her right side than on her left, as well as some swelling with tenderness along the course of the left posterior tendon. The bunion was larger on the right foot. I found a Limb Length Discrepancy of about ⅜ of an inch, with the left leg being shorter and the left hip lower when standing. This improved with a ¼-inch lift for the left side. Both feet were fairly flat.

Not knowing if her Flat Feet also affected possible PseudoStenosis, I treated her with both straps and a heel lift. Three days later, she reported that the back and knee pain, as well as the nighttime pain in her right leg, had disappeared within thirty-six hours. My exam showed no lingering Equinus or nerve sensitivity. Still not knowing if it was the Flat Feet or the discrepancy that needed to be addressed, I gave her a supply of ¼-inch lifts. A month later, with only the use of the lift, there was no recurrence of any of the symptoms, so orthotics were not necessary. (Of course, if her pain had returned despite use of the lifts, then orthotics would have been needed.)

The lesson? Here was a woman who was facing knee replacement surgery. I do not claim that she had no knee arthritis, but many people have arthritis and do not have a lot of pain. Once Barbara started using the lifts, her arthritis did not disappear, but her symptoms did. I am not sure if it was entirely because of the elimination of the nerve sensitivity, or if the mechanics of the knees themselves became so much better once the lift was in place.

I'm aware that my expertise may not seem very impressive with this particular case. I did not know if orthotics would be necessary. I still don't know if the severe pain was caused by mechanics or by the nerve sensitivity from PseudoStenosis. It may have been either one. But that's okay. I'm not writing this to impress anyone. I'm writing this to share methods that can reduce pain.

Here's my advice: Consider the possibilities, and experiment with safe and simple approaches that always work very quickly when they work. If you are not quite sure, but the patient is all better and stays better, that's good enough!

StoryTime: A Great Knee Replacement That Still Hurt

Walter was a 75-year-old man who came in for an ingrown toenail. Physical examination showed signs of LLDx and flexible Flat Feet. An ex-athlete, he could at his initial visit walk only about a block before being forced to stop because of back pain, leg pain, knee pain, and Shortness of Breath. Among the classic findings was severe sensitivity at the left Pes Anserinus. He had had a left knee replacement several years earlier that was helpful, although the knee still ached.

With two treatments—a ¼-inch lift for the short right leg and strapping for Flat Feet—he was significantly better. All back, leg, and knee pain was gone. He was able to go three blocks before he felt Shortness of Breath—which was caused by his cardiac issues.

This story could be in either Chapter 19 (on arthritis) or Chapter 20 (on Shortness of Breath). The Shortness of Breath lesson is obvious. His walking distance increased significantly when his foot pathology was treated. We thereby removed the "25-pound backpack" I describe in Chapter 20.

The other point I want to emphasize is that he had had tenderness of the knee for many years after the replacement. It was not caused by arthritis, or by a poor job by the surgeon, or by age. It was caused by the combination of Limb Length Discrepancy and Flat Feet. Once that was addressed, the knee pain resolved, and so did the sensitivity at the Pes Anserinus.

StoryTime: PseudoStenosis Worsens Genuine Arthritis Pain: Back-to-Back Examples

Greg, aged 40, came in for treatment of severe pain in the back of his left heel, with milder pain in the back of his right heel. He had had difficulty walking for over 5 months. X-rays ordered by his family doctor identified spurs in the back of the heels. Motrin and ice provided minimal help. He had no back, hip, or knee pain. Exam showed Equinus on the right and a severe positive First Interspace Fine Sign on the left. Indirect examination suggested a 5-millimeter (³⁄₁₆-inch) Limb Length Discrepancy. I provided lifts for the short right leg.

Two days later he reported feeling over 80% better, with discomfort on both heels being about the same—only mild. He walked well, and he felt that the heel pain was now a mild annoyance. The Equinus and nerve sensitivity were totally resolved. Indirect exam again showed a 5-millimeter difference. He maintained improvement with lifts.

The next hour . . .

Ilene, aged 67, came in for a follow-up appointment. She had come in 2 weeks earlier with a complaint of arthritic pain on the top of her left foot that had been mild for years but had become much more severe for about 6 months. X-rays showed some arthritis. She had been treated with a removable cast and with anti-inflammatories, both of which provided minimal help. She had no back, hip, or knee pain.

Exam showed Equinus on the right and a severe positive First Interspace Fine Sign on the left. Indirect examination suggested a 5-millimeter (³⁄₁₆-inch) Limb Length Discrepancy. I provided lifts for the short right leg and a prescription for a topical Diclofenac gel. She reported that most pain was gone within 2 days of using the lifts, and that the remainder resolved with subsequent use of the topical gel. Equinus and nerve sensitivity were totally resolved. Indirect exam again showed a 5-millimeter difference.

The lesson? As expounded on in Chapter 18, there is often a conundrum in arthritis: how much of the arthritic pain is from local arthritis, and how much of it is from other factors? I feel that there are three factors affecting local arthritic pain, the local arthritis being only one of them. Two common additional factors affecting osteoarthritis pain are the mechanical stress of the Deforming Force, and the hypersensitivity caused by nerve irritation associated with either Spinal Stenosis or PseudoStenosis. In the cases of Greg and Ilene, I believe that it was only the nerve irritation from PseudoStenosis that caused the pain to be so severe, not a change in the Deforming Force nor the local inflammation. Using a lift that relieved spinal nerve irritation provided relief of the majority of pain. Investigating for SS/PS should be part of the standard treatment protocol for extremity arthritis pain. These two cases demonstrate why.

StoryTime: A Running Career Enabled

Dylan O was a 16-year-old high school student, an avid and competitive runner. He came in for treatment of a wart, but after my exam suggested biomechanical problems, he acknowledged having had back and leg pain aggravated by activity for the last 18 months.

What did the exam show? A slightly flatter foot on the right, with a callus beneath the second metatarsal head, and a callus beneath the fifth metatarsal head of the left foot only. Asymmetric Equinus, -5 degrees on the left and +5 degrees on the right. A positive First Interspace Fine Sign on the right foot only. Discomfort with palpation of the sinus tarsi and plantar aspect of the first metatarsal cuneiform joint on the right side only. The right Iliac Crest was higher and more tender, improved with a 1/16-inch lift under the left heel. Everything pointed to a structural Limb Length Discrepancy, although a small one. I explained my findings and provided several 1/16-inch lifts for all of his right shoes.

When he returned 2 weeks later for follow-up of both the LLDx and the wart, he was doing great. He had some residual neck discomfort, but all back and leg pain had disappeared completely. He could run long distances with no symptoms during or after activity for the first time in 18 months. All signs improved. Indirect exam again suggested a slight LLDx, so I directed him to use 2-millimeter lifts for his left shoes long term. It certainly seems that all of his symptoms were caused by a 2-millimeter Limb Length Discrepancy, including back discomfort, irritation of the nerves in the back, and increased mechanical stress in the longer leg.

The lesson? In most patients I have seen, a small discrepancy like that did not cause the structures of each of the two feet to be so different from each other, let alone in a person so young. I suspect that because he was a runner, the greater changes occurred so early in life. Those of us who have done sports medicine know that at times the feet of 20-year-old ballerinas often show changes that would normally only be seen by middle age. This is attributed to the great stress placed on the feet and ankles by their training. I believe that this applies to this young man as well.

Dylan's enthusiastic interview is available on WalkingWellAgain.com.

StoryTime: I Needed a Second Chance

Stancee is a 48-year-old woman who came in because of severe arthritic right foot pain. This began after multiple rear-foot fractures from an automobile accident 11 years earlier. Told that she might never walk, it took a year before she could walk—with pain—for a few minutes. Now, 11 years later, she could only walk five to ten steps before foot and back pain began. She dragged her right foot and leg after walking just a few minutes. Extensive conservative treatment by multiple podiatrists and orthopedists resulted in no significant improvement. She was advised that surgery might or might not help.

This was my second shot at her symptoms. She had come to me years earlier, and I was one of the many doctors that had had no success. I had injected, provided a brace and medications, but had totally struck out.

This time I recognized the problem—PseudoStenosis caused by LLDx. Her fractures had compressed and shortened her right heel, causing the LLDx. She had Equinus, distal nerve sensitivity, and hip sensitivity. With only a

¼-inch lift in her right shoe, she immediately stood better than she had in years. Within a few days Equinus and hip and nerve sensitivity were resolved. At the next visit a few weeks later, she told me of the extent of her recovery. The day before, she had been on her feet for five hours without pain. She started to dance for me during the interview process, which I plan on including in her interview available on WalkingWellAgain.com.

The lesson? While she certainly had severe arthritis, it is obvious that arthritis was not the cause of her pain. As is presented in detail in Chapters 18 and 19, the first step in evaluating any lower-extremity arthritis is to check for the contribution of Spinal Stenosis or PseudoStenosis to those symptoms. In this case, after a strikeout, my second turn at bat brought a home run, as the true cause was identified. Enjoy her interview!

StoryTime: Radiologic Testing Is Still Evolving!

Carol came in, and my exam suggested a large LLDx that had contributed to the development of symptoms. To further investigate, I ordered both a CT Scanogram and a standing Long Leg Study involving comparative weight-bearing X-rays. One identified an 8-millimeter difference. The other identified a 16-millimeter difference. These tests were taken at the same institution and were read by the same radiologist.

I share this not to negate the value of these tests. They can be helpful. However, there are qualifying factors. First, the two tests do not measure the exact same structural pathology, so clinical examination may be needed to determine which test to use. Second, I want to stress that these tests have not yet reached the level of absolute accuracy that would be needed to make them the final arbiter in a clinical question. Often, radiologists at the same institution give slightly different readings to the same exam, a situation similar to the variability in interpretation of spinal MRI exams.

Radiologic examination for LLDx often has clinical value. I respect the tests and occasionally use the tests, especially for larger LLDx. I am, however, a believer in the value of clinical management, including a detailed examination after intervention, with a detail-oriented clinician having the final say in treatment for LLDx.

StoryTime: Symptoms in Remission but Not Cured

Lisa had resolution of back pain suffered for many years by using a 2-millimeter lift for her left shoe. She maintained improvement at a 1-month follow-up visit, but 6 months later she reported moderate recurrence of pain. She again had asymmetric Equinus and nerve sensitivity.

As weather changed from winter to springtime, she got new shoes *and* returned to old shoes with no lifts. She had run out of 2-millimeter lifts, so she used some other spacers instead. Some shoes had no lift; others had a lift of over 3 millimeters. The old feeling of back pain began to return. I reviewed with her the need to have consistency with both use and height of the lift, and I provided her with several permanent 2-millimeter lifts, thereby setting her back on the path of minimal pain.

The lesson? Women change shoe styles more frequently than men, based upon weather. I have had *so many* patients whose symptoms returned once they stopped using orthotics or lifts. When there is a return of symptoms it is important to think of the factor (orthotics, lifts, ankle braces, walkers, etc.) that originally resolved the problem.

Dr. David Armstrong, an internationally lauded authority on diabetic foot issues, shared the concept of diabetic foot ulcers not necessarily being "cured" but rather being in remission. In a similar vein, symptoms associated with SS/PS may be totally resolved with treatment, but should be regarded as in remission, not cured. If there is recurrence, neither patient nor clinician should be shocked. Rather, they should consider the evaluation and techniques that provided relief in the past. Be sure to be compliant. As always, the devil is in the details.

StoryTime: Shin Splints Subdued

Gary G was a 47-year-old man who came in seeking help for pain in his left leg, diagnosed as shin splints, that had bothered him for about 5 years. The discomfort initially was only brought on by running but was now problematic just with normal standing and walking. He had had mild back discomfort for years as well. Anti-inflammatory medicine provided minimal help. He found himself restricting walking and standing because of pain.

His exam did not show all classic findings, just two. There was no sensitivity along the knee, the nerves, or the hip. He did have greater Equinus on the left side, and his right Iliac Crest was higher, with the two hips evening out with only a 2-millimeter lift under the left heel. I was not sure if the symptoms were from the mild LLDx, or possibly from the tightness of his left Achilles tendon, a symptom that sometimes responds to stretching.

To be honest, in decades past I would have recommended stretching, and he probably would have gotten better. However, this time I initially treated with lifts—2-millimeter lifts for the mild LLDx—but I also demonstrated and provided written instruction sheets for stretching exercises for him to do after a few days if he was not better.

The stretching was not needed. Within 2 days the symptoms were over 95% gone: both back and leg discomfort happened minimally only when he was on his feet for many hours. Note that he had previously had symptoms for 5 years. When he returned for evaluation 2 weeks later, the Equinus was gone, and indirect exam again suggested a minimal LLDx. He reported being more active than he had been in years, with minimal rare discomfort.

Shin splints are often associated with LLDx, Flat Feet, Equinus, or the other causes of PseudoStenosis. Please add shin splints to the list of conditions whose presence should induce checking for these common culprits.

StoryTime: The Fusion Is Perfect; the Foot Is in Agony

Lisa S was a 46-year-old woman with a long story. Part one is kind of standard and reflects the general tone of the book, but part two certainly deserves to be included in the book. .

Lisa had had severe foot, leg, and back pain that was aggravated by limited walking for over 20 years, and she had often been unable to work because of pain. To make this long story shorter, I will only share that she had a Limb Length Discrepancy and severe Flat Feet. Heel lifts helped moderately, strapping to test for orthotics did not help further, but Unna boots as a test for ankle braces did help. I made her ankle braces, incorporating the lift, and she did great. She stopped all pain medication, began to walk for pleasure and exercise, lost 50 pounds, and returned with pleasure to the workforce. A happy ending, or at least a happy middle.

She returned to my office 15 months later a different person. Life is full of curveballs, and she got derailed. She was in an auto accident 8 months before this visit, and she suffered a bad foot injury in the process—a fracture/dislocation of the right midfoot. Optimal treatment included fusion of the damaged joints, which she had done. After months of no weight bearing and healing, she had finally begun to walk on her foot, but she always noted severe pain with walking. X-rays had shown that the fusion had healed solidly. She had been given medication for pain and inflammation, had undergone physical therapy, and had been told that she was fine and could return to work. She came to me with tears flowing, literally, throughout the visit, so much so that I did not video her, even thought I sensed this great story.

Exam showed that her right foot (longer leg) was mildly sensitive at the fusion site but super sensitive along the nerves. (Clinicians, I also considered CRPS/RSD, but there was no temperature change or allodynia.) Exam again showed signs of PseudoStenosis caused by Limb Length Discrepancy, as identified years earlier. There was pain upon palpation of intermetatarsal spaces two, three, and four, the tibial nerve, the Pes Anserinus, and the femoral nerve of the right side only. She had Equinus on the left. Her right Iliac Crest was higher and sensitive, which resolved with a 5-millimeter lift under the left foot. When I added that lift to her left shoe, she stood and walked—and smiled—through the flowing tears. Not all better immediately, but mostly better.

Six days later she returned. I walked into the office and saw the smile on her face. She reported that by the next day, she had felt that the burden of pain had been removed. She walked well, and the day before this follow-up appointment she had spent over two hours on her feet, with only mild discomfort toward the end of the day.

On this visit, I did interview her, which you can see on WalkingWellAgain.com. At the end of the interview, the tears returned, but these were tears of joy.

"Neurogenic Positional Pedal Neuritis" (see the end of Chapter 15) is the term I use for pain in the feet caused or worsened by spinal nerve compression. In her case, severe sensitivity of the spinal nerves caused by PseudoStenosis caused this surgical site to hurt far more than it would have under normal circumstances. Her surgical fusion was successful, but the pain had stayed disabling, until some five-dollar lifts came to the rescue . . .

StoryTime: Full-Time Means Full-Time

Robert was a gentleman in his 60s who came in for diabetic foot care. He acknowledged experiencing pain in his feet and legs when walking for the previous 6 months. He had borrowed his wife's walker but had no improvement. Set too low for him, it hurt his back.

My exam suggested stenosis, so I measured him and prescribed a walker. At the next visit, his symptoms were gone, and he could walk for several blocks without pain.

Robert never did full-time Positional Testing, and his symptoms returned. He was scheduled by another physician to receive physical therapy for his painful legs, but I advised him to put it off for 2 weeks. Two weeks of full-time Positional Testing eliminated all of his symptoms, and he was quite satisfied. He transitioned to Positional Therapy, using the walker only for very long walks, and remained symptom free.

He did ask a unique question. He wanted to use the walker to go for runs! I did not know how that would work, so I advised against it. I suggested that he experiment with different speeds and elevation angles on a treadmill. When people transition to Positional Therapy, it is reasonable that they do a certain amount of experimentation to establish their limits. Each person will eventually find what works best for him or her.

The lesson: Robert did much better after temporary full-time use than he did after only part-time use. The advice presented in Chapters 7 and 10 is not always necessary, but it often makes the difference between good and truly excellent results!

Two of Robert's interviews are available at WalkingWellAgain.com.

StoryTime: Good Habits

Barbara was an 80-year-old diabetic woman who presented with back pain, balance difficulties, and neuropathic pain at night. A lift for her shorter leg brought about improvement in her back pain and balance, and the burning in her feet at night was eliminated by her sleeping with a pillow under her knees. This improvement was maintained until she went into the hospital for Congestive Heart Failure. There, when she tried to walk, she again experienced back pain and instability. The nighttime burning in her feet soon returned as well. Why?

The deterioration in her symptoms had come about because the hospital slippers she wore did not have a lift and because she'd been sleeping without a pillow under her knees. When she returned to the habits that alleviated her pain, relief returned in a couple of days.

The lesson is that the "cure" is actually often a controlling factor. Frequently, to be truly effective, it must be used long term. If symptoms return, the patient should go back to the set of habits that provided relief the first time around.

StoryTime: Relief Is Possible Even with Severe Edema

Leatha was a diabetic with severe edema who'd been unable to walk more than half a block for a few years. Her inability to walk was blamed on her edema, which could not be treated because of tenderness in her legs. Unable to use the steps of her house, she was restricted to the first floor. She had severe sensitivity along the peripheral nerves (a Positive First Interspace Fine Sign) but no loss of sensation, either to light touch or to vibration. Although she used a walker full time, she still suffered from leg pain, back pain, and Shortness of Breath that was blamed on Congestive Heart Failure.

Leatha's walker was set too high, inducing extension rather than flexion. I loaned her a walker set at 30 inches to obtain slight flexion, and she immediately felt more comfortable. After one week, she had less leg pain as well as less leg sensitivity and Shortness of Breath. She could now walk for one and a half blocks—a big improvement, but still quite a limited distance. She was not yet comfortable with steps.

I advised her to practice going up steps one at a time, and to practice going down the steps backward, going one step and then gradually increasing. Within a few weeks she was able to go up and down the stairs of her house. By her next visit two months later, she was able to go to a mall and walk for an hour nonstop with the walker, and at home she could go up and down the stairs a few times each day without difficulty. At her next visit she reported using the walker much less frequently. She was able to go to the mall with only a cane and go up and down her staircase several times over the course of the day. She continued to have the same edema. It just no longer hurt!

The lessons of this story are a reflection of so many ideas presented in this book. Here was a woman with numerous disabilities—including back pain, leg pain, Shortness of Breath, and an inability to climb stairs—all of which had severely limited her for a very long time. All of her symptoms were associated with Spinal Stenosis. After living with her disabilities for years, it took just months to get her back to where she had been before—able to walk miles at a time. She achieved these results through a gradual increase in activity employed with common sense, and through Positional Testing and Adjunct Measures. No other intervention was employed.

Sections of Leatha's four interviews are available at WalkingWellAgain.com.

There is a concept attributed by tradition to King David that says, "Even if a sharp sword rests upon one's neck, one should not refrain from praying for mercy." From a podiatric standpoint, I take this to mean that even when there are many chronic symptoms that seem to have settled in permanently, there is the *possibility* of wonderful relief with the right intervention. I have seen this type of recovery in thousands of people with, I am convinced, Heavenly assistance.

I still see Leatha for routine diabetic foot care. I ask her how she's doing, and I occasionally ask if she has any difficulty walking or standing, just as I routinely ask so many of my patients. She is always effusive and appreciative, so I review my records and remember the reason why she is doing so well: because of the intervention done years ago.

I have many patients who've had similar success stories, and who remind me of the wonderful transitions they've made through the combination of therapies presented in this book. It's a good feeling for me—but it is nothing less than life changing for them.

I hope you have similar success. If you have a good story to share, please send it to me at WalkingWellAgain.com.

CHAPTER 28

Final Thoughts and Moving Forward

As we complete this book, I'd like to share some final thoughts.

I wrote this book to help patients and their families, as well as clinicians, overcome the medical challenges that are addressed in this book. I hope that it was not written in vain. I would love for you to contact me with your successes via my website, WalkingWellAgain.com, for I am sure there will be many. Writing is a lonely pastime, and I would be encouraged to hear from you, both lay readers and colleagues, and to learn that my attempt has been successful.

* * * * *

Physicians, other clinicians, and researchers who read this book (thank you!) may conclude that this effort is not up to contemporary standards. The catch phrase of current medical research is "evidence-based medicine," and what I present are simply the observations of someone who presents himself as having expertise. Of the five levels of evidence, the lowest one—Level 5—is that of expert opinion. While some of the articles that I have published are Level 4, this book is indeed Level 5. You may believe that for me to present my opinions, observations, and brand-new categorizations as established fact is not sufficient in the age of evidence-based medicine. That may be true, but it is not, to my mind, a compelling enough reason to prevent me from sharing the paths to the success that I have had with thousands of patients.

In my introduction I revealed that I have tried to initiate research on my observations for well over a decade. I joke that I've fractured my skull more times than I care to count by running into ivy-covered brick walls. The lack of data to back up my observations is not because of lack of intent or effort. I have many times sought to initiate randomized control studies or large well-managed case series, but I never received the necessary assistance or support from researchers or institutions.

I ask that any communication with me be prefaced by taking a few weeks to investigate if my observations hold water. I welcome communication about clinical observations, implementation, or potential research, but not on the lack of formal documentation for what I have presented here. I have shared this information because of the incredible success I enjoy, and because of my fear that what I have learned would not become broadly available. I know that this book is just one early step.

Which brings me to the main point of this chapter: the broad picture. Let us say that clinical investigation and research validate the observations of this book. What is the potential?

1. Many people with known Spinal Stenosis would have excellent long-term improvement with Positional Testing and Positional Therapy. The incidence of epidural injections, physical therapy, spine surgery, and spinal imaging would all be reduced. These expensive and invasive treatments and tests would not be needed by patients who have a rapid, uncomplicated, inexpensive, and safe set of protocols at their disposal.

2. In many people with diagnosed Spinal Stenosis, it is actually PseudoStenosis that lies at the root of their symptoms. Recognition of the true diagnosis in these individuals, along with proper treatment of them, would preclude the need for Spinal Stenosis treatment that is quite possibly destined to long-term failure. The incidence of epidural injections, physical therapy, spine surgery, and spine imaging would be reduced. Success with

319

Mechanical Testing can make it self-evident that the symptoms of PseudoStenosis, while mediated through the spine, are secondary to lower-extremity mechanical problems. The best long-term management is to treat the cause, not the symptom. The benefit to individuals and the overall cost savings would be great.

3. Arthritis pain is often not only worsened by Spinal Stenosis or PseudoStenosis, but the same causes of PseudoStenosis can actually lead to arthritic degeneration and exacerbated symptoms. Early recognition of the problem MAY reduce development of arthritic changes. Later recognition and treatment can reduce symptoms of arthritis quickly and may prevent worsening of arthritic changes over the years. (I write "may" because, while I strongly suspect that this is true, I do not yet have the experience to state it with the same confidence that I have in the ability of these tools to help reduce symptoms.) *An ounce of prevention is worth a pound of cure:* nowhere does this wise saying of Ben Franklin carry greater potential than in the early recognition and treatment of biomechanical problems.

   Use of these approaches in both investigation and treatment would help myriads of people reduce the spine and lower-extremity pain that is attributed to either degenerative or inflammatory arthritis. It would also provide relief for people suffering from other conditions that may cause pain, conditions such as Fibromyalgia, Multiple Sclerosis, Ehlers-Danlos syndrome, Familial Mediterranean Fever, and many others. Note that I am not saying that these conditions would be cured, only that a great many people would have relief of painful symptoms by identifying and managing Spinal Stenosis and PseudoStenosis.

4. Use of these approaches would reduce pain, mobility restrictions, and medication use for the millions of people whose neuropathic symptoms are in truth caused by or exacerbated by Spinal Stenosis or PseudoStenosis.

5. Use of these approaches would reduce walking limitation in the tens of thousands (or more) of Americans whose claudication symptoms attributed to poor arterial circulation, or leg pain attributed to edema, are in fact caused or exacerbated by Spinal Stenosis or PseudoStenosis.

6. Use of these approaches would reduce the need for medication to control painful symptoms in the above five groups. If only 50% of these patients got better with the techniques I've presented—something I believe easily possible—it follows that millions of people would reduce or eliminate use of medicines and thus save hundreds of millions of dollars each year.

   That number, however, is only the beginning. Anti-inflammatory medications are known to cause gastrointestinal and cardiovascular side effects that can be devastating and even lethal. Pain medication, including narcotics, as well as medicines for neuropathic pain such as Neurontin, Lyrica, Cymbalta, and Tramadol also increase the risk for falls. Hip fractures usually cost the health care system tens of thousands of dollars for each repair and recovery. Tragically, many people live out their days in nursing homes because of such falls. Many medical complications, as well as secondary costs, could be greatly reduced by reducing the need for these medicines.

7. A great many people have poor balance and an increased risk of falls because of the causes of PseudoStenosis or because of the dysfunction associated with Spinal Stenosis. Most could be helped easily and inexpensively.

8. Improving the ambulation of patients who are limited by Spinal Stenosis and PseudoStenosis could greatly improve the management of medical conditions that are aided by activity, including diabetes, heart disease, and the infirmities of aging. Doing so would help aging members of society maintain their independence, and it would reduce the need for assisted-living or nursing-home assistance for seniors who could potentially lead more active and independent lives.

In short, I believe that the information shared in this book has tremendous public-health ramifications, including improved quality of life for millions of Americans and their families, as well as savings of at least $10 billion a year—and probably much more—for Medicare alone, and much more for our health care system as a whole.

However, in order to experience the full benefit of both the public-health issues and the financial ramifications, research must be conducted in respected institutions. If this book has whet the appetite of those in a position to facilitate such research, I strongly encourage pursuing it. I would love to participate in such studies, insofar as this book does not disqualify me from participation. (If such studies are done without my involvement, I ask that the researchers please notify me as well as send me copies of any subsequent publications addressing these issues.) With me or without me, I hope to see the investigations necessary to take this material to a higher and more established level.

Researchers, I end with a quote from the eighteenth-century philosopher Arthur Schopenhauer. He said, "All truth passes through three stages. First, it is ridiculed. Second, it is violently opposed. Third, it is accepted as being self-evident." The techniques I present are so frequently successful in my daily practice, that I am convinced that they will reach Schopenhauer's third stage.

Clinicians, despite the grandiose observations and aspirations presented above, I understand that the direct impact of this book will be limited to much smaller gains. I hope that clinicians who read this will implement changes in their practice by incorporating the tools provided here. Those who do are sure to enjoy the satisfaction of having patients report reduced pain and need for medication, as well as improved walking, standing, sleeping, and even sitting. The effort necessary to incorporate new questions, examination, intervention, and counseling will be amply rewarded by the individual success stories that you will enjoy.

Finally, I want to address the patients, for whom this book was primarily written. I hope that you have found the answers you sought. I hope that you have had relief of symptoms, either by using the techniques presented here, or through the efforts of other clinicians. Relief of symptoms, and the restoration of ability to walk, stand, sleep, and even sit well again, are my main goals. While I greatly enjoy such successes in youngsters and those in middle age, I must confess special satisfaction when hearing of the "Indian summers" reported by senior citizens who had given up hope of regaining the quality of life they had once enjoyed.

Whichever category you fit into, I hope the success is complete and long lasting and allows you to recover and fulfill the maxim often repeated by my dear Uncle David: "You make a living out of what you do for yourself, but a life out of what you do for others." I hope that along with recovery comes the ability to provide additional care for yourself and to again be of assistance to other people in your life.

* * * * *

To all—patients, family and caregivers, clinicians, and researchers, thank you for joining me on my journey. I hope that the information shared helps you on yours.

Stuart Goldman

For the Clinician and the Very Curious

Information on Strapping

As with most of my treatment approaches to biomechanics, I do not claim originality. I add this section on strapping (especially for non-podiatrists) because I want the particular techniques that I use to be clear to anyone who chooses to try them. In contrast to some reports that suggest only short-term effectiveness of foot strapping, I strongly feel that strapping provides persistent benefit. Patients often report resolution of symptoms for several days while strapped, only to have symptoms return quickly after the straps are removed—followed by relief when the straps are reapplied.

As an aside, I have also had patients who experienced relief that lasted for days or weeks, or even long term, after strapping. I believe that improving the mechanics of the feet can reverse the inflammation of areas adversely affected by poor mechanics. Relief is obtained and often maintained until the combination of mechanics and physical challenge combine to cause the inflammation to return. In this same manner, some people successfully treated biomechanically can use the orthotics, braces, or modified shoes only most of the time, when they are most active, and still remain symptom-free even when not using the corrective device.

This point is important to understand, as some patients obtain temporary relief with strapping, and then they decide they do not need the inserts when the symptoms do not rapidly return. They may become upset when the symptoms reappear weeks or months later. This possibility must be communicated clearly. For example, if I apply straps for Flat Feet and a heel lift for Limb Length Discrepancy and the patient experiences relief, it is possible that he does not need orthotics—only lift, which I then provide. However, if symptoms return, it is a signal that the mechanical control of orthotics is indeed needed. Unfortunately, sometimes patients forget this, even if was explained to them well.

Another advantage of the strap or Unna boot is the assurance of one hundred percent compliance. I have seen many patients who reported that treatment such as a lift or insert failed, but who then had good success with a non-removable support such as a strap or Unna boot. This is especially important as people may only wear inserts in certain shoes and not others, and also sometimes go barefoot. Without being strapped, they never achieve the full time compliance for the 1-3 days that may be needed to obtain excellent improvement. Once they experience excellent improvement they are encouraged to make the effort and changes needed to be compliant.

Here is my particular technique in a modified Low Dye strap.

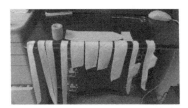

Picture A.1. Supplies include four 1-inch-wide, long strips, three 2-inches-wide, short strips, two 2-inches-wide, long strips cut as a "hat," one piece of Coban long enough to overlap with itself on top of the foot, and one moleskin fascia strap. In this picture, there is also a long, 2-inch strip used to secure a thick heel lift.

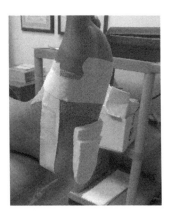

Picture A.2. Coban wrapped around the forefoot, behind the metatarsal heads; a long 1-inch strip applied from just behind the first metatarsal head, behind the heel, to just behind the fifth metatarsal head; and the "hat" strip applied to the ball of the foot, with the thinner parts overlapping on the top of the foot. In this view, a 3/8-inch heel lift to compensate for Limb Length Discrepancy has been applied.

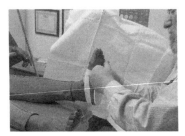

Picture A.3. When overlapping the straps on top, IT IS ESSENTIAL to "load" the foot to make it wide, simulating weight-bearing, to make sure the foot is not bound uncomfortably tightly. I am pushing up on the ball of the foot while wrapping the tape around the top. Coban protects the dorsal skin from pressure and irritation.

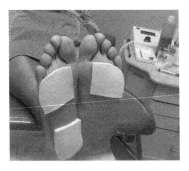

Picture A.4. In this picture, 1/8-inch felt has been applied to effect a reverse Morton's extension to improve first ray function. I put a large Band-Aid on the front of this felt pad to help it stay in place.

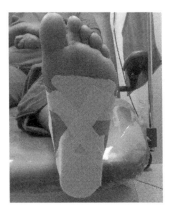

Picture A.5. Apply long strips from the ball of the foot, around the heel, and back to the ball of the foot. I do not place tension on this strap; I just lay it on. If I am applying the strap just to secure the heel lift and not to control pronation, I will actually dorsiflex the forefoot when I apply these straps so as not to reduce pronation. This is important if the heel lift and strap are applied to a normal-arched or High-Arched Foot, which are more common on the side of the shorter leg.

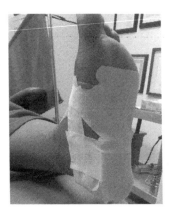

Picture A.6. Apply a single 2-inch strip to the back of the arch, attaching it on the medial and lateral side to the 1-inch strip. Here, a longer strip is needed because of the felt heel lift.

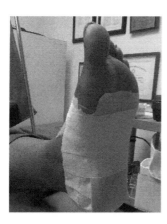

Picture A.7. Apply the moleskin strap from the level of the 1-inch strip in the back of the heel to the ball of the foot. Again, I do not place a lot of tension here; I just lay it on.

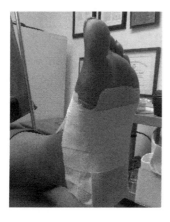

Picture A.8. Apply two 2-inch straps overlapping, over the moleskin, to the level of the 1-inch strip on the sides.

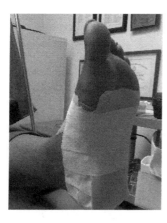

Picture A.9. The long, 1-inch strip overlays the first and is now covering the ends of the 2-inch strips. The "hat" strip, the final locking piece, overlays the first "hat" strip. Again, it is ESSENTIAL to load the foot so that this piece does not bind the foot uncomfortably tight. Occasionally, a patient may stand and find that the top of the strap is too tight, and I will undo this section on top and try to apply it looser.

Direct the patient to stand on the foot and confirm that the strap is tight but not painful. The strap often provides immediate improvement of symptoms, although I caution that full benefit will not be obtained for 1–3 days. I will often strap patients to confirm benefit, and then I'll replace the straps after casting for orthotics. At times, improvement may persist for days or weeks or even for the long term after the straps are removed.

Straps must be kept dry. A commercially available device such as a "Sealtight" may be used. Plastic bags will often leak despite best efforts at taping the top of the bag, so I advise patients to take sponge baths if just plastic bags are used. Another option is to use a plastic or vinyl heel lift under the strap if that is the only important change being effected.

If the patient is allergic to adhesive tape, I apply an under-wrap of Coban to protect the foot, leaving only the skin exposed in the ball of the foot. I have not had people develop rashes in that area with tape. I believe that this modification reduces effectiveness of the strap, but it is still often powerful enough to effectively relieve symptoms.

Information on Unna Boots

If straps are not effective and I suspect that more aggressive control of pronation is needed, I will employ the Unna boot—another form of Mechanical Testing. If this intervention is effective, it strongly suggests that use of a custom ankle brace, such as an Arizona Brace, a Ritchie Brace, or a Platinum Brace, will provide the needed help.

Skill and knowledge of the pitfalls of using an Unna boot are essential. The way the foot is positioned and held while the Unna boot is applied is extremely important. If the wrap is applied at 90 degrees as indicated but the foot is allowed to drop before the wrap is complete, the Unna boot may be quite uncomfortable in the front of the ankle. In addition, at times the Tibialis Anterior tendon is irritated, especially if there is a prominent or "bowstringing" tendon. This irritation may be prevented if felt is placed medial and lateral to the tendon to off-load it.

Occasionally, the Unna boot is not tolerated because the legs are so sensitive from SS-/PS-induced nerve sensitivity. If that is the case, the patient may do Positional Testing for several days with the walker and other Adjunct Measures. Overall sensitivity may then be eliminated, allowing use of the Unna boot. Admittedly, this does somewhat compromise diagnostic clarity, as one cannot see if SS/PS symptoms are helped by the Unna boot, because they have been helped by Positional Testing! However, if either mechanical treatment for arthritic pain or compression therapy for edema is required in addition to PseudoStenosis, this sequence may be needed. In addition, if Positional Testing results in only short-term improvement of SS/PS symptoms, application of an Unna boot after the nerve sensitivity is relieved may prevent recurrence of SS/PS symptoms, suggesting efficacy of an Ankle Foot Orthotic, such as a Platinum Brace or Ritchie Brace, or a gauntlet ankle brace such as an Arizona Brace.

A few tips on applying the Unna boot:

1. The foot must be maintained in a 90-degree or higher position while the Unna boot is applied. Allowing it to plantar-flex, even for a moment, will allow the material to get bunched up in the front of the ankle and become very uncomfortable.

2. Cover the Unna boot with Coban—at least 4 layers on the bottom. This prevents a trail of zinc oxide on the floor and inside the shoes. Keep the foot dorsiflexed until the final Coban layer has been applied.

3. I often include a felt heel lift on both feet for Equinus. A felt lift may be used on only a shorter limb, or a thicker lift on the short limb and a ⅛-inch lift on the longer limb can be used to accommodate both Limb Length Discrepancy and Equinus. For significant first-ray hypermobility, I may include a ⅛-inch felt reverse Morton's extension against the skin.

4. If there is bowstringing of the Tibialis Anterior tendon, I will apply straps of felt on either side to protect against irritation.

5. If there is significant sensitivity of the overall foot and leg—especially if the nerve hypersensitivity suggests SS/PS—the Unna boot may be uncomfortable and the patient may not tolerate it. I may institute Positional Testing with Adjunct Measures for a week to eliminate that sensitivity.

6. If there is nighttime exacerbation of neuropathic symptoms, modify sleep positions as described in Chapter 21.

7. Consider using stockinette and webril above the ankle, especially if there is severe swelling or sensitivity.

8. Do not forget to compensate for Limb Length Discrepancy. Because Posterior Tibial Tendonitis and overall nerve sensitivity are far more common in the longer leg, it is often beneficial to apply a lift with a Low Dye strap on the shorter leg when applying an Unna boot for the longer leg.

9. **Make sure to tell the patient that if the Unna boot is uncomfortable, it is appropriate to remove it. One should not try to put up with pain from an Unna boot.**

10. **I consider it to be a test that suggests success, with value of obtaining a brace, if there is help during the day with standing and walking, even if the Unna boot is uncomfortable at night, and needs to be removed. After all, patients will use a brace during the day, not at night in bed.**

11. Follow up within a few days to ascertain benefit. Check the areas of sensitivity that were identified on clinical examination before treatment.

Full Examination Form

This is the Examination Form that I have used in the past; it may be helpful in clarifying both history and physical examination that has been discussed in this book. For clinicians looking to use my techniques and willing to put the time into using them, this may be helpful. Having the patient fill out the LuSSSExt scale may also be helpful.

Intake Form: Neuropathy, Spinal Stenosis, PseudoStenosis, other Neuro Condition, ASO, or Arthritis

Patient _____ Date _____ Initial eval. Follow up eval.

If diabetic, **duration of diabetes** _____ Yrs Type 1 Type 2 **Other suspected cause** Chemo ETOH Spine _____

ONSET: Sudden Gradual Preceded by _____ **Symptoms are** Improving Getting Worse Stable _____
_____ _____ Yrs _____ _____ Yrs

Meds prev. used for neuro: _____ _____ _____ Now used: _____ _____ Helpful? Very Mod. Mild No

1. **OVERALL estimation of symptoms in feet & legs**   Severe   Moderate   Mild   None   Which involved?

   Numbness O   Paresthesias ☐   10 9 8   7 6 5 4   3 2 1   0   Feet

   Discomfort: Burning O   Pain ☐   Aching ◊   10 9 8   7 6 5 4   3 2 1   0   Legs

   Cold feeling O   Leather / cardboard / stiff ☐   10 9 8   7 6 5 4   3 2 1   0   Thighs

2. **Walking Distance?** Cons Incons _____ Ft   < 1/2 blk   < 1 blk   1-2 blks   3-5 blks   1/2 -1 mile   Over 1 mile   No Limit
   Stopped by symptoms in   FEET LEGS THIGHS HIPS BACK Generalized SOB Other _____

3. **Relief of extremity symptoms by**   N/A   Stand and rest   Lean against something   Sit   Lie Down   None

4. *Grocery Cart* (walker treadmill) status: N/A No better a little better much better unknown **Height** Reported _____ Real _____

5. **Are feet or legs uncomfortable with Standing?** Y N   After how long _____   Relieved by LEANING Y N

6. Are foot symptoms **CONSTANTLY** present Y N   CONSISTENT or VARIABLE in severity

7. **Are symptoms worse lying in bed?** Y N   Nightly _____/wk After how long _____   Feet Legs Thighs Back
   Position: Back side stomach restless **Relieved** in recliner Y N ? Pillow under knees Y N ? Between Thighs Y N ? Other _____

8. **Symmetry**   SAME in each foot /leg   RIGHT worse   LEFT worse   INCONSISTANT
   Toes   L R   TOP of foot   L R   Bottom of foot   L R   Front of leg   L R   Back of leg _____

9. **Most comfortable standing**   Barefoot   flat shoes   standard shoes   high heel shoes   No difference   Unknown

10. Frequently shift from side to side standing?   Yes No   Balance problems or difficult walking straight?   Yes   No

11. Neuropathy in hands?   Yes No   Difficulty buttoning, or drop frequently? Yes No   Lehrmitte's?   Yes   No

12. **Difficult getting up from Chair?** Y N   **Muscle weakness**: N Y _____   **Incontinence** N Y

13 **Back pain** Y N Occ *MRI or CT?* N Y + - Epi N Y FLURO Y N **Helpful** Y N **Back Surg** _____ Decomp fusion Help Y N

14 **NCS**   Y N When _____ Who? _____ Results _____ Status changed since then? Y N

15. **Vasc Studies** Y N When _____ Who? _____ Results _____ Status changed since then? Y N

Focused   EXAM   Left   Right   Left   Right

1. Pulses   DP ____ PT ____   DP ____ PT ____   2. CFT   WNL Slow WNL Slow

3. Skin   WNL   Shiny   Atrophic   Hairless   Rubor   Pallor _____

4. **Equinus** (*Leg cramps* Y N OCC) Y   N   Y   N   5. Significant Biomechanical Problems   Y   N

6. **Pain in Interspace**   1 2 3 4   1 2 3 4   7. VPT 1st MPJ _____ _____

8. Pain/ paresthesias **PT nerve** y L n y R n   **Tib. nerve** y L n y R n   **Fem Nerve** y L n y R n

9. Sensitive **Pes Anserinus** y L n y R n   **Sinus Tarsi** y L n y R n   **1st MC joint** y L n y R n

10. **Muscle wasting**   None   Feet   Legs   Thigh   Hands   11. **Asymmetry of feet**   Y   N

12. **Rotation abnormal**   Y   N _____   **FHL** L R   **Significant Pronation** L R   **Cavus** L R

13 **ASIS** Even Higher L R   **PSIS** Even Higher L R   Iliac Pain Y N   **Relief lift** _____   **LLDx** Shorter L ____ R

Semmes Weinstein Monofilament Record
0= can feel 5.07   1=can feel 6.45   2=cannot feel 6.45
LOPS score includes higher of two scores at each level of the foot. It includes A if *asymmetrical within a foot*
or if greater sensory loss is noted proximally *(atypical)*. It includes (+) if unable to feel the 5.07 above the ankle

Right   **Left**

LOPS Score
0—10

Left _____

Right _____

Malleolus   Malleolus
Lateral Medial   Medial Lateral

Right   Left
Each level is 1.5 inches
Starting above malleolus

Leg LOPS 0-10
Right _____ Left _____

Differential

DPN	Prob	Poss	Unlikely	No
SS -	Prob	Poss	Unlikely	No
PseudoSten	Prob	Poss	Unlikely	No
Biomechanical _____				
Vascular	Prob	Poss	Unlikely	No
Non Diab PN (CIDP?)	Prob	Poss	Unlikely	No

Cervical Sten   Mortons N   TTS   Peroneal

Other P N or Systemic Dis. _____

Other _____

_____ No significant neuropathology

Plan _____

_____ Copyright 1/15

List of Articles by Other Clinicians Supporting Findings of Chapters 12 and 19

As promised, here is a list of articles, in chronological order, which take note of the effect of biomechanics on arthritis of the lower extremity or spine. It is not by any means a complete list, but it is adequate to support some of the information provided in Chapter 12 and especially Chapter 19. I hope clinicians find these articles of interest

1. Langer, S. 1976. "Structural leg shortage: A case report." *Journal of the American Podiatry Association* 66 (1): 38–40.

2. Subotnick, S. I. 1981a. "Limb length discrepancies of the lower extremity (the short leg syndrome)." *Journal of Orthopedic and Sports Physical Therapy* 3 (1): 11–16.

3. Subotnick, S. I. (1981).. "Low-back pain from functionally short leg." *Journal of the American Podiatry Association* 71 (1): 42–42.

4. Hellsing, A. L. 1988. "Leg length inequality: A prospective study of young men during their military service." *Upsala Journal of Medical Sciences* 93 (3): 245–253.

5. McCaw, S. T., and Bates, B. T. 1991. "Biomechanical implications of mild leg length inequality." *British Journal of Sports Medicine* 25 (1): 10–13.

6. Dananberg, H. J., and Guiliano, M. 1999. "Chronic low-back pain and its response to custom-made foot orthoses." *Journal of the American Podiatric Medical Association* 89 (3), 109–117.

7. Dananberg, H. J. 2000. "Sagittal plane biomechanics." *Journal of the American Podiatric Medical Association* 90 (1): 47–50.

8. Gurney, B. 2002. "Leg length discrepancy." *Gait and Posture* 15 (2): 195–206.

9. Hillstrom, H. J., Brower, D. J., Whitney, K., McGuire, J., & Schumacher, H. R. (2002). Lower extremity conservative realignment therapies for knee osteoarthritis. *Physical Medicine and Rehabilitation*, *16*(3), 507-520.

10. Brady, R. J., Dean, J. B., Skinner, T. M., and Gross, M. T. 2003. "Limb length inequality: Clinical implications for assessment and intervention." *Journal of Orthopedic and Sports Physical Therapy* 33 (5): 221–234.

11. Goodman, M. J., Menown, J. L., West Jr, J. M., Barr, K. M., Vander Linden, D. W., and McMulkin, M. L. 2004. "Secondary gait compensations in individuals without neuromuscular involvement following a unilateral imposed Equinus constraint." *Gait and Posture* 20 (3): 238–244.

12. Goss, D. L., and Moore, J. H. 2004. "Compliance wearing a heel lift during eight weeks of military training in cadets with limb length inequality." *Journal of Orthopedic and Sports Physical Therapy* 34 (3): 126–131.

13. Defrin, R., Benyamin, S. B., Aldubi, R. D., and Pick, C. G. 2005. "Conservative correction of leg length discrepancies of ten millimeters or less for the relief of chronic low-back pain." *Archives of Physical Medicine and Rehabilitation* 86 (11): 2075–2080.

14. Clough, J. G. 2005. "Functional hallux limitus and lesser-metatarsal overload." *Journal of the American Podiatric Medical Association* 95 (6): 593–601.

15. Terry MA[1], Winell JJ, Green DW, Schneider R, Peterson M, Marx RG, Widmann RF. 2005 "Measurement variance in limb length discrepancy: clinical and radiographic assessment of interobserver and intraobserver variability." Journal of Pediatric Orthopedics. 2005 Mar-Apr;25(2):197-201.

16. Menz, H. B., and Morris, M. E. 2005. "Determinants of disabling foot pain in retirement village residents." *Journal of the American Podiatric Medical Association* 95 (6): 573–579.

17. Reilly, K. A., Barker, K. L., Shamley, D., and Sandall, S. 2006. "Influence of foot characteristics on the site of lower limb osteoarthritis." *Foot and Ankle International* 27 (3): 206–211.

18. Scherer, P. R., Sanders, J., Eldredge, D. E., Duffy, S. J., and Lee, R. Y. 2006. "Effect of functional foot orthoses on first metatarsophalangeal joint dorsiflexion in stance and gait." *Journal of the American Podiatric Medical Association* 96 (6): 474–481.

19. Khamis, S., and Yizhar, Z. 2007. "Effect of feet hyperpronation on pelvic alignment in a standing position." *Gait and Posture* 25 (1): 127–134.

20. Sabharwal S, Zhao C, McKeon J, Melaghari T, Blacksin M, Wenekor C. 2007 Reliability analysis for radiographic measurement of limb length discrepancy: full-length standing anteroposterior radiograph versus scanogram. J Pediatr Orthop. 27(1):46-50

21. Sabharwal, S., and Kumar, A. 2008. "Methods for assessing leg length discrepancy." *Clinical Orthopedics and Related Research* 466 (12): 2910–2922.

22. Collins, N., Crossley, K., Beller, E., Darnell, R., McPoil, T., and Vicenzino, B. 2008. "Foot orthoses and physiotherapy in the treatment of patellofemoral pain syndrome: Randomized clinical trial. *BMJ* : 337.

23. Grondal, L., Tengstrand, B., Nordmark, B., Wretenberg, P., and Stark, A. 2008. "The foot: Still the most important reason for walking incapacity in rheumatoid arthritis: Distribution of symptomatic joints in one thousand RA patients." *Acta Orthopaedica* 79 (2): 257–261.

24. Lee, Y. C., and Shmerling, R. H. 2008. "The benefit of nonpharmacologic therapy to treat symptomatic osteoarthritis." *Current Rheumatology Reports* 10 (1): 5–10.

25. Zeifang, F., Schiltenwolf, M., Abel, R., and Moradi, B. 2008. "Gait analysis does not correlate with clinical and MR imaging parameters in patients with symptomatic lumbar spinal stenosis." *BMC Musculoskeletal Disorders* 9 (1): 89.

26. Reilly, K., Barker, K., Shamley, D., Newman, M., Oskrochi, G. R., and Sandall, S. 2009. "The role of foot and ankle assessment of patients with lower limb osteoarthritis." *Physiotherapy* 95 (3): 164–169.

27. Block, J. A., and Shakoor, N. 2010. Lower limb osteoarthritis: Biomechanical alterations and implications for therapy." *Current Opinion in Rheumatology* 22 (5): 544–550.

28. Vaidya, S. V., Patel, M. R., Panghate, A. N., and Rathod, P. A. 2010. "Total knee arthroplasty: Limb length discrepancy and functional outcome." *Indian Journal of Orthopaedics* 44 (3): 300.

29. Gross, K. D., Felson, D. T., Niu, J., Hunter, D. J., Guermazi, A., Roemer, F. W., Dufour, A. B., Gensure, R. H., and Hannan, M. T. 2011. "Association of flat feet with knee pain and cartilage damage in older adults." *Arthritis Care and Research* 63 (7): 937–944.

30. Franettovich, M., Chapman, A. R., Blanch, P., and Vicenzino, B. 2010. Augmented low-dye tape alters foot mobility and neuromotor control of gait in individuals with and without exercise-related leg pain." *Journal of Foot and Ankle Research* 3 (5).

List of Articles Published by the Author That Are Relevant to This Book

My Publications on Spinal Stenosis, PseudoStenosis, and their Relationship with Lower-Extremity Symptoms

1. Goldman, S. M., Funk, J. D., and Christensen, V. M. 1997. "Spinal stenosis: A common cause of podiatric symptoms." *Journal of the American Podiatric Medical Association* 87 (3): 117–124. This article stresses the prevalence of Spinal Stenosis in causing or exacerbating many foot and leg symptoms.

2. Goldman, S. M. 2003. "Neurogenic positional pedal neuritis: common pedal manifestations of spinal stenosis." *Journal of the American Podiatric Medical Association* 93 (3): 174–184. This article provides details on the symptoms of Spinal Stenosis as they present in the foot, and includes an introduction to physical findings and to what will later be labeled "Positional History" and "Positional Testing."

3. Goldman, S. M. 2003. "Value of a grocery cart and walker in identification and management of symptomatic spinal stenosis in diabetic patients presenting with peripheral neuropathy or claudication." *Diabetes Care* 26 (6): 1943–1943. This letter presents an introduction to what will later be labeled "Positional History" and "Positional Testing" in differentiating both neuropathic and arterial symptoms from those of Spinal Stenosis in diabetic patients.

4. Goldman, S. M. 2004. "Diabetic peripheral neuropathy and spinal stenosis: Prevalence of overlap and misdiagnosis. An introductory report." *Diabetic Medicine* 21 (4): 394–396. This letter presents an introduction to what will later be labeled "Positional History" and "Positional Testing" in differentiating

both neuropathic and arterial symptoms from those of Spinal Stenosis in diabetic patients.

5. Goldman, S. M. 2005. "Nocturnal neuropathic pain in diabetic patients may be caused by spinal stenosis." *Diabetic Medicine* 22 (12): 1763–1765. This article identifies the pattern of Spinal Stenosis frequently causing nocturnal symptoms mistaken for neuropathy, and it reports insights on differentiation and management.

6. Goldman, S. M., Barice, E. J., Schneider, W. R., and Hennekens, C. H. 2008. "Lumbar spinal stenosis: Can positional therapy alleviate pain?" *Journal of Family Practice* 57 (4): 257–260. This article provides then-current details in both Positional History and Testing, and results of a retrospective review of fifty-three patients treated in my office with documented Spinal Stenosis and symptoms. Coauthored by Dr. Charles Hennekens, author of *Epidemiology in Medicine*, at that time the fifth-most quoted medical author in the world over the prior five years.

7. Goldman, S. M. 2013. "The professor position and the single stance flexion test may clarify the effect of lumbar spinal stenosis or pseudostenosis on lower-extremity symptoms." *Journal of the American Podiatric Medical Association* 103 (2): 156–160. This article explains two immediate forms of Positional Testing and also presents the concepts and introductory details of PseudoStenosis, including its ability to mimic or exacerbate all lower-extremity symptoms of Spinal Stenosis.

Acknowledgments

Sixty years of living and 34 years of practicing podiatric medicine, have taught me that so much in life depends on the efforts and kindness of others. I have great appreciation for the many people who have done so much for me personally and professionally, and I want to take this opportunity to acknowledge them. This is not a complete list, but it includes some of those who have had a great impact.

First, thanks to my parents, Minnie and Al Goldman, may they rest in peace. The gift of a loving and secure home goes a long way in building a life of decency and happiness. The loving family they brought me into exuded values that I can only hope to emulate.

My Aunt Laikee Zelitch, who seamlessly took on the role of providing deep motherly love for over forty years, after her best friend could no longer give it to her children. Her late husband, my Uncle David, lived the maxim he shared: "You make a living out of what you do for yourself, but a life out of what you do for others." He cost me a lot of money. If he were not such a good example of the value of giving charity . . .

My big brother, Roy, who always treated me as an equal even when young, and whose lifetime love has given me the gift of believing that I could accomplish great things. A great brother, a great uncle, a great host, a great husband and father, a great person. Also a great barbecuer.

My mother-in-law, Bernice Sir, has, with absolute loving consistency, provided a vacation haven for us to visit in Florida. Thanks, Grandma, we'll try to visit more often.

My teachers who became colleagues in Orlando. Two stand out, thirty-plus years later. Bill Silverman, a dedicated and honorable family doctor, who taught by example the need to be a medical Don Quixote, striving to find the best diagnosis and treatment even when it was outside standard practice. His inspiration is felt in this book. Terry Ballard, a fine surgeon, who handled so many different kinds of cases in a small community hospital, always with great deliberation and dedication, teaching by example. Also, I am grateful that many lifelong friendships that began there, with the Hara, Schwab, Singer, and Kronfeld families.

Rabbis who shared lessons of infinite value, including R Noach Weinberg Z"L, R. Haskel Wachsman AKA Zaide Haskel Z"L, R. Abraham Twerski, The Lubavitcher Rebbe Rabbi Menachem Mendel Shneerson, R Kalman Packouz, R. Pesach Krohn, R. Menachem Goldberger, R. Joel Feldman, R. Josh Fass, R. Shalom Dubov, R. Zalman Bukiet, R. Kenneth Brander, R Shimon Apisdorf , and many others. Those paying attention may note that the list is in alphabetical order, if one reads right to left.

Colleagues or friends in Boca Raton, whom I still miss, including Dave Levinson (Thank David), Meyer Cohen, Danny Ettedgui, Alan Berger, Bob Spoont, Baruch Plotkin, Bob Dabrow, and Stuart Rubin. Also Dr. Bret Ribotsky, a visionary podiatrist, who shared the lesson of sacrificing precious office time in order to accomplish a precious project.

Special thanks to Dr. Charlie Hennekens. One of the most important researchers in medical history, he inspired me, through a brief collaboration, to think globally in the goal of helping people.

Here in Baltimore, Dr. Brad Lamm of the Rubin Institute of Sinai Hospital. As I gave up surgery in order to write this book, I have been able to refer to him with great confidence. At the office of Dr. Anil Uberoi, who hosted my first office home in Baltimore. Tash and Ms. Grady for being such levelheaded straight shooters. My office staff, including Linda, Cecelia, Natalie, and Nicole, who keep my office flowing as I think about distant matters.

My medical colleagues in Pikesville, Drs. Milan Wister, Miguel Sadovnik, Dave Roggen, and especially my dear friend Dr. Elliot Rothschild. I have known other internists who were as good, but none better. I am grateful for the welcome I've enjoyed for these six years. Other physicians, including Drs. Alan Friedman, Julian Jakobovits and Yaniv Berger have blessed me with their confidence, a privilege I treasure. Dr. Mark Young, a talented physiatrist, author, and scholar, and a good friend. Dr. Marian Lamonte, the first neurologist to embrace use of my techniques. Awareness of the success she had encouraged me to strive to publicize. My friends and neighbors, including the Katzes, Blums and Elashvilis, who make the neighborhood feel like home.

My first editor, the talented author Libby Lazewnik. Like a voice teacher preparing a singer, she helped me to develop a better way to share my stories and to ensure that this book was prepared for the general audience. Karen Toso, who helped greatly in organization and refinement, and Chana Frank, who lovingly attacked my book and found a great many minor errors, both ensured that the book would have a more professional presentation. I am grateful to all three editors.

The Journal of the American Podiatric Medical Association, and the APMA itself. JAPMA, led by Dr. Warren Joseph, by publishing three articles, provided the opportunity to refine and share findings, and the encouragement to continue exploring "outside the box". They also kindly allowed me to include copyrighted pictures and charts in this book. The APMA graciously allowed me the privilege to lecture at a few National Scientific Meeting. It is an organization that fills the dual role of looking out for the needs of our profession but always with an eye toward the best interests of the American public that we serve.

The Beacon, a senior citizen newspaper that serves the Baltimore area. In that it provides excellent content of interest to seniors, it seems to encourages active readership. Advertising in the Beacon brought me many patients with unusual or chronic pain, which allowed me to help many people I would not otherwise have reached, and also helped me to refine my understanding and thus this book.

I am maintained by the love of my family. My children, Nechama, Ary, Goldie, Shoshana, and Avi, all bring a special light to my life. I so much enjoy being with them—I forget that they are or recently were teenagers! The most important person for me to thank is Debbie, my wife and partner for life. She guides a loving home for my kids as did my parents for me, and I believe that her love has gone a long way in helping them develop so well. She has tolerated without complaint my focus on this project for over twenty years, knowing full well that it was not intended for fame or fortune nor would make our day-to-day challenges any easier. She understands that it was reflective of what Viktor Frankl wrote in *Man's Search for Meaning*, and that it was part of me. Without her love and support, I could not have reached this stage. Anyone who benefits from the articles I have published or from this book owes her a debt of thanks.

Finally, in that all wisdom and success is guided by Heaven, I would like to thank G-d. He has blessed me with good health and a loving family in a wonderful and safe country. He has led me to a profession that I love, has provided me with necessary opportunities and teachers, has fortified my persistence, and has given me all the original insights that I share in this book.

Index